Applied Mindfulness

Approaches in Mental Health
for
CHILDREN AND
ADOLESCENTS

Editorial Board

Applied Mindfulness

Approaches in Mental Health
for
CHILDREN AND ADOLESCENTS

Edited by

**Victor G. Carrión, M.D., and
John Rettger, Ph.D.**

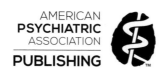

AMERICAN
PSYCHIATRIC
ASSOCIATION
PUBLISHING

Copyright © 2019 American Psychiatric Association Publishing
ALL RIGHTS RESERVED
First Edition
Manufactured in the United States of America on acid-free paper
23 22 21 20 19   5 4 3 2 1

American Psychiatric Association Publishing
800 Maine Avenue SW
Suite 900
Washington, DC 20024-2812
www.appi.org

Library of Congress Cataloging-in-Publication Data
Names: Carrión, Victor G., editor. | Rettger, John, editor. | American Psychiatric Association Publishing, publisher.
Title: Applied mindfulness : approaches in mental health for children and adolescents / edited by Victor G. Carrión, and John Rettger.
Description: Washington, D.C. : American Psychiatric Association Publishing, [2019] | Includes bibliographical references and index.
Identifiers: LCCN 2018048941 (print) | LCCN 2018050433 (ebook) | ISBN 9781615372461 (eb) | ISBN 9781615372126 (pb : alk. paper)
Subjects: | MESH: Mindfulness—methods | Psychology, Adolescent | Evidence-Based Practice—methods
Classification: LCC BF724 (ebook) | LCC BF724 (print) | NLM WS 465 | DDC 155.5—dc23
LC record available at https://lccn.loc.gov/2018048941

British Library Cataloguing in Publication Data
A CIP record is available from the British Library.

Contents

Part 1
Introduction to Mindfulness

Part II
Mindfulness Application to Specific Clinical Diagnoses

Part III
Mindfulness Application to Specific Clinical Populations

Contributors

Karen Bluth, Ph.D.
Assistant Professor, Department of Psychiatry, Frank Porter Graham Child Development Institute, School of Medicine, University of North Carolina, Chapel Hill, North Carolina

Michael Bready, M.A.P.P.
Founder and Director, Youth Mindfulness, Glasgow, Glasgow, Scotland, UK

Catherine Cook-Cottone, Ph.D.
Professor and Director, Advanced Certificate in Mindful Counseling, Department of Counseling, School, and Educational Psychology, University at Buffalo, State University of New York, Buffalo, New York

Tara Cousineau, Ph.D.
Community Leadership Fellow, Center for Mindfulness and Compassion, Cambridge Health Alliance, Cambridge, Massachusetts

Susan Delaney, Psy.D.
Bereavement Consultant, Irish Hospice Foundation, Dublin, Ireland

Sayyed Mohsen Fatemi, Ph.D.
Associate Professor of Psychology and Chair of the Desk of North America, Department of Psychology, Ferdowsi University of Mashhad, Mashhad, Iran; Fellow, Department of Psychology, Harvard University, Cambridge, Massachusetts

Lisa Flook, Ph.D.
Associate Scientist, Center for Healthy Minds, University of Wisconsin-Madison, Madison, Wisconsin

Matthew S. Goodman, M.A.
Ph.D. candidate in Clinical Psychology, California School of Professional Psychology, Alliant International University, San Diego, California; Predoctoral intern, Providence Family Medicine Center/Alaska Family Medicine Residency, Anchorage, Alaska

Sam Himelstein, Ph.D.
Licensed Psychologist, Center for Adolescent Studies, Oakland, California

Lorraine Hobbs, M.A.
Director, Family Programs, University of California, San Diego Center for Mindfulness, San Diego, California

Erik Jacobson, Ph.D.
Chief Psychologist, Upstate Cerebral Palsy, Utica, New York

Mari Janikian, Ph.D.
Assistant Professor, Department of Psychology, American College of Greece, Athens, Greece

Bridget Kiley, M.Sc.
Senior Research Center Coordinator, Center for Mindfulness and Compassion, Cambridge Health Alliance, Cambridge, Massachusetts

Mari Kurahashi, M.D., M.P.H.
Clinical Assistant Professor, Stanford School of Medicine, Stanford, California

Ellen J. Langer, Ph.D.
Professor, Department of Psychology, Harvard University, Cambridge, Massachusetts

Christine Lathren, M.D.
Postdoctoral Fellow, Program on Integrative Medicine, Department of Physical Medicine and Rehabilitation, School of Medicine, University of North Carolina, Chapel Hill, North Carolina

Pamela Lozoff, M.S.W., RYT
Founder and Director, Spirit of Youth Yoga, Los Gatos, California

Laila A. Madni, Psy.D.
Adjunct Faculty, Graduate Psychology Department, Antioch University Los Angeles, Culver City, California

Kristina C. Mendez, M.S.
Doctoral candidate in Clinical Psychology, Pacific Graduate School of Psychology, Palo Alto University, Palo Alto, California

Stewart Mercer, Ph.D.
Professor of Primary Care Research, Institute of Health and Wellbeing, General Practice and Primary Care, University of Glasgow, Glasgow; Usher Institute of Population Health Sciences and Informatics, Medical School, University of Edinburgh, Edinburgh Scotland, UK

Allison Morgan, M.A., OTR, E-RYT
Founder and Director, Zensational Kids, Montvale, New Jersey

Alejandro Nunez, B.A.
Research Coordinator, Department of Psychiatry and Behavioral Science, Stanford University School of Medicine, Stanford, California

Sita G. Patel, Ph.D.
Associate Professor, Pacific Graduate School of Psychology, Palo Alto University, Palo Alto, California

Celeste H. Poe, LMFT
Graduate student in Clinical Psychology, Pacific Graduate School of Psychology, Palo Alto University, Palo Alto, California

John P. Rettger, Ph.D.
Mindfulness Program Director, Early Life Stress and Pediatric Anxiety Program, School of Medicine, Stanford University, Stanford, California

Amy Saltzman, M.D.
Founder and Director, Still Quiet Place, Meno Park, California; Cofounder and Director, Association for Mindfulness in Education, Menlo Park, California

Randye J. Semple, Ph.D.
Associate Professor, Department of Psychiatry and Behavioral Sciences, Keck School of Medicine, University of Southern California, Los Angeles, California

Zev Schuman-Olivier, M.D.
Executive and Research Director, CHA Center for Mindfulness and Compassion; Medical Director, Addictions, Cambridge Health Alliance; Instructor in Psychiatry, Harvard Medical School, Cambridge, Massachusetts; Investigator, Center for Technology and Behavioral Health at Dartmouth; Instructor in Psychiatry and Biomedical Data Sciences, Geisel School of Medicine at Dartmouth, Hanover, New Hampshire

Sharon Simpson, Ph.D.
Trainee Clinical Psychologist, Institute of Health and Wellbeing, University of Glasgow, Glasgow, Scotland, UK

Meena Srinivasan
Program Manager, Office of Social and Emotional Learning, Oakland Unified School District, Oakland, California

Eleni Vousoura, Ph.D.
Associate Lecturer, Department of Psychology, American College of Greece; Research Associate, First Department of Psychiatry, University of Athens, Athens, Greece

Nicole Ward, M.S.
Clinical Psychology Ph.D. candidate, Palo Alto University, Palo Alto, California

Sally Wyke, Ph.D.
Interdisciplinary Professor of Health and Wellbeing, Institute of Health and Wellbeing, College of Social Science, University of Glasgow, Glasgow, Scotland, UK

Sarah Zoogman, Ph.D.
Fellow, Harvard Vanguard Medical Associates, Atrius Health, Cambridge, Massachusetts

Disclosure of Interests

The following contributors to this book have indicated a financial interest in or other affiliation with a commercial supporter, a manufacturer of a commercial product, a provider of a commercial service, a nongovernmental organization, and/or a government agency, as listed below:

Karen Bluth, Ph.D.   *Intellectual property rights/training monies:* Making Friends with Yourself: A Mindful Self-Compassion Program for Teens
Tara Cousineau, Ph.D.   *Intellectual property rights/training monies:* Making Friends with Yourself: A Mindful Self-Compassion Program for Teens
Lorraine Hobbs, M.A.   *Scientific advisor/consultant:* Whil Concepts Inc., a workplace wellness platform. *Founder and principal investigator:* BodiMojo Inc., with research and development and grants related to technology interventions in adolescent and family health
Allison Morgan, M.A., OTR, E-RYT   *Founder:* Zensational Kids. *Developer:* Educate 2B program.
John P. Rettger, Ph.D.   *Educator:* Summit Professional Education workshops and online mindfulness-based intervention course.
Randye J. Semple, Ph.D.   *Royalties:* New Harbinger Publications.

The following contributors have indicated that they have no financial interests or other affiliations that represent or could appear to represent a competing interest with the contributions to this book:

Victor G. Carrión, M.D.; Susan Delaney, Psy.D.; Sayyed Mohsen Fatemi, Ph.D.; Matthew S. Goodman, M.A.; Erik Jacobson, Ph.D.; Mari Janikian, Ph.D.; Bridget Kiley, M.Sc.; Mari Kurahashi, M.D., M.P.H.; Pamela Lozoff, M.S.W., RYT; Laila A. Madni, Psy.D.; Alejandro Nunez, B.A.; Celeste H. Poe, LMFT; Amy Saltzman, M.D.; Zev Schuman-Olivier, M.D.; Sharon Simpson, Ph.D.; Eleni Vousoura, Ph.D.; Nicole Ward, M.S.; Sarah Zoogman, Ph.D.

Preface

To cultivate the healing power of mindfulness requires much more than mechanistically following a recipe or set of instructions.... In practicing mindfulness you will have to bring your whole being to the process.

—Kabat-Zinn 2005

In the spirit of the above teaching, it is important to point out that this book is not a cookbook or an easy instructional manual that the reader can simply pick up and read and be ready to start implementing and teaching mindfulness to youth. As Jon Kabat-Zinn taught, "you will have to bring your whole being to the process" (Kabat-Zinn 2005). This primarily involves being willing to dedicate oneself to a path of mindfulness where the learning of the practices comes from the "inside out." One must be willing to practice diligently every day.

Therefore, this book is more of a map that presents you with a bit of the vast terrain that many researchers and clinicians have begun charting from a Western and clinical perspective over the past few decades. To reflect the teaching of Alfred Korzybski, who remarked that "the map is not the territory," the meditations and yoga postures represented here in this text cannot be comprehended through reading them alone, nor can they be meaningfully taught by reading the words aloud in a peaceful tone (Korzybski 1995). They must be practiced, felt, experienced, lived, and reflected on. The full territory of which these practices are maps can never be fully revealed in a completed form because the human being is always an unfolding. The outward journey of becoming a mindfulness teacher must begin from within your own heart. As Kabat-Zinn notes, in Asian languages the word for mind and heart are the same. Therefore, this book is about the application of heartfulness in your therapeutic work. We hope that this text will provide the inspiration for readers to initiate or continue their mindfulness journey.

This work collects a select range of topics that the editors believe have wide therapeutic application, and accordingly, the text brings together leading and emerging thinkers on these subjects. The book is divided into four parts. Part I ("Introduction to Mindfulness") provides an essential foundation of knowledge in the field of clinical mindfulness for youth. As highlighted above, it is vital to begin the journey through this book with the understanding that in order to become a mindfulness facilitator for youth, one must have an inside-out perspective by developing a dedicated, daily personal practice of mindfulness. Chapter 1 ("Developing a Personal Mindfulness Practice") gives the reader introductory knowledge on how to get started with a practice. There are specific mindfulness scripts throughout the book that you may try out in service of your own practice development. Some of the authors include audio practices and/or clear written descriptions of practices to offer support for readers endeavoring to learn how to meditate and move mindfully in the adaptation of these skills into their clinical practice. Case examples are included in some chapters; the names and background information of the patients have been modified to protect their privacy.

After internalizing the practices and establishing a committed practice, you can begin to take steps toward leading others. Part II ("Mindfulness Application to Specific Clinical Diagnosis") offers mindfulness strategies and protocols directed toward specific clinical scenarios. Part III ("Mindfulness Application to Specific Clinical Populations") addresses specific populations. Last, Part IV ("Mindfulness Settings") offers examples of how to integrate mindfulness into a variety of settings, including home and work, and how to incorporate nature into your practice of mindfulness.

Because the main motivation for this book is to help counteract the high levels of stress that our youth are facing, we must ask ourselves whether the current generation of youth is experiencing more stress than earlier generations. We like to think we have moved beyond the eras of poverty, illness, exploitative labor, and lack of protections, but are we really providing youth with more opportunities than they had in the past? The answer is yes, but not for all, and for those for whom we provide opportunities, we have limited their life experience and provided excessive expectations regarding their accomplishments, thus replacing one stress with another.

Think about a ratio of stress experienced (numerator) and coping abilities (denominator). Past generations of youth may have struggled even more than today's youth with issues such as war, illness, and shorter life spans, but their coping abilities may have been tested, developed, and relied on for their own survival. Today, overprotection and too-focused expectations may limit the development of coping skills, altering the ratio toward a higher form of personal dissatisfaction and even functional impairment. Achievement is now expected across many domains of a young person's life. Youth are expected to excel academically, socially, and athletically and to be involved in numerous extracurricular activities.

The advance of technological applications in social media may offer opportunities that were nonexistent for younger generations, but it has also exposed current youth to undesired and/or premature experiences, which they still may not have developed the ability to manage. Another important and, perhaps, unanticipated consequence of the rise in technology is a reduction in healthy play, time spent outside, and physical wellness. In fact, according to the Centers for Disease Control and Prevention, during the past 50 years or so, the obesity rate has tripled among youth in the United States, from 4%–5% in the 1960s (Centers for Disease Control and Prevention 2010) to 18.5% in 2015–2016 (Hales et al. 2017). Certainly, numerous variables, such as diet and nutrition, are also likely contributors to this adverse change, but the increase in screen time and the resulting lack of exercise, sleep, and the joys of playing outdoors are also likely influencers. Other countries experience a similar kind of crisis of technology addiction among youth. The relationship among these variables is complex and multifaceted. We must feel compassion for today's youth, whose experience can be understood as a product of the complexity that is expected for an interim generation learning to adapt technology into everyday life. They are our "test" on how civilization will handle advanced technology in the future.

We, as parents and caretakers, are also being challenged on how to provide the right balance between exposure and protection—a demanding task even during periods of stability. In this scenario, it is not surprising that society has searched for approaches that can help us anchor or center ourselves. People are identifying ways to improve self-health and wellness, such as exercise, yoga, and meditation. This brings us to this book. We have found it critical to summarize some of the existing practice and investigation work in the field of mindfulness, specifically as it applies to youth. The spread of mindfulness in clinical practice, as well as in other settings, reflects the need to find an antidote to the highly stressful, disconnected lives youth complain about today. Even for youth who are not facing or experiencing difficulties with stress, learning mindful coping as a preventive approach may prepare them for unforeseen experiences ahead.

The spread of mindfulness is not a fad; mindfulness is actually an "ancient technology" that has become a necessary human response to our current lifestyle. This spread will not subside. We must, then, be vigilant of its proper application and appropriate developmental and cultural adaptations, and we must examine current and new approaches on how to evaluate the effectiveness of these interventions with well-designed studies. Mindfulness must be applied with validity by qualified facilitators. Quick, unsupervised dissemination may result in the delivery of inappropriate techniques, and this may jeopardize the use of mindfulness as a tool.

At the Stanford Early Life Stress and Pediatric Anxiety Program, we have been engaged in ongoing community-based work delivering mindfulness and yoga programming to underserved youth and their helpers in our neighboring community. Most recently, we have been investigating how a structured approach (a curriculum) provided in a significant dosage (two classes per week) to large settings (all elementary grades of a school district) in a comprehensive manner (yoga, mindfulness, and related socioemotional and neurobiological learning themes) could be scientifically studied in terms of biological, psychological, social, and academic outcomes. We partnered with Pure Edge, Inc., an educational nonprofit organization dedicated to cultivating success in schools through training focus. Our shared aim was to train school staff to deliver their curriculum (Pure Power) in a school district, with a demographically similar school district as a control site.

We became interested in the Pure Power curriculum (available free of charge at pureedgeinc.com to all schools and to those affiliated with nonprofit organizations working with youth) because of the feasibility of implementation and because of its appealing dosage and comprehensiveness, which we felt were needed to create change. The Pure Power approach emphasizes what we believe are the important ingredients of change in contemplative approaches: essentially, training the breath, conditioning the body through yoga movement (which is the centerpiece of the curriculum), the inclusion of intentional rest practice, and understanding themes related to the foundations of mindfulness—kindness, compassion, and growth—and how we can, through our behavior, transform the brain through neuroplasticity. To investigate the effects of this curriculum, we designed a longitudinal, multimethod study. We are now on our third year of the study and collecting data on the control group. This research is designed to offer meaningful insights and build on the current research understanding of youth mindfulness by including physiological and neurobiological domains across time (baseline, 1-year follow-up, and 2-year follow-up). Data collection is ongoing. Please refer to our website, med.stanford.edu/elspap.html, for the study's findings.

In order to help our children maintain and develop their natural mindfulness, we must first serve as models. No matter how sophisticated the science of mindfulness may become, its authentic and inspired delivery can spring forth only from one's own practice. Our call to action for you is to first build your own personal mindfulness practice.

If you have already established a mindfulness practice, we encourage you to move forward with identifying areas in your work with youth where you can begin to incorporate the practices you will learn in this book. That may mean scaffolding your approach to beginning with your colleagues or trainees, then, when you feel ready, inviting youth to the experience of mindfulness. You may be surprised to learn they are more expert than we are. As your practice grows and develops, we invite you to come back to this book, time and time again, to revisit the insights offered here. Mindfulness continuously invites us to examine our place in the world and our work. It is our hope that as you grow in your practice of mindfulness, you, too, will become a mindful innovator and leader for youth.

Last, it is customary in various contemplative traditions to acknowledge with love and gratitude the many teachers and guides who have taught over the years, and their ancestor teachers stretching back across time, for their dedication to establishing practices that cultivate wisdom, peace, love, and compassion. May there be an honoring and a space of gratitude for all of the first peoples across the Earth who were pioneers in shedding a light on the various contemplative practices and to those who preserved the teachings so that they may be handed down through generations. Along with being a map to the heart, this book is a celebration of the hard work of the many researchers, scholars, educators, and clinicians who have contributed to its publication. Their dedication to this project and their wisdom and courage in shining a new light on how to come into the present moment with youth is inspiring. The editors are grateful to these individuals as well as for the support of our project manager, Elizabeth Santana, and our student assistant, Avery Rogers, for administrative support. We are also grateful to the youth who in exemplary ways teach all of us therapists how to be heartful and to master the present moment.

It makes sense to pause here and set an intention: the intention that this journey into mindfulness may provide the skills, knowledge, courage, wisdom, and energy for practitioners to become conservationists of this Earth such that our generation clears a more peaceful path for youth. May all heartful and mindful practices consolidate in the purpose of advancing needed policy changes to protect the future and leave our youth with a world that is a much cleaner, healthier, and safer than it is today. It is everyone's duty.

We think David W. Orr, an environmental studies and politics professor, is on to something with his reflection:

> The plain fact is that the planet does not need more successful people. But it does desperately need more peacemakers, healers, restorers, storytellers and lovers of every kind. It needs people who live well in their places. It needs people of moral courage willing to join the fight to make the world habitable and humane.

The time to show our youth the skills of health and wellness and how to kindle the compassion of their hearts so they can become the next generation of caretakers of this world is now. We encourage you to carry on, practice, and teach.

Victor Carrión, M.D.
John P. Rettger, Ph.D.
Chi Kim, M.Ed.

References

Centers for Disease Control and Prevention: Prevalence of Overweight Among Children and Adolescents: United States, 1999–2002. Atlanta, GA, Centers for Disease Control and Prevention, 2010. Available at: www.cdc.gov/nchs/data/hestat/overweight/overweight99.htm. Accessed October 26, 2018.

Hales CM, Carroll MD, Fryar CD, Ogden CL: Prevalence of obesity among adults and youth: United States, 2015–2016. NCHS Data Brief Oct(288): 1–8, 2017 29155689

Kabat-Zinn J: The foundations of mindfulness practice: attitudes and commitment, in Full Catastrophe Living: Using the Wisdom of Your Body and Mind to Face Stress, Pain, and Illness. New York, Bantam Dell, 2005, pp 31–46

Korzybski A: Science and Sanity: An Introduction to Non-Aristotelian Systems and General Semantics, 5th Edition. Brooklyn, NY, Institute of General Semantics, 1995

Orr D: Earth in Mind? On Education, Environment, and the Human Prospect, 10th Anniversary Edition. Island Press, 2004

Audio Files

The brief guided meditations that are included in this book provide the listener with basic instructions on how to engage in a simple mindfulness meditation. These instructions include guidance on how to establish your seated posture, how to initiate breath awareness, and how to pay attention to sensations of the breath moving through the body. Additionally, the listener is instructed on how to work with the natural tendency of the mind to wander during meditation. The recordings includes optional cues for listeners to pause the recording in order to practice sitting on their own. The meditations conclude with a relaxing breath and the inclusion of brief gratitude practice. The audio files can be accessed online by navigating to www.appi.org/Carrion.

Audio 1: Breath Awareness Practice (Chapter 1)
Length: 5:28
Description: This simple breath awareness practice can be used to help you get a feel for what it is like to practice mindfulness. You can listen to this file to guide your seated meditation.

Audio 2: Breath Awareness Practice for Individuals With Attention-Deficit/Hyperactivity Disorder (Chapter 6)
Length: 5:39
Description: This breath awareness practice has been adapted for use with youth with attention-deficit/hyperactivity disorder.

Audio 3: Ocean Breath (Chapter 10)
Length: 6:41
Description: This guided meditation is intended to help youth develop a self-regulated, self-soothing practice through breathing.

Audio 4: Earth Body Scan (Chapter 10)
Length: 9:29
Description: This guided meditation is intended to help youth establish a sense of grounding, security, and release.

Part I

Introduction to Mindfulness

Chapter

1

Developing a Personal Mindfulness Practice

John P. Rettger, Ph.D.

JON KABAT-ZINN, the founder of mindfulness-based stress reduction (MBSR), one of the most well researched and widely implemented mindfulness programs across the globe, defines *mindfulness* as paying attention in a way: on purpose, in the present moment, and nonjudgmentally (Kabat-Zinn 2013). As my understanding of mindfulness has expanded and evolved over the past 15 years, I have come to think that the practice is enhanced by an explicit acknowledgment of the importance of self and other—that is, compassion. I would like to include compassion (see Chapter 2, "Mindful Self-Compassion") as part of our definition of mindfulness for this book.

A long-held virtue among mindfulness and yoga instructors is the importance of one's personal practice. This chapter is a how-to guide: how to begin, what you will need, what to do, and how to manage obstacles and challenges and stay on the "path." This topic is worthy of its own book. Given the limited space of a single chapter, I will have to be precise and therefore point you to other resources that can provide a more complete explanation and serve as a more comprehensive guide. I would recommend Jon Kabat-Zinn's *Full Catastrophe Living* (Kabat-Zinn 2013) as an excellent manual for cultivating a mindful lifestyle. The intention of this chapter is to provide you with the initial support to get you started with mindfulness. My call to action for you after reading this chapter is to start to practice and take the further steps necessary to deepen your practice by getting involved in a local mindfulness or yoga community.

As mental health professionals, we often must wear many hats and juggle busy professional and personal lives. Therefore, I think it is important to remember that mindfulness practice is as much a safe refuge for us as it is an offering for our patients. Our own self-care ought to be a priority, and so, too, must be our personal mindfulness practice. This is how to become an authentic guide: to practice and live what you aim to teach. Certainly, if we are going to encourage our patients to explore their vast and likely unchartered internal environment, we must be dedicated to making our own exploration.

This is not easy, and there will always be a constant pull toward other "to-dos" given the demands of our work and personal life and what we traditionally hold as priorities. Self-care has not been valued and supported enough in our profession. There is a difference between saying it is a value and actually engaging in the time and efforts to live out the value of self-care every single day. We must put mindfulness at the top of the list. I recall once either hearing or reading Jon Kabat-Zinn teach something to the effect of "we must sit as if our life depends on it, because it does!" Stress and burnout can and will end careers early and have costs with respect to the quality of patient care. Perhaps in your role as a therapist or educator you have come to see that those things that truly transform us often do not come easy. Mindfulness is no different—we must dedicate ourselves to it and reshape the perspective we have about how we want to approach the moments in our lives. This is where the attitudinal foundations of mindfulness (Kabat-Zinn 2013) can be of support to us.

Attitudinal Foundations

There are nine foundations of mindfulness taught by Jon Kabat-Zinn (2013). I list them here in an order that makes sense to me in terms of approaching, building, or strengthening a mindfulness practice. They also apply more generally to how you can approach the moments of your life. The nine foundations are all naturally interrelated and overlap with each other.

The first is *beginner's mind.* This involves an orientation to our present-moment experiences that is free of preconceptions and judgments. Mindfulness trains us to experience the reality of the moment as it is, not as we would like it to be.

To approach the moment in this way requires us to be able to unearth our perpetual flow of wants, desires, likes, and dislikes and even neutral reactions that we form toward ourselves, others, and our experiences. These judgments serve to shut down possibilities in our lives. The classic book *Zen Mind, Beginner's Mind: Informal Talks on Zen Meditation and Practice* (Suzuki et al. 2011, p. 1) opens with the now famous line "In the beginner's mind there are many possibilities, but in the expert's there are few." Mindfulness invites us to stay open to our experience and welcome in as many possibilities as we can. This type of realization is helpful in developing your practice because there will be times when you are bored and frustrated, and meditation feels like a chore or task to check off your daily to-do list. This is the moment to connect to your own heart and your original intention of beginning the mindfulness journey. Come back to beginner's mind time and time again. The more you carefully observe your experiences in meditation, the more you will discover that each moment has a unique flavor and that you can come to live each day with as much aliveness as a fresh perspective can give you. In fact, if you notice your breath, every single breath you take is like a snowflake; breaths are precious in that as humans we have a finite number of them.

The second foundation is *patience*. As previously noted, you will have periods of frustration, and there will be days when you feel no solace from having meditated and may even end a meditation feeling more anxious than when you started. This may be an indication that you have introduced goals into your experience and have gotten caught up in striving toward achieving an outcome. It is okay to wish for meditation to bring about a sense of relaxation. However, you cannot let that desire interfere with what your reality is.

Therefore, *nonstriving* is an essential ingredient and foundation to include in your practice and life. Along with patience and nonstriving come elements of *letting go* and *acceptance*. As human beings, we have a natural tendency to wish to cling to pleasant experiences and avoid those that are unpleasant. As a result, we perpetuate suffering by desiring our experiences to be other than what they are. Acceptance plays a central role in learning to embrace experience. Rather than being passive, avoidant, and/or compliant, acceptance is the active and complete acknowledgment and naming of what truth or reality exists in the moment. We cannot move to initiate and sustain genuine change when we are not able to correctly identify and be with what is occurring now.

In terms of your personal practice, the acceptance piece comes in when you embrace both pleasure and pain and everything between. This means that even on the days when the last thing you feel like doing is taking time to sit and notice your breath, you still come to the practice, even if that means for that day it is about stringing together one or however many more single mindful breaths at a time. These are the moments when the practice of self-compassion can come in (for more on self-compassion, see Chapter 12, "Trauma-Informed Yoga"). This means to be kind to yourself in the moments when you are caught in struggle.

Yoga practice is a powerful teacher of how to move with and through struggles with gracefulness. The most basic way to do this is to take a bigger breath in the moments of intensity when it feels as if you can't stay with a challenging pose any longer. Usually, that bigger breath brings in the freedom and ease that is needed to stay with and even embrace the challenge of the moment. Learning this on the yoga mat usually translates to everyday life. Taking that big breath in and a long, deep, feeling breath out when one is having difficulty can make all the difference, especially for youth who may struggle with self-regulation and subsequently make poor choices.

Along with self-compassion comes the practice of self-kindness. This is key to staying on the meditation and yoga path. If you have been disconnected from your body for some time, it can be incredibly challenging to connect to a yoga practice or feel into the body in meditation. Yoga can be challenging even for high-performing athletes who are not accustomed to the kind of breathing, stretching, and fine motor coordination and balance that a physical yoga practice requires. In our culture we tend to emphasize "strength" over "flexibility." I put these terms in quotation marks because I do not mean them just in the context of the physical body. For too long we have been caught up in powering through things, achieving, and "sucking it up." Now is the time to recognize that we must exercise new flexibility in our thinking and realize that what is needed more now is a "sacred pause": a time to stop all the doing and remember what it is to be a human being on this Earth. We are beings destined toward love. We are beings desperately in need of greater community and caring.

With respect to implementing your practice, you must determine what is the smallest step forward and start with that. This is where *nonjudgmental* awareness is a helpful perspective. Mindfulness calls us toward a space where we put aside any focus on our shortcomings and the internal dialogue that can sound something like "if only." An example of this pertaining to the practice of mindfulness is "If only I could still my mind and relax" or "If only I could get into that yoga pose." You can likely think of plenty of examples of how this may play out in your personal and professional life.

A helpful remedy to the judgments and the moments of doubt is the practice of *trust*. In this context, trust refers to a couple of different things. The most basic form of trust is self-trust. You must come to a healthy realization that you have what it takes to be committed to this path of mindfulness. This translates into having the belief that you have what it takes to be successful in your life. Mindfulness holds the potential to unlock your strengths and inner wisdom that enable you to work with or relate in a healthy way to the challenges in your life. You may even be surprised at what you can do and may overcome substantial barriers that you have been working with. Trust also enables us to discern, as is taught in the Serenity Prayer, what are the changeable and the unchangeable experiences in life and how to make peace with them. The other dimension of trust is to trust in the practices of yoga and mindfulness and the related teachings. Aside from all the contemporary and emerging scientific investigations into mindfulness and yoga, we must recognize that these practices have been around for centuries—if they weren't effective, then surely they would have faded into oblivion.

There is a certain *generosity* of the spirit that we all possess as human beings. Mindfulness cultivates this generosity by enabling us to "give ourselves over to life" (Kabat-Zinn 2013) and to care for ourselves such that we are then able to offer our compassion and care to others. It is a way of giving to others. A way of connecting to generosity in the practice of mindfulness is through the breathing. Most of us tend to not use the full capacity of the breath, and the result of shallow breathing is a disconnection from our natural ability to relax and feel grounded and connected. By practicing generosity of the breath, we expand our capacity to breathe and essentially let life in.

The last foundation presented by Jon Kabat-Zinn is *gratitude*, which can be expressed simply through a thankfulness for having this breath right here, right now. Another simple way to experience gratitude is to remember to take a moment to thank yourself every day for taking any amount of time, no matter how small, to arrive on the meditation cushion or yoga mat. It is essential to acknowledge that your efforts in the practice will serve to awaken compassion in your heart and that compassion will extend outward as a warm embrace toward your patients and loved ones.

What I hope you are taking away from these foundations is that mindfulness is more than meditation and yoga. Mindfulness has a lot to do with how you approach your life and interpret your experiences. The techniques that are practiced on the meditation cushion or yoga mat help you to grow the "muscles" to do the heavy lifting of living a truly compassionate life. What I am describing here is the distinction between formal and informal mindfulness practices. The formal practice of mindfulness consists of those structured techniques such as seated meditation or various forms of physical yoga, among many other mind-body practices. Informal mindfulness practices are everyday activities that we can perform with a directed attention toward the present-moment activity. A good example of this is washing the dishes. You can wash the dishes while having music or the television on and do the task without ever really noticing much about the experience. You are simply doing it to get it done. Or you can wash the dishes without any other stimuli and simply notice the sounds of the dishes clanking, the smell of the soap, the feel of the warm or hot water on your skin, the sight of the floating bubbles, and even any lingering taste from your meal. This is how you transform a chore into an opportunity for practice. There are practice opportunities happening all the time around you.

Mindfulness Practices

There are many distinct styles of meditation and of yoga. Although I cannot discuss all of these styles in this chapter, you will find many examples of how to practice in subsequent chapters. I also maintain a mindfulness practice blog at mindful.stanford.edu where you can go to find many practices that are suitable for youth. I strongly advise you to try all practices for yourself first before offering them to others. Additionally, I suggest you be willing to try different meditation practices and styles of yoga to find one that resonates most with you. You can find a description of various yoga postures in Chapter 12.

Breath Awareness Practice

Here is a simple breath awareness practice for you to begin to get a feel for what it is like to practice. You can also listen to these instructions while you are seated and ready to begin your mindfulness practice (Audio 1, available online at www.appi.org/Carrion).

 Audio 1: Breath Awareness Practice (5:28)

> Come to a comfortable sitting position in your chair. Sit a bit forward so that your back is not touching the chair back; this is helpful in lengthening up through the spine to ensure that the breath can travel freely through the body. Do your best to see that both of your sitting bones are evenly resting on the flat of the chair and both of your feet are firmly grounded to the floor. Breathe in through your nose and sense the air flowing through the nostrils and down through the collar bones, rib cage, and into the low belly. Feel your lower belly expand and stay connected to yourself, to your body, as the inhale becomes the exhale. Feel the awareness that follows the exhale from the low belly all the way through the rib cage, the collar bones, and up and out through the nostrils. Let the breath flow naturally one breath to the next in a way that feels good for you. It is likely you will notice your mind wandering, and when it does, from a place of self-compassion, simply bring this wandering mind back to the breathing. Continue in this way for a few minutes. After a few minutes—you can set a timer for any length of time—gently bring your awareness back to the breath, back to the body, and slowly let go of the meditation as you exhale. Open your eyes, reorienting yourself to the room. Take a moment of gratitude; it is optional to place your hands over your heart as a symbolic gesture of thankfulness to yourself for taking the time to complete this meditation.

Take a few moments here to reflect on your experience and perhaps make some notes in a journal.

In the remainder of this chapter, I offer a few practices and suggestions that stem from student questions I have received over the years. Space limitations do not allow a comprehensive presentation; readers interested in a more complete discussion of this topic can refer to meditation teacher and psychologist Tara Brach's "FAQ for Meditation" (Brach 2018).

Practice Suggestions

Meditation Posture

I do not hold any traditional view on what is the best posture in which to practice. You can practice meditation sitting down in a chair or on the floor. You can stand or lie down. You can even practice a walking meditation.

When practicing seated meditation, an important postural alignment point is to do your best to sit with an elongated spine. The spine has natural curves in it, so there isn't technically a "straight" back position, as you will hear many teachers say. It is important to sit "tall" so that you are not collapsing through the torso and so that your breathing can flow more easily. The other point I focus on when I am in a seated position on the floor is to use a prop such as a meditation cushion, which is called a zafu. Or you can use a yoga bolster (a big cylinder-shaped or rectangular pillow) or rolled blanket, yoga block, or any pillow sturdy enough to support you. There are also meditation benches that support a kneeling position. The key is to sit with your hips at the same level with or higher than your knees.

Physical Preparation

In my view, it is vital to have some sort of physical workout regime or a yoga practice to support meditation. As clinicians and researchers, naturally we spend quite of bit of time sitting down. Therefore, we need to find ways of caring for the physical body and clearing out excess energy to allow the body to feel more tranquil and the mind to be calmer when it is time to sit for meditation. Yoga is particularly well suited for this purpose because of the emphasis on both strengthening and stretching the body. To sustain a long period of seated meditation in the more classical postures, such as seated with legs crossed on a zafu, it is helpful to open the hips and strengthen the core of the body. This suggestion is not a requirement for seated meditation, but I believe you will find it much easier to sit longer periods of time with a stronger body.

Mental Environment

It is beneficial to choose a time of day when your mind feels awake and mostly settled. This may be helpful in reducing the amount of mind "chatter" that may be happening during the practice. In my perspective, however, I am OK with meditating with a busy mind. I view it as part of the practice for the day. I do my best to not get caught up in the business of the mind but to observe that thinking is happening and then calling my focus back onto my breath, body, or some other physical anchor. A common misperception regarding meditation practice is that it must involve a kind of emptying of the mind. My viewpoint is that there may be moments of this kind of mental stillness, but for the most part, the average person will likely have to learn to embrace the mind chatter rather than rather than resist it.

The time in which the mind will be most settled will vary from person to person. Some enjoy meditating early in the morning before the day gets busy. It can be particularly pleasant to meditate around the time the sun is rising be-cause it is a beautiful metaphor for the meditation practice as being a process of illumination—although it does not always feel that way! Other people may wish to meditate at the end of the day when they have completed all their im-portant daily activities. They feel that they can be more with the practice and less concerned about what is coming up the rest of the day. However, it is im-portant to recognize that the mind may already jump to tomorrow. Do your best to stay present to what's happening in the here and now, and the meditation practice will grow and unfold.

Emotional Environment

Your emotional state can impact your ability to sit for meditation or the level of commitment that you bring to the yoga practice. Specific breathing strategies can be used to help settle one's emotions and facilitate a deepened state of re-laxation. For specific practices, the reader can refer to Chapter 12 and try out the breathing practices detailed there. As an experiment, you can try noticing your level of emotional arousal prior to engaging in the breath work and then after. Typically, you will achieve noticeable results if there is a sufficient level of hyperarousal prior to engaging in the breathing.

Practice Environment

It is helpful and important to establish a dedicated space in your home and, if possible, your office to support your mindfulness practice. If your mindfulness practice is seated meditation, then having a special corner in a room can suffice. I suggest you keep this area clear from any distractions and excess objects or ma-terials—it should be a clutter-free space where the only activity that is performed is meditation. In creating a yoga space, you will need a bit more room so you can move through the postures. It is inspiring to decorate the space with images or objects that you consider to be sacred or special to you. For example, some practitioners will put traditional images, such as pictures of their meditation or yoga teacher, or devotional images or cultural artifacts from their particular religious tradition in their practice space. These images and artifacts serve as sources of motivation and inspiration and as a reminder of the core teachings of the mindfulness or contemplative path.

If you work in a shared space, you can be creative about using objects that are more portable and smaller so you can take them out when it is time to sit. Another helpful tip for those with limited space is to minimize the use of heavy furniture that you have to move to create a yoga space; you might resist practicing because of the added burden of having to move the furniture. Ideally, the practice space should be kept clean, organized, and free of distractions or stress cues (e.g., computers or other digital devices used for work, invoices, pending work items). Take steps to tidy the space up and do your best to make it a desirable place to practice; I have worked in community clinics and schools where the space was not very clean, which was not conducive to practicing mindfulness.

For those who are new to learning the practice of mindfulness or are working on developing a home practice, you may need to rely on apps or videos to support your practice. In this case, it is OK to use a device, such as a tablet, if you turn off any notifications or alerts that would redirect your attention away from the practice. It is challenging when you are newer to mindfulness to maintain the necessary disciplined attention to not abandon the practice for other household demands. It is not uncommon to hear that, for example, the laundry got in the way of the meditation. Therefore, early in development of your practice, it may be advantageous to seek out a community, such as those at meditation centers or yoga studios. Being around others who are on a similar path can be helpful in staying dedicated. This requires an ongoing and daily commitment to practicing, even when you do not want to.

Meditation Dosage

Dosage can be thought of and conceptualized as number of minutes per day and a count of practice sessions per week. One may wonder, is it better to sit, for example, for 10 minutes three times per day or once for 30 minutes per day? I think this answer will vary according to the unique needs and goals of the practitioner. Tara Brach suggests between 15 and 45 minutes per day (Brach 2018). In one study, the researchers reported positive effects after participants practiced an average of 27 minutes per day over an 8-week MBSR program (Hölzel et al. 2011). In my work with patients and students, on numerous occasions students reported that the 3-minute breathing space in mindfulness-based cognitive therapy has been a meaningful and useful practice. I do believe there is a benefit to both longer and shorter practice periods when applied with discernment.

Working With Obstacles

As you continue to practice, it is likely that you will encounter obstacles along the way. These obstacles may include aversion, laziness, desires, worry, and doubt (for a more in-depth exploration, see Saraswati 2003). A number of these have been written about in Buddhist and Yogic texts. Such challenges are considered universal and are encountered by all practitioners of yoga and meditation at some point.

A helpful mindfulness practice that you can use in working with the above obstacles is to move toward, rather than away from, them to develop a healthy "friendship" with them by using the RAIN practice (Brach 2018). The acronym RAIN stands for recognizing the obstacle, accepting it as being part of your present-moment experience, investigating it with kindness and curiosity, and practicing non-identification with it. Another form of the "N" in the RAIN practice is self-nurturing. Brach teaches that the addition of the self-nourishment piece forms the practice of the "RAIN of self-compassion." Using the RAIN process can help to shift your energy enough to move through the obstacles and create increased insight. For those readers wishing to learn more about this practice, see my blog post on establishing a clear mind in meditation (Rettger 2016).

Practice Schedule

Having considered all the above information, you may be wondering how to structure a practice schedule. To give you an idea of what a weekly practice might look like, I have put together a sample weekly schedule (Table 1–1). The schedule includes multiple practices per day that you can choose from depending on how you are feeling on any given day. At least one meditation and one yoga practice are suggested. Ideally, each day would include a bit of both yoga posture and meditation.

You can use the audio practices included with this book or search for online resources such as video websites or audio directories to find guided practices that you will enjoy. I wish you the best in establishing your mindfulness practice and trying out the many wonderful practices that are included in this book.

TABLE 1-1. Sample weekly practice table

	Monday	Tuesday	Wednesday	Thursday	Friday	Saturday	Sunday[a]
Gentle yoga—yin or restorative			X				X
Active yoga—Vinyasa or power	X	X		X		X	
Awareness of breathing (group at beginning or ending of yoga or body scan practice)		X		X		X	
Lovingkindness or self-compassion focused meditation	X		X				X
Body scan—brief (less than 5 minutes)	X		X		X		X
Body scan—long		X		X		X	
Extended mindfulness meditation (45 minutes or longer)	X		X		X		X
Shorter meditation period—work to accumulate to 25 minutes		X		X		X	

[a]Sunday can be a rest day or used for gentler restorative practices. You can also choose another day that can serve as a rest and recovery day from physical practices.

KEY POINTS

- The attitudinal foundations provide a framework to apply to your meditation and yoga practice and everyday life experiences.
- Commit to a daily mindfulness practice, including both formal and informal practices.
- Seek out the support of a meditation and/or yoga community to support your practice and learning.

References

Brach T: FAQ for Meditation, 2018. Available at: www.tarabrach.com/faq-for-meditation2. Accessed May 4, 2018.

Hölzel BK, Carmody J, Vangel M, et al: Mindfulness practice leads to increases in regional brain gray matter density. Psychiatry Res 191(1):36–43, 2011 21071182

Kabat-Zinn J: Full Catastrophe Living: Using the Wisdom of Your Body and Mind to Face Stress, Pain, and Illness. New York, Bantam, 2013

Rettger J: I'm a longtime meditator and still don't have a clear mind. New York, Sonima, June 27, 2016. Available at: www.sonima.com/meditation/clear-mind. Accessed May 4, 2018.

Saraswati S: The Yoga-Sutras of Patanjali. Boston, MA, Shambhala, 2003

Suzuki S, Dixon T, Smith H, et al: Zen Mind, Beginner's Mind: Informal Talks on Zen Meditation and Practice. Boston, MA, Shambhala, 2011

Chapter

2

Mindful Self-Compassion for Teens and Young Adults

Karen Bluth, Ph.D.
Christine Lathren, M.D.
Lorraine Hobbs, M.A.

ALTHOUGH compassion is a well-studied phenomenon that can be defined as the awareness of another person's suffering coupled with the deep desire to help (Goetz et al. 2010), emotional health research also explores the benefits of taking a compassionate stance toward one's own personal suffering. Self-compassion originates in Buddhist philosophy, whereby the interconnectedness of all beings makes no distinction between *others* and *self* (Neff 2003a). However, researchers and clinicians alike have found the concept of self-compassion to be relevant to present-day Western culture and, in particular, to successful navigation of the often self-critical and tumultuous adolescence phase.

Self-compassion is described as treating oneself with the same kindness, understanding, and support during a difficult time that one would give to a good friend. A more formal definition of self-compassion as conceptualized by Neff (2003a) is that it is a state of mind or attitude characterized by three components: self-kindness, common humanity, and mindfulness. *Self-kindness* refers to responding to one's imperfections, setbacks, mistakes, or any situation causing distress with care and encouragement as opposed to criticism. *Common humanity* entails recognizing that imperfections and difficulties are part of life. Thus, difficulties are not isolating but rather are an experience that unifies all people. Finally, *mindfulness* in the context of self-compassion refers to having a balanced awareness of painful emotions. In this case, difficulties are neither avoided nor overexaggerated; instead, they are tended to with attention and care. When these three components are taken together, a self-compassionate person is able to acknowledge and forgive personal weaknesses in difficult times while simultaneously maintaining healthy motivation to address the problematic situation at hand (Barnard and Curry 2011).

Self-compassion can be considered an adaptive coping mechanism and bears similarities to self-esteem (Neff et al. 2007) but with important distinctions that highlight its unique relevance to common adolescent issues. From a developmental standpoint, sizable physical, physiological, socioemotional, and cognitive shifts leave adolescents particularly vulnerable to stress and mental health problems such as anxiety and depression (Lee et al. 2014). Although forming close friendships and an achieving a sense of "belonging" within peer groups are important aspects of healthy adolescent development, some teens become highly self-evaluative, which can lead to self-criticism and negative self-views when they feel that they do not measure up (Neff and McGehee 2010). Moreover, increased introspection and egocentric tendencies can lead adolescents to feel extremely self-conscious (as if they are being scrutinized), inadequate, and alone in their difficulties (Elkind 1985). Elkind has labeled this phenomenon, in which adolescents feel that they are continually being observed and evaluated, as the *imaginary audience* (Elkind 1985).

Whereas self-esteem promotes self-worth by comparing oneself with peers, self-compassion promotes commonality, nonjudgmental connection to others, and self-soothing when one feels that one falls short (Neff 2003a). In a longitudinal study of high-school students, self-compassion buffered against the negative impact of low self-esteem (Marshall et al. 2014). Additionally, self-compassion is associated with more stable feelings of self-worth, is negatively correlated with social comparison (Neff and Vonk 2009), and is positively correlated with a sense of social connectedness (Akin and Akin 2015). Self-compassion may be particularly relevant to older adolescent females, who report lower self-compassion levels compared with both younger adolescent females and all-age adolescent males (Bluth et al. 2017) and who suffer twice the rate of depression compared with males (Nolen-Hoeksema and Girgus 1994). Regardless of gender, self-compassion may combat precisely the types of developmental difficulties adolescents face.

In adults, correlational research has confirmed self-compassion's robust positive association with multiple measures of well-being (Zessin et al. 2015) and negative correlation with psychopathology (MacBeth and Gumley 2012), with mirrored findings in adolescents (Marsh et al. 2017). In an effort to cultivate self-compassion and its positive correlates, Neff and Germer (2013) created an adult mindful self-compassion (MSC) intervention that follows an 8-week group-based format similar to that of mindfulness-based stress reduction. In a clinical trial, adult MSC participants made significant gains in self-compassion, mindfulness, and well-being measures posttraining that were maintained a year later. Following this lead, we created Making Friends with Yourself: A Mindful Self-Compassion Program for Teens and Young Adults (MFY; Bluth et al. 2016), an adapted MSC intervention tailored for adolescents ages 11–20. In general, this program differs from the adult program in that classes are shorter and developmentally appropriate (e.g., they are more activity based, incorporate mindful movement and an opening art activity, have shorter guided meditations) and include a component about the adolescent brain. As discussed more fully later in this chapter, empirical evidence supports this adapted program as effective in promoting adolescent emotional well-being and resilience while decreasing psychological distress and related symptomatology (e.g., anxiety, depression) (Bluth and Eisenlohr-Moul 2017; Bluth et al. 2016).

Program Structure and Therapeutic Process

Given the numerous mental health benefits of self-compassion, the main purpose of MFY is to strengthen skills that increase self-compassion. Mindfulness is foundational to self-compassion; therefore, mindfulness skills such as mindful art and movement are included. Through this program, teens become open to the possibility that self-kindness and self-care can be more motivating than "beating themselves up." This awareness presents a radically different understanding to teens of how they view themselves and the way in which they approach their lives. Most importantly, engaging in this program begins a lifelong practice in transforming the way in which they relate to themselves.

MFY is typically taught in a group format, optimally with 8–14 teens and two instructors, using an 8-week curriculum of weekly meetings that last 1 hour and 45 minutes. A version for schools that includes the same content is formatted into sixteen 50-minute classes. A more intensive version is offered as a summer camp and is scheduled over 4 days, 4 hours each day. Two instructors are recommended to allow flexibility during the sessions should a participant require one-on-one attention for any reason.

Each of the eight MFY sessions follows a routine format. To facilitate the transition from the fast-paced school day into the slower-paced, self-reflective MFY class, each session opens with a mindful art activity. During this time, teens are asked to notice physical sensations (e.g., the feeling of their pen in their hand, the sounds of the pen on the paper) as well as any thoughts that might be arising (e.g., any judgment about how the art is turning out). Often, the art activity also offers a hands-on introduction to a concept or exercise that is fully explored later in the session.

Next, the instructor guides the group in an opening meditation, followed by a discussion of the previous week's home practice. During this time, teens have the opportunity to hear how others may be struggling in the same ways they are, reinforcing their common humanity. Teens also share any successes in integrating the self-compassion skills into their daily lives. Often, this portion of the class reiterates the self-compassionate response; if participants share that they practiced less than they should have, the instructor encourages them not to judge themselves harshly but rather to respond with warmth and kindness.

The main topic of the week is then introduced through a combination of didactics, discussion, exercises, and video clips. The topics for each of the 8 weeks are as follows: discovering mindful self-compassion, paying attention on purpose (mindfulness), lovingkindness, self-compassion, self-compassion versus self-esteem, living deeply (core values), managing difficult emotions, and embracing your life with gratitude. As part of each topic, relevant formal and informal practices are introduced (see "Core Techniques" section of this chapter). These practices form the foundation of mindful self-compassion practice in daily life and are to be used as home practice during the subsequent week.

Of note, halfway through each class, the instructor guides the teens in mindful movement practice. This serves to reinforce mindfulness concepts while also providing teens with the opportunity to stretch their bodies. The class always ends with the teens having an opportunity to share their "takeaway" for the class; this helps to provide closure as well as to reinforce what they have learned. Home practice for the upcoming week is also discussed.

Assessment tools are available to measure self-compassion over the course of treatment. A 26-item self-compassion scale (Neff 2003b) and a brief 12-item version (Raes et al. 2011) have a 0.97 correlation, indicating that the brief scale measures the same construct as the original scale. The full scale allows investigation of the three components of self-compassion (self-kindness, common humanity, and mindfulness), but the shorter scale is less burdensome and therefore appropriate when you are not exploring subscales. A youth version with simpler wording is in the process of being developed (K.D. Neff, personal communication, 2018). Depending on the research questions and participant population, any one of these measurement tools can be used to assess self-compassion prior to and after implementing the MFY program. Additionally, given that increases in self-compassion can have a positive impact on many other aspects of life, including stress, emotional health (e.g., anxiety, depression, affect), life satisfaction, and resilience, these constructs are often simultaneously measured before and after the intervention as well.

Teaching Making Friends With Yourself: Instructors' Personal Practice and Role

In order for the MFY curriculum to be maximally beneficial for the teens, it is critical that instructors have a well-established personal mindfulness and self-compassion practice; in other words, instructors must embody self-compassion. Without this, the practices come across as being empty of any real depth or value.

An experienced instructor who has a regular mindfulness and self-compassion practice will be sensitive to the needs of the teens with whom he or she is working and will respond to those needs with *loving, connected presence*. For example, when a teen is experiencing a difficult emotion, the instructor may encourage the teen to engage in a soothing self-touch gesture (e.g., placing his or her hands on the heart) or to silently name the emotion, which activates the prefrontal cortex (the executive function center of the brain) and inhibits the amygdala (the fight-or-flight or emotion center of the brain), thereby downregulating the intensity of the emotion. The experienced instructor will recognize when practices become too intense and may suggest that the teen "close" by bringing his or her attention to an object outside of his or her body or by thinking about something else entirely. If the instructor senses that the teen feels safe enough to proceed with exploring emotions, he or she may encourage locating the associated sensation in the body and "softening," or relaxing, that area, further easing the heightened emotions. This process empowers teens; the teens develop strength and resilience as they gain skills in emotional self-regulation.

The challenge that many therapists face in teaching self-compassion, then, is learning to differentiate between the role of therapist and that of self-compassion instructor. A therapist enters into the therapeutic relationship with an ethical responsibility to help heal patients. This contract is oriented toward change—whether it is changing specific behaviors, changing patients' attitudes toward themselves, or changing patients' attitudes to the way in which they approach life. This is in direct conflict with the role of the self-compassion instructor, whose main responsibility is to guide the teen to be nonjudgmentally aware of his or her experience and, when painful feelings arise, to engage in self-soothing behaviors. In certain therapy approaches, the therapist may have a greater focus on the "neck up," noticing negative thought patterns, investigating why emotions occur, and subsequently making suggestions about how to change those thoughts and emotions. In contrast, the self-compassion instructor works more from "the neck down," asking teens to investigate where anger resides in the body, for example, and then introducing ways to soothe this sensation. Because physical sensations are intricately linked to emotions, soothing physical sensations will ease the difficult emotion, lessening its strength.

Thus, therapists who are trained to "fix" the patient must learn to let go of the outcome of the therapeutic relationship and, first and most important, be present and connected with the teen, in touch with a felt sense of both their own and the teen's emotional experience in the moment. When teaching self-compassion, the instructor is planting seeds that will take root and flourish when the time is right for the teen. Letting go of the outcome is akin to preparing the soil; the instructor is setting the groundwork for the seeds to germinate and grow.

Case Example

Rachel, an 18-year-old entering college with a history of eating disorders and hospitalization, attended a mindful self-compassion group. Her boundaries were clear from the outset. She repeated the words "Don't touch me" in the first three classes. In class four, she indicated that she awoke in the middle of the night, experiencing great anxiety on the verge of becoming a panic attack. She recalled the soothing touch of placing a hand on the heart and recited a few lovingkindness practices she had learned. This helped relieve some of the anxiety, and she was able to avoid a panic attack and return to sleep. During the group discussion, she began to weep. The instructor, Molly, facing Rachel with her own hand on her heart (exhibiting loving, connected presence), could see that Rachel was beginning to get increasingly upset, in part because of the vulnerability of sharing. Moving directly across from Rachel, Molly guided her through inquiry, or the process of tracking her own experience, which helped Rachel identify and explore her direct experience of suffering and what support she might need in that moment. Although Rachel likely would have preferred to leave the room and escape her own vulnerability, the experience of being held by the acceptance of the instructor and the group allowed her to feel safe enough to be present with her feelings and therefore move through them. In the end, she was able to find a soothing touch gesture that offered comfort in the moment. The connection between Molly and Rachel enabled Rachel to make the necessary shift so that she was able to attend to her own experience and respond to her own suffering with compassion.

Core Techniques

Both formal and informal practices are offered in MFY. Formal practices involve setting aside a period of time each day (5–20 minutes) to practice a specific meditation or exercise. Informal practices are those that are implemented in the moment when one is experiencing difficulty, such as a moment of feeling anxious or stressed. In this moment, the teen can engage in a short informal practice (10 seconds to 3 minutes) that serves to remind him or her of the principles of self-compassion and initiates a self-soothing behavior. Although participants are expected to engage in both formal and informal home practice as a way to reinforce skills that are taught in class, most teens prefer and use informal practice most often, and preliminary research shows that informal practice supports positive outcomes (R. Campo, unpublished data, 2017). In the following subsections, we describe an opening course exercise and several core formal and informal practices that form the foundation of the MFY curriculum.

Opening Exercise: How Would I Treat a Friend?

Similar to the adult MSC program, the MFY program begins with an exercise called *How would I treat a friend?* that highlights the purpose of the course and defines self-compassion in a meaningful and understandable way. The exercise begins by asking teens to imagine how they would treat a good friend who had encountered an emotionally challenging experience, such as missing a key goal in a soccer game or being excluded from an important social event. Together, a small group (i.e., two or three teens) brainstorms what they would say to their friend and how they would act toward him or her. Next, the teens imagine themselves in the same situation. In small groups, the teens discuss how they would treat themselves, including the words they would say to themselves and the tone of voice they would use. The entire group then reconvenes to report their small-group findings and to discuss this astonishing statistic: 78% of adults report treating friends much more kindly than they do themselves during similar challenging circumstances (Knox and Neff 2016). In fact, most of us are quite judgmental and harsh with ourselves. Neff's (2003a) informal definition of self-compassion is then offered: *Self-compassion is treating yourself with the same kindness and care as we treat our friends at times of suffering.* The goal of MFY then is articulated to the teens as learning how to treat yourself with the same kindness and care as you treat your good friends.

Informal Practice

SOOTHING TOUCH

Soothing touch is the first self-compassion tool introduced to teens, and as an informal practice, it can be used at any time throughout the day. First, the instructor describes the physiology behind soothing touch: just as petting a dog or cat is comforting, engaging in a soothing touch gesture for oneself promotes the release of the hormone oxytocin, which eases stress, relieves tension, and stimulates social bonding. It is important to provide this scientific explanation because teens might otherwise consider this practice as "touchy-feely," which can be a turn-off to many skeptical teens. The instructor then introduces the various ways in which teens can soothe themselves through gestures (e.g., putting a hand on the heart, cradling one's face in one's hands, folding one's arms and giving oneself a gentle squeeze) for teens to try out, and teens are encouraged to find one that is comforting for them. Teens generally respond well to this exercise and report that they use soothing touch regularly throughout their daily interactions and activities either alone or in combination with other mindfulness or self-compassion exercises.

A MOMENT FOR ME

A moment for me is a second core practice that can be combined with soothing touch practice and used immediately when one is struggling or experiencing difficulty. This practice uses all three components of self-compassion: mindfulness, common humanity, and self-kindness. First, the teen begins with a statement that acknowledges the difficulty, such as "This is a moment of struggle." Although it may seem obvious that this moment is emotionally challenging, often teens (and adults as well) tend to resist or push away difficult emotions. Further, fully recognizing that the moment is challenging by stating it out loud in this way engages the prefrontal cortex, which then lessens the activation of the amygdala, the part of the brain responsible for heightened emotions, such as anger and fear. Stating emotions with a calm and matter-of-fact tone represents the mindfulness component of self-compassion, which brings a balanced perspective and awareness to the situation.

The second part of a moment for me is acknowledging that this experience is not unique to the teen, and this occurs through stating to oneself, "Having struggles is part of life." This is the common humanity component of self-compassion and tends to be particularly impactful for teens as they reframe their emotional difficulty as part of the normal human experience. This can be a radical turning point for many teens, who often feel that they are the only ones who are struggling with feelings of inadequacy, worthlessness, and self-loathing. Thus, knowing that this is part of the growth process and common among most—if not all—teens is often extremely powerful.

Finally, the third and last part of the a moment for me practice is self-kindness, or taking an active role in being kind to oneself. This begins with a soothing touch gesture—putting a hand over one's heart or stroking one's cheek, for example. Next, teens say something to themselves that is soothing, such as "May I be kind to myself in this moment." Teens are encouraged to personalize the practice by thinking about the particular words that resonate with them, such as "I love you" or "I'm here for you" or "Don't worry; everything is going to be OK." Because teens (and also adults) do not generally say kind and comforting words to themselves, this can feel awkward or uncomfortable at first. Teens are reassured that it is normal to experience some discomfort when speaking to themselves kindly because this is a new way of relating to oneself, and it would therefore be expected to feel somewhat odd. With practice, this last part of a moment for me becomes not only more comfortable but eventually quite soothing.

Formal Practice

MUSIC MEDITATION

In *music meditation*, often a favorite among teens, a melodic, relaxing instrumental music piece between 5 and 10 minutes in length is introduced as a mindful listening practice. In the music meditation, selections without lyrics are chosen because instrumental music promotes "feeling" the music within the body as opposed to thinking about the words.

To begin the practice, teens are instructed to find a comfortable place to sit or lie down and to close their eyes if they are comfortable doing so. They are then asked to listen closely to each tone of the music that will be played, to hear the different instruments and the pitch of the music, and to pay attention to each tone as it is being played. When they find that their mind has wandered, which will happen generally after a few seconds to a minute, they are instructed to gently guide their attention back to the tones of the music. Following this practice, teens can share what the experience was like for them. Finally, teens are encouraged to find their own music that meets the guidelines of music meditation (i.e., instrumental and melodic) for home practice.

COMPASSIONATE BODY SCAN

Similar to a traditional mindfulness body scan, *compassionate body scan* begins by bringing attention to different parts of the body, starting with the feet and slowly proceeding upward to the legs, torso, arms, and head. Unlike the traditional body scan, however, as each part of the body is brought into one's attention, guidance in the compassionate body scan reminds teens to be grateful for how each part of the body supports them, whether it is helping to keep them alive (e.g., heart, lungs) or making it possible for them to get around (e.g., legs, feet). If aversion or resistance arises when one focuses on a particular body part, the instructor encourages teens to be open to the possibility of gradually accepting these parts of the body. Because many teens are focused on their body image and how they appear to others (Steinberg and Morris 2001) and because the media offer images of perfect and often unattainable bodies, one's body is often a source of tremendous self-judgment for many teens. For this reason, a compassionate body scan, one that cultivates acceptance for one's body, can help reduce anxiety.

Exercise and Informal Practice: Here-And-Now Stone

Because mindfulness is a foundational component of self-compassion, mindfulness skills are also included in the MFY curriculum. One of the favorite mindfulness exercises among teens is the *here-and-now stone*, which is derived directly from the adult MSC curriculum (Neff and Germer 2013). Each teen selects a polished stone from a basket of stones and is encouraged to study it carefully by holding it up to the light; noticing the different lines, colors, and markings that it may have; and noticing the feel of the stone (e.g., whether it is warm or cool to the touch). Teens are encouraged to get to know their stone well enough so that "if it were in a pile of similar polished stones you would find it in an instant." For an added effect, the room is darkened, and teens are given mini-flashlights to use to explore their stones. After a few minutes, the teens are asked, "Did any of you notice that you weren't particularly stressed, anxious, or depressed when you were exploring your stone?" The explanation is then provided that when we bring our attention to our physical sensations, as we do through our senses, our attention is in the present moment, and, as such, our minds are not dwelling in the past (i.e., ruminating) or worrying about the future. Only the present exists in these moments, and our minds are surprisingly free of worry and stress. For this reason, when we are mindful, we are less anxious and depressed. Teens are then encouraged to keep their stone with them to hold and explore informally during times of distress as a way of bringing attention out of thinking mode and into the physical experience. Teens have described this informal practice as being particularly useful during academic testing situations.

Adaptations

MFY is appropriate for youth ages 11–20 and has been empirically tested with participants ages 11–18 (Bluth and Eisenlohr-Moul 2017; Bluth et al. 2016). However, because developmental needs and interests vary considerably across this age range, we suggest that the age range for any given group be no more than 4 years. Also, to accommodate these developmental needs, slight variations in the curriculum should be made for younger teens. For example, most groups of younger teens benefit from a movement break partway through the 1.75-hour class. Frequently, however, older teens not only do not need a movement break but would prefer not to have one. For this reason, many of the mindful movement activities in the curriculum are optional.

One pilot-tested and published MFY adaptation combined elements of MFY and the adult MSC curricula to offer an online 8-week course (using the WebEx platform) for young adult cancer survivors from across the country (Campo et al. 2017). In this group video chat version, games requiring physical group interaction (e.g., tossing a bean bag around the group) were not feasible and therefore were omitted. Also, some exercises and meditations from the adult MSC program were substituted for those of MFY to ensure that the curriculum was appropriate for a slightly older age group (mean age 27), and other elements were omitted entirely (e.g., explanation of adolescent brain development).

Finally, several other MFY adaptations have been piloted or are under way to meet the unique needs of special subpopulations of teens. In fall 2017, an MFY adaptation was delivered to teens undergoing inpatient treatment for eating disorders. Posttraining feedback was positive, with participants reporting that the program was "eye-opening" and "the best program [they had] received so far" in their hospital stay (K. Bluth, M. Hill, and S. Zerwas, unpublished data, 2017). Additional adaptations are under way for teens with gender dysphoria and for Inuit teens of northern Quebec, who suffer from suicide rates 11 times the national average. Additionally, plans are under way to adapt MFY for youth ages 8–11. With time, we anticipate further adaptations for other cultures and subpopulations of youth.

Empirical Evaluation of Making Friends With Yourself

Two published studies support the feasibility, acceptability, and positive emotional well-being outcomes of MFY. A third study supports the feasibility, acceptability, and preliminary outcomes of the modified version created for the online program for young adult cancer survivors. The first study, published in 2016, was designed as a waitlist crossover study for teens ages 14–17; the first cohort ($n=16$) received the intervention, and the waitlist group ($n=18$) was evaluated (Bluth et al. 2016). The waitlist group then received the intervention. Analyses were conducted in two ways: First, between-group analyses compared outcomes of the intervention group with that of the waitlist group. Second, the two groups that received the intervention were combined, and within-group analyses were conducted to assess postintervention outcomes of this larger sample; both analyses controlled for pretest scores. Findings indicated that the intervention group had greater life satisfaction and self-compassion and lower depression than the waitlist control group, with trends toward greater mindfulness and social connectedness and lower anxiety. When the two cohorts were combined ($n=29$), findings indicated significantly greater mindfulness and self-compassion and lower anxiety, depression, perceived stress, and negative affect postintervention. Further, both mindfulness and self-compassion separately predicted, or explained, decreases in anxiety while controlling for the other. Increases in mindfulness also predicted decreases in depression, and increases in self-compassion predicted decreases in perceived stress and increases in life satisfaction (Bluth et al. 2016).

Further, as an exploratory analysis, formal home practice was investigated as a predictor of increases in mindfulness and self-compassion (Bluth et al. 2016). Interestingly, findings indicated that home practice was not a significant predictor of these outcomes. In other words, although the teens had greater mindfulness and self-compassion at the end of the intervention, this was not necessarily because they engaged in home practice. Increases in mindfulness and self-compassion, and related increases in emotional well-being, may be a result of in-class activities or discussions, informal "in the moment" practices integrated into daily life, and perhaps a shift in perspective that occurs as a result of the class meetings and informal practice.

Indeed, qualitative data support the importance of informal practices and perspective shifts (Bluth et al. 2016). Practices such as the here-and-now stone that use tangible objects to promote calmness and clarity appeared beneficial during stressful school encounters. Other teens discussed benefits from understanding common humanity, which helped teens to realize that most of their peers also experience emotional challenges. As one teen commented at the end of the course, "You know, I haven't really done much practice at home this whole time...or any at all, actually...but this course has changed how I see life" (K. Bluth, S. Gaylord, R. Campo, M. Mullarkey, and L. Hobbs, unpublished data, 2016). These findings are preliminary, and little research has been conducted investigating the role of home practice in predicting outcomes of mindfulness and self-compassion interventions with youth; therefore, more research is needed to explore the role of home practice in predicting outcomes.

Feasibility and acceptability of MFY was further confirmed by attendance and retention data, which were higher than expected. Attendance averaged 84% over the two cohorts, and 87% of the participants completed the program (Bluth et al. 2016). Qualitative data in which participants articulated their favorite practices, how they implemented the practices in their daily lives, how they had a better understanding of the concepts of mindfulness and self-compassion, and that they felt they were not alone in their struggles, confirmed acceptability of the program. One teen summed up her experience as follows:

> I guess I'm thankful for the tools that I've learned, because I get a lot of anxiety about school, especially. I feel like in the last few weeks my anxiety in the moment has decreased because I'm mindful and compassionate toward myself, and I don't know, I feel much better about a lot of stuff I have to do, because I know it's not the end of the world if I don't do it or whatever. (Bluth et al. 2016, p. 488)

Another pilot study for teens ages 11–17 (N=47) included five cohorts of students and took place over the course of several years (Bluth and Eisenlohr-Moul 2017). Findings indicated that postintervention, adolescents who attended the MFY curriculum perceived that they had lower stress after the program and self-reported greater resilience, curiosity and exploration (defined as a tendency to attempt and embrace new learning opportunities), and gratitude. Further, both mindfulness and self-compassion covaried with perceived stress and depressive symptoms, such that as mindfulness and self-compassion increased from preinvervention to postintervention, perceived stress and depressive symptoms decreased. Mindfulness also covaried with anxiety, and self-compassion covaried with resilience and curiosity and exploration. When examining demographic factors, results indicated that high-school participants demonstrated greater improvements in self-compassion than did middle-school participants and also greater decreases in depressive symptoms. However, this may be largely due to the greater level of depressive symptoms in high-school students at baseline. Further, there were trends demonstrating that females increased slightly more in self-compassion than did their male counterparts, also potentially because of lower self-compassion at baseline (Bluth and Eisenlohr-Moul 2017).

A third study implemented an adapted version of the adult MSC and adolescent MFY curricula to pilot an online video chat intervention for young adult cancer survivors from across the country (Campo et al. 2017). This 8-week intervention was delivered in five cohorts (n=25, mean age=27) to these young adults, who typically suffer from high rates of distress, including anxiety and depression, related to facing a life-threatening illness. Quantitative findings indicated that this mode of delivery was feasible; 84% attended at least six of the eight sessions. Additionally, the young adult participants rated acceptability as high, with a score of 4.36 out of 5. Psychosocial outcomes (anxiety, depression, social isolation, body image, posttraumatic growth, mindfulness, and self-compassion) changed significantly from preintervention to postintervention, with medium to high effect sizes (Campo et al. 2017).

Furthermore, a qualitative analysis of the recorded intervention sessions examined the relevance of self-compassion skills in addressing the unique psychosocial needs of a subset of these young adult cancer survivors (n=20, mean age = 27) (Lathren et al. 2018). Participants found self-compassion skills helpful in coping with three main stressors: isolation from peers, body concerns, and ongoing health-related anxiety. Regarding isolation, it appeared that although participants often felt misunderstood or unsupported by peers, self-compassion skills helped them to realize their inner wisdom and ability to provide emotional self-care. In other words, participants could provide their own self-directed support rather than relying on others who "don't get it." Additionally, participants noted benefiting from connectedness with other young cancer survivors and increased gratitude for those relationships in their lives that were supportive.

Participants also noted improved appreciation for their bodies (i.e., they felt gratitude for the parts that were working well instead of focusing on parts that were negatively impacted by cancer) and decreased anxiety during health-related experiences such as oncology procedures. Importantly, participants reported many instances of tailoring self-compassion practices to make them relevant and useful during stressful encounters, as highlighted by this quotation that demonstrates the use of phrases from a lovingkindness meditation that was taught in class:

> And I've actually throughout the week found myself adapting the phrases that I'm using kind of based on how I'm feeling. So, I had an oncology check-up on Friday and so the whole time I was thinking—"May I be healthy, may I be healthy." (Lathren et al. 2018, p. 653)

Although some participants found tapping into physical sensations challenging at first because of reminders of cancer side effects or worries about recurrence, this distress appeared to subside with instructor guidance and with practice. Overall, qualitative analysis shed light on the positive quantitative findings and points to the relevance of self-compassion to well-being for youth with serious illness.

Conclusion and Future Directions

The first training for teachers of MFY was in spring 2016, and since then interest in the program has spread internationally. Depression, anxiety, stress, and suicidality among teens are increasing at an alarming rate (Twenge 2017), and there is a tremendous need for adolescents to learn coping resources. MFY offers a toolbox of practices that help, and as the research base for MFY continues to strengthen and grow, we anticipate an increasing need for MFY teacher trainings as well as trainings for similar mindfulness and compassion programs. It is our ethical obligation to offer teens an array of skills that help them to navigate the challenging adolescent period.

In the future, we expect to develop adaptations of MFY for younger populations, various types of school-based programs, programs for families, and programs that meet the needs of different cultures and subpopulations of teens, such as teens who are particularly at risk for poor mental health trajectories. Armed with the skills provided by MFY and other similar programs, teens will be able to traverse life's inevitable challenges knowing they can count on themselves to respond with kindness and support whenever they need it.

KEY POINTS

- The effective instruction of mindful self-compassion stems from the instructor's own established mindfulness and self-compassion practice.
- Letting go of outcomes is critical in teaching teens mindful self-compassion in order to provide them the opportunity to find their own pace and pathway to learning the tools that work for them.
- Research on mindful self-compassion interventions in adolescents and adults is burgeoning and showing positive outcomes.

Discussion Questions

1. What are some of the emotional well-being challenges that adolescents face today? In what ways can self-compassion help to alleviate these challenges?

2. What does the recent research on self-compassion report? How does this compare with the evidence on adults?

3. What are some of the key ways in which a self-compassion therapist must "change hats" when teaching Making Friends with Yourself?

Suggested Readings

Bluth K: The Self-Compassion Workbook for Teens: Mindfulness and Compassion Skills to Overcome Self-Criticism and Embrace Who You Are. Oakland CA, New Harbinger, 2017

Siegel D: Brainstorm: The Power and Purpose of the Teenage Brain. New York, TarcherPerigee, 2014

Vo D: The Mindful Teen. Oakland CA, New Harbinger, 2015

References

Akin U, Akin A: Examining the predictive role of self-compassion on sense of community in Turkish adolescents. Soc Indic Res 123(1):29–38, 2015

Barnard LK, Curry JF: Self-compassion: conceptualizations, correlates, and interventions. Rev Gen Psychol 15(4):289–303, 2011

Bluth K, Eisenlohr-Moul TA: Response to a mindful self-compassion intervention in teens: a within-person association of mindfulness, self-compassion, and emotional well-being outcomes. J Adolesc 57:108–118, 2017 28414965

Bluth K, Gaylord SA, Campo RA, et al: Making Friends with Yourself: A mixed methods pilot study of a mindful self-compassion program for adolescents. Mindfulness (N Y) 7(2):479–492, 2016 27110301

Bluth K, Campo RA, Futch WS, et al: Age and gender differences in the associations of self-compassion and emotional well-being in a large adolescent sample. J Youth Adolesc 46(4):840–853, 2017 27632177

Campo RA, Bluth K, Santacroce SJ, et al: A mindful self-compassion videoconference intervention for nationally recruited posttreatment young adult cancer survivors: feasibility, acceptability, and psychosocial outcomes. Support Care Cancer 25(6):1759–1768, 2017 28105523

Elkind D: Egocentrism redux. Dev Rev 5:218–226, 1985

Goetz JL, Keltner D, Simon-Thomas E: Compassion: an evolutionary analysis and empirical review. Psychol Bull 136(3):351–374, 2010 20438142

Knox M, Neff K: Comparing compassion for self and others: impacts on personal and interpersonal well-being. Paper presented at the 14th Annual Association for Contextual Behavioral Science World Conference, Seattle, WA, Association for Contextual Behavioral Science, June 2016

Lathren C, Bluth K, Campo R, et al: Young adult cancer survivors' experiences with a mindful self-compassion (MSC) video-chat intervention: a qualitative analysis. Self and Identity 17(6):646–665, 2018

Lee FS, Heimer H, Giedd JN, et al: Mental health: adolescent mental health—opportunity and obligation. Science 346(6209):547–549, 2014 25359951

MacBeth A, Gumley A: Exploring compassion: a meta-analysis of the association between self-compassion and psychopathology. Clin Psychol Rev 32(6):545–552, 2012 22796446

Marsh IC, Chan SWY, MacBeth A: Self-compassion and psychological distress in adolescents—a meta-analysis. Mindfulness 25(11):1–17, 2017

Marshall SL, Parker PD, Ciarrochi J, et al: Self-compassion protects against the negative effects of low self-esteem: a longitudinal study in a large adolescent sample. Journal of Personality and Individual Differences 74:116–121, 2014

Neff KD: Self-compassion: an alternative conceptualization of a healthy attitude toward oneself. Self Ident 2(2):85–101, 2003a

Neff KD: The development and validation of a scale to measure self-compassion. Self Ident 2:223–250, 2003b

Neff KD, Germer CK: A pilot study and randomized controlled trial of the mindful self-compassion program. J Clin Psychol 69(1):28–44, 2013 23070875

Neff KD, McGehee P: Self-compassion and psychological resilience among adolescents and young adults. Self Ident 9(3):225–240, 2010

Neff KD, Vonk R: Self-compassion versus global self-esteem: two different ways of relating to oneself. J Pers 77(1):23–50, 2009 19076996

Neff KD, Kirkpatrick K, Rude S: Self-compassion and its link to adaptive psychological functioning. J Res Pers 41:139–154, 2007

Nolen-Hoeksema S, Girgus JS: The emergence of gender differences in depression during adolescence. Psychol Bull 115(3):424–443, 1994 8016286

Raes F, Pommier E, Neff KD, et al: Construction and factorial validation of a short form of the Self-Compassion Scale. Clin Psychol Psychother 18(3):250–255, 2011 21584907

Steinberg L, Morris AS: Adolescent development. Annu Rev Psychol 52(1):83–110, 2001 11148300

Twenge JM: Have smartphones destroyed a generation? The Atlantic, September 2017. Available at: www.theatlantic.com/magazine/archive/2017/09/has-the-smartphone-destroyed-a-generation/534198. Accessed May 16, 2018.

Zessin U, Dickhäuser O, Garbade S: The relationship between self-compassion and well-being: a meta-analysis. Appl Psychol Health Well-Being 7(3):340–364, 2015 26311196

Chapter

3

State of the Research on Youth Mindfulness

Sarah Zoogman, Ph.D.
Eleni Vousoura, Ph.D.
Mari Janikian, Ph.D.

THERE is now burgeoning clinical evidence for the efficacy of mindfulness-based interventions (MBIs) in targeting a variety of common mental disorders in adults, including depression, anxiety, and pain-related disorders, accompanied by promising evidence in addressing attention-deficit/hyperactivity disorder (ADHD), trauma-related disorders, severe mental illness, disordered eating, and addictive behaviors. Meta-analyses of clinical trials of mindfulness interventions have yielded moderate effect sizes across a range of physiological and psychological health outcomes (for an overview, see Khoury et al. 2013).

Research on MBIs in the youth population is limited compared with the adult literature, but in recent years there has been a clear effort to increase available research. A considerable number of feasibility studies and randomized controlled trials (RCTs) have been conducted since the 2010s. This interest is also reflected by the sharp increase of systematic and meta-analytic reviews of MBI research published since 2013 focusing on child and adolescent populations.

The overarching aim of this chapter is to provide an overview of the current research status of MBIs in the child and adolescent population. Our focus will be only on evidence coming from interventions that contain mindfulness as part of their core training, in the form of formal meditation practice. Thus, interventions incorporating aspects of mindfulness secondary to other treatment components (e.g., dialectical behavioral therapy, acceptance and commitment therapy) will not be discussed in this review.

Specifically, in this chapter we critically review available research evidence on the effectiveness of mindfulness interventions targeting different mental disorders across different contexts of implementation. Because this research is still preliminary, one of the primary goals of this chapter is to identify limitations and directions for future studies.

Overview of Existing Mindfulness-Based Programs

The two most common adult MBIs are mindfulness-based stress reduction (MBSR) and mindfulness-based cognitive therapy (MBCT). A comprehensive review of these interventions is offered by Baer (2014). Briefly, MBSR is an evidence-based 8-week intervention developed in the 1970s by Jon Kabat-Zinn. MBSR is a group-based mind-body intervention program of varying duration and intensity that aims to decrease stress and improve coping skills through training in formal practices. The intervention consists of four major strategies geared toward increasing mindful awareness, including body scan exercises, mental exercises focusing attention on breathing, physical exercises focusing on the awareness of bodily sensations, and the practice of being fully aware during everyday activities.

MBCT grew out of cognitive-behavioral therapy (CBT) for depression in combination with several MBSR elements. Similar to MBSR, MBCT is brief and structured and focuses on increasing mindful awareness and cultivating a nonjudgmental attitude toward one's thinking and feeling. Its unique focus on decreasing ruminative processing aims at preventing depressive relapse. MBCT combines MBSR techniques (e.g., meditation, breathing exercises, yoga stretching) with CBT modules, including psychoeducation on the nature of depression and relapse prevention and linking thoughts and behaviors with feelings.

Several mindfulness-based programs are available for youth. Most programs are adapted from adult MBIs but contain important modifications in content and format to match the developmental stage of children and adolescents. The majority of the mindfulness programs require shorter meditation practices and have no daylong retreats, which are commonly found in adult MBIs. In MBSR, mindfulness exercises are modified to adopt more age-appropriate language and incorporate developmentally appropriate guided practice with the use of visual imagery and exercises that are more fun and engaging. The format of mindfulness exercises has also been adapted but varies depending on the program and the setting in which MBSR is implemented.

On the other hand, the adaptation of MBCT for children (MBCT-C) targets both depression and anxiety symptoms (Semple et al. 2010). The joint targeting of anxiety and depression is established on the basis of the idea that anxiety and depression may represent one underlying disorder with a common trajectory and age-dependent expression, and rumination appears to be a transdiagnostic mechanism found in both disorders. MBCT-C shares similar goals and therapeutic strategies with the original adult version. That said, it has undergone multiple logistic adaptations to match children's differing attentional and memory abilities: sessions are reduced from the 2-hour weekly sessions of the 8-week adult program to weekly 90-minute sessions over the course of 12 weeks, and meditative practices are shorter and more frequent during sessions. In addition, adaptations on the content of exercises include linguistic changes to match children's limited verbal fluency and the use of more experiential techniques focusing on body sensations and perceptions.

An important element in MBIs with youth is the involvement of parents or other family members. Parental involvement may vary significantly across curricula, from assistance with homework, to participation in family sessions along the MBI implementation, to even full participation in treatment (i.e., parent-child MBI programs).

Several MBI programs have been implemented in mental health, medical, and school-based settings. Depending on the context of delivery, mindfulness and related concepts (e.g., compassion, yoga, cognitive behavior therapy) vary significantly in the degree they are emphasized in each program.

Current State of Evidence Base of Mindfulness-Based Interventions

In recent years, there has been an increase in the numbers of systematic reviews and meta-analyses evaluating the efficacy of MBIs in youth. To our knowledge, there are so far four comprehensive meta-analyses looking into the effects of MBIs across a range of mental health, health, cognitive, socioemotional, and relationship outcomes.

The first published meta-analysis was conducted by Zenner et al. (2014). This meta-analysis focused specifically on school-based interventions for children and adolescents. The authors identified 24 group-design studies (N=1,348) completed through August 2012, including several unpublished studies (k=8). Findings from this analysis indicated that MBI had a moderate overall effect size (g=0.40) across domains of stress, emotional problems, and coping, with an additional large effect size for areas of cognitive performance, such as attention, inhibition, and grades (g=0.80).

Subsequently, Zoogman et al. (2015) conducted a second meta-analysis of MBI studies published between 2004 and 2011. A sample of 20 group-design studies targeting MBI with youth ages 6–21 years in school and other community settings was included in the meta-analysis. The study yielded similar results to those of Zenner et al. (2014), showing that MBI had small to moderate therapeutic effect for a variety of outcomes (emotion and behavioral regulation, depressive and anxiety symptoms, stress, attention, and cognitive functioning). Follow-up, exploratory analyses indicated that MBI had consistently small positive effects across three more targeted outcome domains: mindfulness (*del*=0.28), psychological symptoms (*del*=0.37), and non-symptom-oriented outcomes (*del*=0.21). In addition, a significantly larger effect size was found on psychological symptoms compared with other dependent variable types (*del*=0.37 vs. *del*=1-0.21) and for studies drawn from clinical samples compared with nonclinical samples (*del*=0.50 vs. *del*=0.20).

A third meta-analysis was published the same year by Kallapiran et al. (2015), who used a different methodology by including only randomized controlled designs published through 2014. The authors confirmed previous meta-analytic findings, reporting small to large therapeutic effects for each mental health outcome domain.

More recently, Klingbeil et al. (2017b) completed a meta-analysis of a sample of 76 group-design studies testing MBI with youth in both school and nonschool settings published prior to January 2016. Their analysis yielded small effect sizes for either precomparisons or postcomparisons (g=0.31) and controlled comparisons (g=0.32), which were maintained over time, as evidenced by results of the 12 controlled studies that included follow-up assessments (g=0.40). Uniformly small to moderate effects were reported across a range of mental health outcomes, such as internalizing problems (g=0.39), negative emotion and subjective distress (g=0.25), externalizing problems (g=0.30), attention (g=0.29), and emotional and behavioral regulation (g=0.32), along with physical health (g=0.28), academic achievement and school functioning (g=0.39), positive emotion and self-appraisal (g=0.28), and social competence and prosocial behavior (g=0.37). Moderate effects were reported for mindfulness (g=0.51) and metacognition and cognitive flexibility (g=0.40). Interestingly, therapeutic setting (school vs. other) did not moderate findings.

The findings from these meta-analyses suggest that MBIs are safe, feasible, and efficacious, yielding at least small positive effects across various outcome domains, such as academic performance, cognitive skills, and psychological and physiological health. MBIs seem to be beneficial and effective in diverse settings (i.e., school and community) with both general and clinical populations of children and adolescents. There is, however, significant heterogeneity among the studies included in the meta-analyses in terms of patient profiles, implementation setting, and outcome measures. To overcome this, in the following section we will review the empirical evidence of MBIs implemented in different settings and, separately, for each disorder category.

Mindfulness-Based Interventions in Mental Health Settings

MBIs are being increasingly integrated into mental health settings. A growing body of literature supports its promising use for a variety of psychological symptoms. In the following subsection, we discuss empirical evidence for the efficacy and utility of MBIs across a wide range of disorders and symptoms and also address some applications to specialty populations.

Mindfulness-Based Interventions for Acute Anxiety and Depression Symptoms

Depressive and anxiety symptoms are highly prevalent among youth and are associated with significant functional impairment and often detrimental developmental outcomes. Anxiety is the most frequently occurring mental disorder in childhood and adolescence, and it is often a precursor to depression in adolescents, which is constitutes a leading cause of disability in this age group (American Psychiatric Association 2013).

MBIs are a valuable therapeutic tool for addressing and preventing the recurrence of depressive symptomatology. One of the putative mechanisms of action in MBIs is the reduction in rumination, a passive and repetitive focusing on depressive symptoms and their causes and consequences, which is commonly found in depressive disorders. Mindfulness entails purposefully nonjudgmental awareness and acceptance of the present moment, which can decrease ruminative processing, thus resulting in reduction of depressive symptoms.

MBIs are also effective in reducing stress and anxiety symptoms. The nonjudgmental stance cultivated in MBIs allows participants to mindfully observe and accept anxious thoughts and enables them to attend to unpleasant, anxiety-provoking sensations and thoughts instead of engaging in experiential avoidance. In addition, MBIs address the impaired attention commonly associated with high levels of anxiety symptoms by improving attentional focus.

A significant number of studies support the use of MBIs among youth with internalizing symptomatology. One of the first methodologically strong trials testing the efficacy of MBIs with clinical youth populations was conducted by Biegel et al. (2009). The authors randomly assigned a sample of 102 adolescents ages 14–18 with various psychiatric diagnoses receiving community mental health support to either MBSR for teenagers (MBSR-T, consisting of eight 2-hour classes) or treatment as usual (psychotherapy and/or medication management). Findings showed that adolescents in the MBSR-T group reported significant reductions in perceived stress, anxiety, and depression by the 3-month follow-up and demonstrated diagnostic improvements. Additional improvements were reported in interpersonal conflict, global functioning, self-esteem, and sleep routines.

The preliminary efficacy of MBCT-C has been examined in several feasibility studies, with studies reporting significant symptom reduction in internalizing and externalizing problems and improvements in attention and self-control. More recently, Semple et al. (2010) conducted the first RCT of MBCT-C with 25 low-income, inner-city clinic-referred children (ages 9–13). Youth treated with MBCT-C showed greater reductions in anxiety and inattention compared with waitlist control, although no posttreatment differences were reported in behavior problems.

The effectiveness of MBIs in reducing internalizing symptoms is supported by several meta-analyses. For instance, meta-analytic evidence by Zoogman et al. (2015), Kallapiran et al. (2015), and Klingbeil et al. (2017b) support the efficacy of MBIs in reducing a variety of mental health outcomes, including stress, anxiety, and depression, while improving quality of life and well-being.

Mindfulness-Based Interventions for Recurrent Internalizing Symptoms

Youth depression tends to follow an enduring trajectory, with a course that often continues into adulthood. With relapse rates in depression reaching as high as 50%–80%, there is a need for psychosocial interventions as a prophylactic against recurrence of mood disorders (American Psychiatric Association 2013). MBCT was developed to address the relapsing nature of depression by building awareness of negative thoughts and feelings at times of potential relapse or recurrence of mood symptoms and cultivates a different way of relating to unpleasant thoughts and bodily sensations as transient phenomena of the mind rather than accurate reflections of reality. Although data from adult trials support MBCT as a well-established treatment for recurrent depression, especially when accompanied by residual symptoms, it has not been extensively studied in the context of youth depression.

One small pilot study by Ames et al. (2014) implemented an 8-week MBCT group program for adolescents (12–18 years) with residual symptoms of depression. Findings revealed significant reductions in depressive symptoms and improvements in rumination and quality of life, as well as a high level of treatment acceptability, as evidenced by low dropout rates and qualitative insight by completers. Results, albeit promising, are limited by the very small sample size ($N=11$), absence of a control condition, and lack of long-term follow-up assessment. Further evaluation of the efficacy of MBIs in the maintenance and prophylaxis of recurrent mood disorder is needed with more methodologically robust designs.

Mindfulness-Based Interventions for Externalizing Symptoms

MBIs appear to be useful as targeted interventions for decreasing disruptive behavior in youth. Recently, a meta-analysis of single-case MBIs published between 2006 and 2014 analyzed findings from 10 studies ($N=48$) targeting disruptive behavioral problems among adolescents with psychiatric diagnoses (e.g., ADHD, autism spectrum disorder [ASD]; Klingbeil et al. (2017a). The authors found moderate effects of mindfulness interventions on disruptive behavior not only during the active treatment phase but also during maintenance. Moreover, the efficacy of MBIs was not context dependent, with participants responding equally well to school- and home-based interventions. Together with the results from the meta-analytic studies discussed earlier, there is significant evidence supporting the use of MBIs to decrease externalizing symptoms such as oppositional defiant behavior and behaviors resulting from conduct disorder. In this section, we look into evidence on ADHD.

ADHD is a neurodevelopmental disorder characterized by persistent symptoms of inattention, hyperactivity, and impulsivity that result in significant impairment across major areas of daily functioning (American Psychiatric Association 2013). Core symptoms of ADHD include significant impairments in organizing and planning activities, pronounced distractibility, and marked difficulty with sustaining attention, along with excessive talkativeness, fidgety motor behavior, and reduced tolerance of frustration.

Mindfulness-based programs for ADHD aim to reduce inattention symptoms but also the accompanying anxiety and depressive symptomatology, which are very common in individuals with the disorder. The most basic technique involves self-regulation of attention, which allows the individual to be oriented toward the present in an authentic way. In addition, breathing techniques help participants enhance their attention and concentration skills. These techniques help individuals gain a gradual focus on their inner experiences, such as their feelings and affections. Focusing on more neutral stimuli, such as breathing, helps people with ADHD distract themselves from negative thoughts.

Several mindfulness-based interventions have been implemented for children and adolescents with ADHD, with and without parallel interventions for their parents, and the results are quite encouraging. MBIs not only are effective in reducing the primary symptoms of ADHD, such as inattention, impulsivity, and lack of self-monitoring skills; they also target coexisting symptoms of internalizing (e.g., anxiety, depression) and externalizing (e.g., conduct problems) disorders.

Evans et al. (2018) recently conducted a comprehensive meta-analysis, investigating the use of a wide range of meditation-based interventions (including MBIs) with children with ADHD up to age 18 years. The authors identified 16 meditation-based studies; of these, 7 were MBIs, the majority of which included parents along with children. Overall, large effect sizes were found for core ADHD symptoms among MBIs, although one of the studies reported small effect sizes in favor of the control group. These findings are consistent with reports from another recent systematic review evaluating the efficacy of MBIs and yoga-based interventions among youth, which reported moderate to large effect sizes on executive function and attention measures (Mak et al. 2018).

Regarding externalizing symptoms, findings were mixed, with some studies showing small to moderate reductions in disruptive behaviors along with preliminary evidence that MBIs may increase child compliance, whereas others found no effect on child externalizing symptoms. Evidence on improvements in well-being and functioning was limited and had significant discrepancies, reflecting heterogeneity in measurements, particularly regarding child report versus parent report measurement tools. Finally, there was evidence (albeit inconsistent) showing significant decrease of parental stress and preliminary support for increasing satisfaction and happiness among parents and improving parent-child relationships (Evans et al. 2018).

There are several limitations in the empirical literature for the effectiveness of MBIs for ADHD. Most studies are severely underpowered and use uncontrolled designs, with significant risk biases. There is significant heterogeneity in measures employed, most importantly the mixed use of child report versus parent report questionnaires. Notwithstanding these limitations, mindfulness training appears to have been successfully implemented for children and adolescents with ADHD. One interesting question that remains to be tested is whether combined interventions that include concurrent parent training in the treatment modality are more beneficial than child-focused interventions that target only children. The underlying rationale for such a claim is that involving parents allows them to support both the maintenance and generalizability of therapeutic gains posttreatment.

Mindfulness-Based Interventions for Autism Spectrum Disorder

Mindfulness interventions have been adapted for children with ASD. Autism constitutes a highly heterogeneous clinical disorder characterized by socioemotional deficits related to social communication and interaction, accompanied by a range of cognitive and motor symptoms (American Psychiatric Association 2013). Mindfulness training can be a useful adjunct to behavioral management interventions in addressing core ASD symptoms. In addition, it may help alleviate symptoms of anxiety, depression, and disrupted sleep patterns that are frequently comorbid in children with ASD.

Despite the fact that MBIs hold significant promise for autism, evidence for their efficacy is limited. In a recent systematic review conducted by Hourston and Atchley (2017) investigating the effect of various mind-body therapies for ASD, the authors identified nine studies of either MBSR, MBCT, or MYmind (i.e., a 9-week group mindfulness training program with parallel mindful parenting training) used with children with autism. Didactic content emphasized mindfulness instruction as a tool for coping with ADHD symptoms, stress, difficult emotions, and family relationships.

In almost all of the studies, MBIs were delivered to parents in some form; either as mindful parenting training with or without parallel mindfulness training in their children or through a training-of-trainers model, in which parents were trained to deliver the intervention to their children. The majority of studies had a small sample size, with only one study adopting a randomized controlled design. Results, albeit preliminary and empirically weak, showed improvements in internalizing and externalizing symptoms and attention problems, and parent-based MBIs appeared to improve children's comorbid symptoms of hyperactivity.

Interventions must undergo several adaptations to increase feasibility and acceptability of mindfulness techniques in this clinical population, given the cognitive and socioemotional deficits encountered in patients with ASD. For instance, treatment protocols use less metaphorical and ambiguous language, keeping in mind that children with ASD might be challenged by the figurative language typically adopted by MBIs, and provide clear description of the goals and tasks of each mindfulness session to best address inflexibility and the preference for strict routines commonly seen in individuals with ASD. Other adaptations included increasing the amount of time for breathing exercise and weeks of training to account for possibly slow information processing (Hourston and Atchley 2017).

Mindfulness-Based Interventions for Substance Use Disorders

Substance use disorders (SUDs) are characterized by chronic and excessive use of substances or behavioral patterns that cause extreme stress and become uncontrollable. SUDs result in an inability to meet major social, school- or work-related, or interpersonal responsibilities. They tend to follow a chronic course with frequent relapses and are linked to increased morbidity and high mortality rates (American Psychiatric Association 2013).

The principles of mindfulness are highly relevant for the treatment of addictive disorders. Individuals struggling with SUDs engage in pronounced escapist behavior, described in MBIs as running on "autopilot," to avoid coming to terms with unpleasant thoughts or emotions, including cravings for the substance. MBIs target this maladaptive emotional coping style by cultivating an intentional and accepting focus of one's attention on present-moment experience. Meditative practice teaches participants to "surf the urge" rather than respond to cravings in an either suppressing or reactive manner. In addition, dispositional mindfulness—mindfulness as a personality trait rather than a learned skill—is inversely correlated with impulsivity.

Accumulating evidence supports the efficacy of MBIs both as treatment and as relapse prevention for SUDs in adults. Research in youth substance-related disorders is less extensive and robust, although in recent years a line of studies has tested the adaptation of MBIs for at-risk populations, such as homeless and incarcerated youth, as well as youth with sleeping problems.

Among youth, sleep plays a pivotal role in SUDs. MBIs have been implemented as sleep intervention to prevent relapse by improving sleep hygiene and regularizing biorhythms. Bootzin and Stevens (2005) found that completion of four or more sessions in a treatment program resulted in improved sleep among participants, and, in turn, improving sleep contributed to the reduction of substance abuse at a 12-month follow-up. In a subsequent trial, Britton et al. (2010) reported preliminary results with 18 adolescent outpatients who completed a six-session mindfulness-based sleep intervention with mindfulness meditation (MM). Completion of the MM program resulted in improvements in sleep duration, psychological distress, and relapse resistance and reduced substance use. Of note, frequent MM practice was associated with longer sleep duration and greater improvement in self-efficacy about substance use.

Mindfulness-Based Interventions for Sleep Disorders

MBIs have been adapted for the treatment of discrete sleep disorders. Blake and colleagues (2016) tested the efficacy of a multicomponent group sleep intervention combining CBT and MBI elements in an RCT with 144 adolescents (12–17 years) exhibiting high levels of anxiety disorders and sleep disturbances. Following completion of the intervention, participants showed improvements in sleep induction difficulties and related daytime dysfunction, and intervention was also associated with small effects on concomitant anxiety symptoms.

Mindfulness-Based Interventions for Eating Disorders

Eating disorders (EDs) are a group of mental health conditions characterized by significantly disturbed eating patterns, ranging from excessive diet restrictions and maladaptive weight-loss strategies to compulsive eating and overeating. EDs often have their onset in adolescence, when issues pertaining to body image peak, and are associated with significant distress and functional impairment, increased morbidity, and high rates of comorbid disorders and substance abuse.

Mindfulness interventions have been adapted for EDs, particularly binge eating and overeating or emotional eating. EDs have been linked with underlying deficits in emotion regulation; overeating is thought to be an escapist and maladaptive strategy for coping with psychological distress. Mindfulness works at the core of these emotion regulation deficits by cultivating awareness of internal experiences (e.g., emotions, physical sensations), improving one's ability to cope adaptively with emotions and building compassion and self-acceptance. Evidence from the adult literature shows promising treatment effects of MBIs for binge-eating disorder and obesity-related eating behaviors (Kristeller et al. 2014). On the other hand, MBIs have yielded weak effects for anorexia nervosa and bulimia, but third-wave CBT interventions that contain elements of mindfulness practice, such as dialectical behavior therapy and acceptance and commitment therapy, hold promise as treatments for these disorders.

The evidence base for the use of MBIs in youth targeting binge eating and obesity is promising but limited. A pilot study tested the efficacy of mindfulness-based eating awareness training for adolescents (MB-EAT-A) with 40 ninth-graders recruited from high school health physical education classes randomly assigned to 12 weekly sessions of MB-EAT-A or health education control. After 6 months, adolescents participating in the MB-EAT-A program had moderately increased intense aerobic exercise and improved dietary habits

(Barnes and Kristeller 2016). Moreover, Atkinson and Wade (2015) conducted a school-based cluster randomized controlled trial in 19 classes of adolescent girls (*N*=347) allocated to a 3-session MBI, a dissonance-based intervention, or classes-as-usual control. Significant improvements were found in a broad range of eating disorder variables, with moderate between-group effect sizes ranging from 0.47 to 0.67 at 6-month follow-up. Taken together, these results demonstrate the feasibility and preliminary efficacy of MBIs in school settings. Methodologically stronger studies are needed to evaluate the potential of school-based mindful eating programs as a means of improving eating patterns and preventing obesity among high-risk youth.

Mindfulness-Based Interventions in Medical Settings

There is ample evidence for the use of MBIs in patients managing various medical conditions, including chronic illnesses, pain, and other medical conditions. Research points to significant benefits of mindfulness-based practices for adults undergoing treatment for or recovering from cancer, with a variety of documented effects, including reductions in pain, anxiety, depression, stress, and sexual difficulties, as well as improvements in self-perceived well-being and physiological markers of stress and immune function.

Research on the effects of MBIs for pediatric patients is limited. A recent systematic review of the literature identified eight trials targeting various chronic illnesses, including HIV infection, cardiac disease, headache, obesity, and mixed chronic pain conditions (Brown et al. 2017). Findings from these studies support the utility of MBIs for managing a range of physiological and psychological symptoms, but the soundness of the research is weak. The majority of existing trials are feasibility studies, with only one study including a control group, and none of the studies included inpatient participants; all participants were recruited from academic or hospital-affiliated outpatient centers. More research is required to determine whether the same effects can be transferred to children and pediatric medicine.

Evidence on the effectiveness of MBIs adapted for cancer-related pain in children and adolescents is scarce. To our knowledge, there is no published trial of MBIs for youth with cancer, aside from a study protocol for a randomized controlled trial examining the effectiveness of MBIs among adolescents with cancer. Evidence from other chronic medical conditions is also limited. Taken together, MBIs for medical pediatric patients are promising but underresearched.

Mindfulness-Based Interventions in Educational Settings

MBIs have been increasingly integrated in schools because interventions can be implemented directly with groups of children and adolescents in areas of need at little cost. Consequently, several MBIs for schools have been developed and applied since 2000, targeting a heterogeneous group of students, from pre-schoolers to high school students. Examples of training curricula are MindUp, Inner Kids, Stressed Teens, and Learning to Breathe. For a comprehensive review, see Baelen et al. (in press) and Meiklejohn et al. (2012).

Research evaluating MBIs in educational settings is also growing. Meta-analytic evidence supports the effectiveness of MBIs in school settings (Zenner et al. 2014). School-based mindfulness training appears to help students cultivate awareness and other skills that may enhance their coping capacities in dealing with psychosocial as well as academic challenges (Baelen et al., in press; Meiklejohn et al. 2012). Both uncontrolled studies and RCTs have documented improvements in important cognitive (e.g., executive function, attention), mental health (e.g., anxiety and depression, stress), and interpersonal outcomes.

Flook et al. (2010) evaluated the efficacy of mindful awareness practices in a group of second- and third-grade children and found improvement in executive functioning capacities, including attention shifting, monitoring, and initiating. Schonert-Reichl and Lawlor (2010) conducted an RCT to examine the effectiveness of a mindfulness education program and found increased optimism and improved teacher-rated behavior and social competence. In a recent qualitative study, Dariotis et al. (2016) conducted focus group discussions with 22 middle school students from urban schools who participated in a 16-week mindfulness and yoga intervention. Youth reported improved emotional appraisal and emotional regulation skills following the intervention.

In a systematic review of MBIs for youth in school settings, Felver et al. (2016) reviewed 28 studies published through June 2014. Half of the studies assigned students to different conditions (e.g., MBI group or waitlist control) to evaluate intervention effects designs ($N=16$), including both experimental ($n=10$) and quasi-experimental ($n=6$) designs. The authors concluded that MBIs are acceptable and possibly effective interventions for various target behaviors. Maynard et al. (2017) conducted a systematic review of 61 trials investigating the effects of MBIs in primary and secondary schools and the impact they had on cognitive, behavioral, socioemotional, and academic achievement outcomes. Results indicated that MBIs have small, positive effects on cognitive and socioemotional processes, but these effects were not seen for behavioral or academic outcomes.

Overall, although MBIs in school settings seem to be effective, the results reported in the literature should be interpreted with caution because of the diversity of programs and outcome measures combined with the pilot character of most studies. Critical reviews of existing research have underscored the importance of additional large-scale studies using rigorous experimental methodology on normative student populations to enhance the empirical support for MBI in school settings.

Mindfulness-Based Interventions in Community Settings for Specialty Populations

Mindfulness training has been implemented in community settings for at-risk youth facing grave psychosocial problems. Such populations include homeless youth living in shelters, foster homes, or juvenile detention centers or on the streets, as well as incarcerated minors. Research has shown that these populations have significantly higher rates of mental health problems, such as mood, anxiety, and conduct disorders. Often having endured traumatic experiences and considerable stress due to their volatile living arrangement, they are at increased risk for developing posttraumatic stress disorder and substance use problems and are at particular risk for suicide attempts.

To date, no large-scale randomized controlled study has been conducted in this field, but there is preliminary evidence for the feasibility and clinical utility of MBIs based on open trials. One adaptation of MBIs for homeless youth was Youth Education in Spiritual Self-Schema (YESSS), a 4-week, peer-led group-based mindfulness meditation program held twice weekly aiming at fostering spirituality, meaning, and positive emotions and reducing negative self-schemas. In a study by Grabbe et al. (2012), 39 young people living in a shelter participated in the YESSS program. Following completion of the program, the youth showed decreased symptoms of depression, anxiety, and stress; increased spirituality; and strengthened resilience. However, despite salutary effects across these outcomes, no decreases in impulsivity were observed following the intervention.

Himelstein (2011) implemented and pilot tested an 8-week mindfulness-based substance use intervention with 60 incarcerated youth. The program was based on MBSR with some adjustments to group discussions and exercises tailored to the unique issues faced by incarcerated youth (e.g., youth poverty, community violence, substance misuse). Using a mixed-method approach, Himelstein found a significant decrease in impulsivity, along with an increase in the perceived risk of drug use, but no changes in reported self-regulation after completion of the program.

The findings from such pilot studies are promising, suggesting that the application of mindfulness in at-risk, underserved populations that have limited access to mental health interventions can be feasible, acceptable, and potentially effective. With appropriate modifications to increase acceptability among users, MBIs have the potential to decrease the risk of substance use and related internalizing and externalizing symptoms while empowering youth and increasing their resilience. However, similar to other applications of MBIs in youth, these preliminary findings are yet to be confirmed with large-scale controlled designs.

Critical Assessment of Empirical Base of Mindfulness-Based Interventions for Youth

The number of mindfulness intervention studies in children and adolescents is growing quickly, and as a result, there are many research challenges to be addressed to strengthen the empirical status of MBIs. In this section, we summarize current limitations in existing empirical literature of MBIs in children and adolescents. Issues pertaining to measurement, research design methodology, and developmental adaptation of interventions are discussed at length.

Measuring Mindfulness in Youth

There is marked variability in the measurement of mindfulness in youth. A recent comprehensive review of existing measurement tools for assessing mindfulness in children and adolescents (Goodman et al. 2017) identified seven self-report measures: 1) the Child and Adolescent Mindfulness Measure (CAMM); 2) the Mindful Attention Awareness Scale for Adolescents (MAAS-A) or 3) Children (MAAS-C); 4) Comprehensive Inventory of Mindfulness Experiences-Adolescents (CHIME-A); 5) Mindful Thinking and Action Scale for Adolescents (MTASA); 6) Mindfulness Scale for Pre-Teens, Teens, and Adults (MSPTA); and 7) Mindfulness Inventory for Children and Adolescents (MICA). Of note, only four of these measures have published validation information.

Each one of these tools assesses one or more of the putative core mindfulness skills, including observation of present-moment experience; acting with awareness rather than mindlessly or on "automatic pilot"; and adopting a nonjudgmental stance toward internal experiences such as cognitions, emotions, and bodily sensations. However, the psychometric properties of these tools vary considerably, and intercorrelations among the measures are generally low, suggesting low convergent validity. Moreover, there is controversy as to whether mindfulness is a unidimensional or multifaceted construct and, if the latter, which and how many facets exist. Even more complex is the age sensitivity of the construct: as children's metacognitive skills rapidly shift and develop over time, so do mindfulness skills evolve, and this must be accounted for by the various existing mindfulness measures. These issues reflect the overall lack of consensus on how mindfulness is operationalized and assessed (for more information, see Goodman et al. 2017).

Although self-reports are undoubtedly useful in measuring clinical outcomes, alternative assessments should be considered to offer a more comprehensive account of the construct of mindfulness. For instance, objective measures (i.e., physiological or experimental tools) and third-person accounts (i.e., parent, clinician, or teacher reports) should be used in tandem with youth self-reports. Another promising approach is ambulatory measurement of mindfulness through *ecological momentary assessment* (EMA), a procedure in which participants report on their feelings and behaviors as they experience them in real time during a specific period. EMA has not been adopted in youth trials yet, but it is only a matter of time, given the increasing interest in technology-assisted interventions and use of mental health apps. It is anticipated that such an approach will be instrumental in increasing the sensitivity of mindfulness measures, which are currently limited by the retrospective nature of self-report methods.

Reliable and valid measures of mindfulness for children and adolescents not only will allow researchers to accurately detect changes in mindfulness skills and dispositional traits following completion of MBIs; they are also much needed to elucidate the mechanisms of action of various mindfulness training programs. Although it is assumed that reductions in symptoms are mediated by increase of mindful awareness and the cultivation of an accepting, nonjudgmental attitude toward inner experience, these assumptions have not yet been supported empirically (see discussion of mechanisms of action in the next subsection).

Methodological Limitations of Existing Trials

The current evidence base of mindfulness interventions for children and adolescents, as promising and exciting as it may be, remains quite limited, fragmented, and methodologically weak. Across clinical disorders and populations, research studies of mindfulness interventions are underpowered and rarely adopt a randomized control design.

Additionally, significant heterogeneity exists among mindfulness programs. Training curricula range in duration and intensity of mindfulness practice, which may introduce dosage issues. Studies also differ with regard to patient inclusion criteria, particularly comorbid mental health and health conditions. The considerable methodological heterogeneity of existing studies may explain inconsistencies in effect sizes reported among meta-analyses: Zenner et al. (2014) found larger effects on cognitive outcomes compared with emotional ones, and Zoogman et al. (2015) found larger effects for psychological symptoms compared with other outcomes, but Klingbeil et al. (2017a, 2017b) found comparable effects for all outcomes across different delivery contexts.

Research on factors moderating treatment effectiveness of youth MBIs is very limited. Treatment moderators are pretreatment factors that help determine which aspects of MBIs are particularly effective and for which subgroup of youth patients. It is possible that clinical characteristics of the disorder, along with comorbidity, functional impairment, and premorbid cognitive functioning, may influence the efficacy of MBIs. Other factors may involve patient characteristics, such as demographic characteristics (age, gender, ethnicity), personality traits, and dispositional mindfulness. Another factor that has been identified in the adult literature as potentially moderating results is the mindfulness training of the therapists. In addition, studies should investigate the effects of certain aspects of the mindfulness training curriculum, such as duration of the intervention, type of developmental adaptations, mode of delivery (home, clinic, school), intensity of homework practice, and modality and parental involvement (group vs. individual vs. family), on treatment effectiveness.

Equally underresearched are the treatment mediators of youth MBIs. Knowledge of mediators and biological markers of therapeutic change is limited in the adult literature as well; however, in recent years, several putative mechanisms have been investigated (for a review, see Zoogman et al. 2017). It is possible, however, that youth interventions may have different mechanisms of change.

Recommendations for Future Studies: Where to Go From Here?

To address the methodologically weak areas of the existing research base of MBIs, future studies should aim at replication of previous findings by testing MBIs in larger, controlled studies. For MBIs targeting clinical populations, there should be consensus on appropriate diagnostic tools (structured clinical interviews and questionnaires) to determine study entry eligibility. Standardization of mindfulness training protocols is also required because there is notable variability in types of MBI programs employed in various studies.

Once methods for sampling, assessments, procedures, and design become more streamlined and consistent among studies, testing for treatment moderators should be the next step. Inclusion of mixed methods (quantitative methodology in conjunction with qualitative methodology) is also vital to allow for assessment of safety, feasibility, and acceptability of interventions. In addition, prior to efforts to disseminate interventions on a large-scale level, particularly in universal school-based intervention, studies should conduct cost-effectiveness analysis in parallel with treatment efficacy and effectiveness analysis. To date, very few studies have investigated the cost-effectiveness of MBIs in youth.

Finally, it is vital that the research community begin to explicitly examine the mechanisms of change (e.g., what are the pathways and mediators?) along with unique biological markers of change. Such research has the unique capacity to build a better understanding of how and why mindfulness works for a variety of symptoms in children and adolescents.

Conclusion

Research on the therapeutic effects of mindfulness training for youth is rapidly expanding. The past two decades have witnessed a booming interest in various applications of mindfulness interventions for a variety of health and mental health conditions across a range of setting with youth of all ages. Data from a large body of open trials suggest that MBIs for youth are safe; when adapted appropriately to meet the unique developmental needs of each age group and/or population type, MBIs are useful and unlikely to cause harm to recipients. Mounting evidence from implementation of youth mindfulness training across different settings suggests that MBIs are versatile and can be successfully delivered in clinical, home, and school contexts with comparable therapeutic success.

That said, the current state of the evidence base of MBIs for youth is limited and has evident gaps and remaining questions. The current body of empirical evidence testing the efficacy of MBIs in youth presents serious methodological limitations. Evidence described in this chapter derives from small, uncontrolled studies, and there is a dearth of high-quality RCTs that would help establish a solid empirical base for MBIs in this population.

Most mental disorders have their onset in childhood and adolescence and tend to follow a chronic course; thus, targeting mental health symptoms during that period is a critical window of opportunity. Nevertheless, research on empirically based treatments and practices for child and adolescent mental health interventions is underdeveloped, and there is a limited understanding for whom and why psychotherapy works best. Mindfulness training holds undoubted therapeutic promise for youth, but we must strengthen our understanding of its mechanisms of action and indicated applications. More robust research is very much needed to leverage the therapeutic benefits of mindfulness.

KEY POINTS

- Existing mindfulness-based programs for youth are modified versions of MBSR and MBCT but with shorter meditation sessions, developmentally appropriate language, and parental involvement.
- Meta-analytic studies of mindfulness-based interventions for youth show significant effects. Other studies show promising use for a variety of internalizing and externalizing psychological conditions, in addition to neurodevelopmental, substance, sleep, and eating disorders.
- Existing research into the use of mindfulness with children and adolescents is limited by variability in mindfulness measurement tools, poor study methodology, heterogeneity in mindfulness programs used, and limited research on moderators and mediators of therapeutic effects.

Discussion Questions

1. Are mindfulness-based interventions effective in targeting symptoms of specific psychological disorders, or are they more effective *transdiagnostically*, that is, across a range of symptoms?

2. Do children and adolescents benefit more from mindfulness-based interventions implemented in clinical settings or school-based settings?

3. With mindfulness-based interventions being extensively adapted for use in children and adolescents, are they changed to such an extent that they no longer have fidelity and similarity to the original adult treatments?

Suggested Readings

Greenberg MT, Harris AR: Nurturing mindfulness in children and youth: current state of research. Child Dev Perspect 6(2):161–166, 2012

Tan LB: A critical review of adolescent mindfulness-based programmes. Clin Child Psychol Psychiatry 21(2):193–207, 201625810416

Zoogman S, Goldberg SB, Hoyt WT, et al: Mindfulness interventions with youth: a meta-analysis. Mindfulness 6(2):290–302, 2015

References

American Psychiatric Association: Diagnostic and Statistical Manual of Mental Disorders, 5th Edition. Arlington, VA, American Psychiatric Association, 2013

Ames CS, Richardson J, Payne S, et al: Mindfulness-based cognitive therapy for depression in adolescents. Child Adolesc Ment Health 19(1):74–78, 2014

Atkinson MJ, Wade TD: Mindfulness-based prevention for eating disorders: a school-based cluster randomized controlled study. Int J Eat Disord 48(7):1024–1037, 2015 26052831

Baelen RN, Esposito MV, Galla BM: A selective review of mindfulness training programs for children and adolescents in school settings, in Transforming School Culture With Mindfulness and Compassion. Edited by Jennings PA, DeMauro AA, Mischenko P. New York, Guilford (in press)

Baer RA: Mindfulness-Based Treatment Approaches: Clinician's Guide to Evidence Base and Applications, 2nd Edition. New York, Elsevier, 2014

Barnes VA, Kristeller JL: Impact of mindfulness-based eating awareness on diet and exercise habits in adolescents. Int J Complement Altern Med 3(2):00070, 2016

Biegel GM, Brown KW, Shapiro SL, et al: Mindfulness-based stress reduction for the treatment of adolescent psychiatric outpatients: a randomized clinical trial. J Consult Clin Psychol 77(5):855–866, 2009 19803566

Blake M, Waloszek JM, Schwartz O, et al: The SENSE study: post intervention effects of a randomized controlled trial of a cognitive-behavioral and mindfulness-based group sleep improvement intervention among at-risk adolescents. J Consult Clin Psychol 84(12):1039–1051, 2016 27775416

Bootzin RR, Stevens SJ: Adolescents, substance abuse, and the treatment of insomnia and daytime sleepiness. Clin Psychol Rev 25(5):629–644, 2005 15953666

Britton WB, Bootzin RR, Cousins JC, et al: The contribution of mindfulness practice to a multicomponent behavioral sleep intervention following substance abuse treatment in adolescents: a treatment-development study. Subst Abus 31(2):86–97, 2010 20408060

Brown ML, Rojas E, Gouda S: A mind-body approach to pediatric pain management. Children (Basel) 4(6):50, 2017 28632194

Dariotis JK, Cluxton-Keller F, Mirabal-Beltran R, et al: "The program affects me 'cause it gives away stress": urban students' qualitative perspectives on stress and a school-based mindful yoga intervention. Explore (NY) 12(6):443–450, 2016 27688017

Evans S, Ling M, Hill B, et al: Systematic review of meditation-based interventions for children with ADHD. Eur Child Adolesc Psychiatry 27(1):9–27, 2017 28547119

Felver JC, Celis-de Hoyos CE, Tezanos K, et al: A systematic review of mindfulness-based interventions for youth in school settings. Mindfulness 7(1):34–45, 2016

Flook L, Smalley SL, Kitil MJ, et al: Effects of mindful awareness practices on executive functions in elementary school children. J Appl Sch Psychol 26(1):70–95, 2010

Goodman MS, Madni LA, Semple RJ: Measuring mindfulness in youth: review of current assessments, challenges, and future directions. Mindfulness 8(6):1409–1420, 2017

Grabbe L, Nguy ST, Higgins MK: Spirituality development for homeless youth: a mindfulness meditation feasibility pilot. J Child Fam Stud 21(6):925–937, 2012

Himelstein S: Mindfulness-based substance abuse treatment for incarcerated youth: a mixed method pilot study. International Journal of Transpersonal Studies 30(1–2):1–10, 2011

Hourston S, Atchley R: Autism and mind-body therapies: a systematic review. J Altern Complement Med 23(5):331–339, 2017 28437148

Kallapiran K, Koo S, Kirubakaran R, et al: Effectiveness of mindfulness in improving mental health symptoms of children and adolescents: a meta-analysis. Child Adolesc Ment Health 20(4):182–194, 2015

Khoury B, Lecomte T, Fortin G, et al: Mindfulness-based therapy: a comprehensive meta-analysis. Clin Psychol Rev 33(6):763–771, 2013 23796855

Klingbeil DA, Fischer AJ, Renshaw TL, et al: Effects of mindfulness-based interventions on disruptive behavior: a meta-analysis of single-case research. Psychol Sch 54(1):70–87, 2017a

Klingbeil DA, Renshaw TL, Willenbrink JB, et al: Mindfulness-based interventions with youth: a comprehensive meta-analysis of group-design studies. J Sch Psychol 63:77–103, 2017b 28633940

Kristeller J, Wolever RQ, Sheets V: Mindfulness-based eating awareness training (MB-EAT) for binge eating: a randomized clinical trial. Mindfulness 5(3):282–297, 2014

Mak C, Whittingham K, Cunnington R, et al: Efficacy of mindfulness-based interventions for attention and executive function in children and adolescents—a systematic review. Mindfulness 9(1):59–78, 2018

Maynard BR, Solis MR, Miller VL, et al: Mindfulness-based interventions for improving cognition, academic achievement, behavior and socio-emotional functioning of primary and secondary students. Oslo, Campbell Collaboration, 2017. Available at: https://campbellcollaboration.org/media/k2/attachments/Campbell_systematic_review_-_Mindfulness_and_school_students.pdf. Accessed May 3, 2018.

Meiklejohn J, Phillips C, Freedman ML, et al: Integrating mindfulness training into K-12 education: fostering the resilience of teachers and students. Mindfulness 3(4):291–307, 2012

Schonert-Reichl KA, Lawlor MS: The effects of a mindfulness-based education program on pre- and early adolescents' well-being and social and emotional competence. Mindfulness 1(3):137–151, 2010

Semple RJ, Lee J, Rosa D, et al: A randomized trial of mindfulness-based cognitive therapy for children: Promoting mindful attention to enhance social-emotional resiliency in children. J Child Fam Stud 19(2):218–229, 2010

Zenner C, Herrnleben-Kurz S, Walach H: Mindfulness-based interventions in schools—a systematic review and meta-analysis. Front Psychol 5(JUN):603, 2014 25071620

Zoogman S, Goldberg SB, Hoyt WT, et al: Mindfulness interventions with youth: a meta-analysis. Mindfulness 6(2):290–302, 2015

Zoogman S, Foskolos E, Vousoura E: Mindfulness as an intervention in the treatment of psychopathology, in Becoming Mindful: Integrating Mindfulness Into Your Psychiatric Practice. Edited by Zerbo E, Schlechter A, Desai S, et al. Arlington, VA, American Psychiatric Association Publishing, 2017, pp 80–102

Chapter

4

Measuring Mindfulness

Matthew S. Goodman, M.A.
Laila A. Madni, Psy.D.
Randye J. Semple, Ph.D.

IMAGINE looking into a foggy mirror. Your reflection waits on the other side, but it is not until you wipe away the fog that you can see yourself clearly. This is one benefit of mindfulness practice—the ability to observe our thoughts, feelings, and sensations with more clarity. Before we begin cultivating mindful awareness, however, we must consider the degree to which we have clear access to the nature of our minds. The answer seems to be: not as well as we think we do. The challenge of *seeing the mind clearly* is one of the central problems that we face in asking people to self-report how mindful they are. This can be especially challenging in youth, whose brain networks devoted to metacognitive or higher-level awareness and abstraction are not fully developed (Gogtay et al. 2004). Consider this vignette:

A researcher read aloud a self-report mindfulness questionnaire to a group of elementary school students while he was collecting research data. One item on the questionnaire was "I find it difficult to stay focused on what's happening in the present." One student, who appeared to be distracted by external stimuli, asked, "Could you repeat the question?" After the researcher repeated the question, the student responded aloud, "Oh, no—that never happens to me!" and marked the corresponding response choice.

As this vignette illustrates, asking children to be mindful of how unmindful they actually are is not an easy task. In this chapter, we discuss some of the challenges and limitations of assessing mindfulness in youth, review current validated assessment instruments, and offer suggestions for assessing mindfulness in different settings (e.g., clinic vs. school) and with youth at different developmental stages. We close by proposing alternative methods of assessment.

Challenges of and Limitations to Assessment

The self-report conundrum illustrated in the vignette has been discussed by several authors (for in-depth discussions of this topic, see Goodman et al. 2017; Grossman 2011). This challenge is underscored by some studies demonstrating that adolescents with prior meditation or yoga experience score *lower* than their meditation-naïve peers on self-report measures of mindfulness (e.g., de Bruin et al. 2014). This is not to suggest that children and adolescents will invariably exhibit this trend but simply offers one example of what some readers may discover when assessing mindfulness in youth.

Before we attempt to assess mindfulness, however, it is prudent to ascertain what we are measuring. Most scholars and practitioners agree that the construct of mindfulness involves some component of *present-focused, nonjudgmental attention*. Many other qualities are associated with mindfulness, however, including concentration, compassion, lovingkindness, emotional equanimity, somatic awareness, skillful decision making, nonattachment, and wisdom. Should these qualities also be included in the definition and assessment of mindfulness? Indeed, scholars across many disciplines continue to debate the exact meaning of mindfulness. Developing a consensus operational definition remains an ongoing task for academics. To assess mindfulness outside a research context, discerning the specific components of interest can help focus one's choice of assessments. Some of the mindfulness measures reviewed in this chapter offer both a global measure of mindfulness (i.e., as a single, unitary construct) and assessment of its constituent parts (e.g., awareness, decentering, acceptance, openness). Some practitioners may find it more useful to select a measure with close proximity to mindfulness. A school counselor, for example, might choose a compassion or executive functioning measure to assess interpersonal or attention problems, respectively.

In assessing mindfulness, we must also decide whether we wish to measure state or trait mindfulness. *State mindfulness* refers to the ability to cultivate a particular quality of mind in a particular moment, such as during meditation, whereas *trait mindfulness* refers to a more stable, dispositional quality. Existing validated mindfulness measures favor the assessment of trait mindfulness. Some researchers have found a relationship between state and trait mindfulness (Brown and Ryan 2003), whereas others have suggested that there may actually be little overlap between the two (Thompson and Waltz 2007). Thus, asking youth to self-report their tendency to be mindful not only introduces the foggy mirror problem but may also be a poor reflection of their ability to cultivate a mindful state within a given moment. Practitioners attempting to measure mindfulness might therefore consider whether the assessment of state mindfulness or trait mindfulness is most salient to their particular purposes.

Self-Report Measures of Mindfulness for Youth

In this section, we offer a brief overview of existing validated mindfulness measures for youth ages 9–18. A summary of each measure is provided in Table 4–1. All seven measures are self-report instruments. Strengths and limitations of each are discussed, with reference to their utility in specific settings (e.g., clinics, schools, community). Readers are referred to Goodman et al. (2017) for a more detailed discussion of theoretical foundations, validation studies, and psychometric properties of these measures.

Child and Adolescent Mindfulness Measure

The Child and Adolescent Mindfulness Measure (CAMM) is a 10-item self-report measure of "present-moment awareness, and nonjudgmental, nonavoidant responses to thoughts and feelings" in 10- to 17-year-old children and adolescents (Greco et al. 2011, p. 610). Respondents rank on a 5-point scale (0=never true; 4=always true) how true each item is for them. All items are negatively worded and reverse scored, with higher scores indicating greater mindfulness. The CAMM has correlated positively with academic competence, social skills, happiness, quality of life, self-esteem, and self-regulation and correlated negatively with externalizing problems, internalizing symptoms, stress, rumination, catastrophizing, self-blame, and somatic complaints (de Bruin et al. 2014; Greco et al. 2011).

The CAMM has been validated in several languages and cultures, including English-speaking children and adolescents in the United States, Dutch-speaking

TABLE 4–1. Self-report measures of mindfulness in youth

Measure	Age range (years)	Number of items	Time to complete	Measure validated?	Factors	Areas of positive correlation	Areas of negative correlation
CAMM	10–17	10	Less than 5 minutes	Yes	Present-moment awareness and nonjudgmental, nonavoidant responses to thoughts and feelings	Mindfulness (MAAS-A), well-being, effortful control, self-esteem, academic competence, quality of life, social skills, happiness, self-regulation	Externalizing problems, internalizing symptoms, stress, somatic complaints, rumination, self-blame, catastrophizing, worry, negative affect
MAAS-A	14–18	14	Less than 5 minutes	Yes	Receptive state of attention that, informed by an awareness of present experience, simply observes what is taking place	Mindfulness (CAMM), life satisfaction, positive affect, happiness, quality of life, wellness, self-regulation, agreeableness, conscientiousness, openness to experience	Neuroticism, negative affect, stress, substance abuse to cope with stress, rumination, catastrophizing
MAAS-C	9–13	15	Less than 5 minutes	Yes	Receptive state of attention that, informed by an awareness of present experience, simply observes what is taking place	School self-concept, optimism, perceived autonomy in classroom, positive affect, academic efficacy, academic achievement goals	Negative affect, depression, rumination, anxiety

TABLE 4–1.	Self-report measures of mindfulness in youth *(continued)*						
Measure	Age range (years)	Number of items	Time to complete	Measure validated?	Factors	Areas of positive correlation	Areas of negative correlation
CHIME-A	12–14	25	Less than 10 minutes	Yes	1. Awareness of internal experiences 2. Awareness of external experiences 3. Acting with awareness 4. Accepting and nonjudgmental orientation 5. Decentering and nonreactivity 6. Openness to experience 7. Relativity of thoughts 8. Insightful understanding	Mindfulness (CAMM), well-being	Emotional dysregulation, perfectionism, negative affect, depression, anxiety, weight and shape concerns
MTASA	13–17	32	Less than 15 minutes	Yes	1. Healthy self-regulation 2. Active attention 3. Awareness and observation 4. Accepting experience	Mindfulness (MAAS, KIMS, FFMQ), positive affect, life satisfaction	Negative affect

TABLE 4–1. Self-report measures of mindfulness in youth (continued)

Measure	Age range (years)	Number of items	Time to complete	Measure validated?	Factors	Areas of positive correlation	Areas of negative correlation
AAMS	11–19	19	Less than 10 minutes	Yes	1. Focus on the present moment 2. Being nonreactive 3. Being nonjudgmental 4. Self-accepting	Self-compassion, emotion regulation	NA
MSQ	10–14	15	Less than 5 minutes	Yes	1. Mindful attention 2. Mindful acceptance 3. Approach and persistence	Joy of learning, school connectedness, educational purpose, academic efficiency, academic achievement	NA

Abbreviations. AAMS = Adolescent and Adult Mindfulness Scale; CAMM = Child and Adolescent Mindfulness Measure; CHIME-A = Comprehensive Inventory of Mindfulness Experiences–Adolescents; FFMQ = Five Facet Mindfulness Questionnaire; KIMS = Kentucky Inventory of Mindfulness Skills; MAAS = Mindful Attention Awareness Scale; MAAS-A = Mindful Attention Awareness Scale for Adolescents; MAAS-C = Mindful Attention Awareness Scale for Children; MSQ = Mindfulness School Questionnaire; MTASA = Mindful Thinking and Action Scale for Adolescents; NA = not available.

children and adolescents in the Netherlands, Catalan-speaking adolescents in Spain, and Italian-speaking children and adolescents in Italy. Each of these studies used nonclinical samples; the CAMM's validity in clinical populations is still unknown. A single-factor construct of mindfulness appears to be favored, which does not allow for the parsing out of discrete components of mindfulness.

Mindful Attention Awareness Scale for Adolescents

The Mindful Attention Awareness Scale for Adolescents (MAAS-A; Brown et al. 2011) is a measure of dispositional (trait) mindfulness for adolescents ages 14–18 that was adapted from the adult MAAS (Brown and Ryan 2003). It contains 14 items, all of which are negatively worded. Respondents rate the absence, rather than presence, of mindfulness in their daily life—with particular emphasis on present-focused attention (e.g., "I rush through activities without being really attentive to them"). Responses are based on a 6-point scale (1=almost always; 6=almost never) in which higher total scores reflect greater mindfulness. MAAS-A scores have correlated positively with positive affect, happiness, life satisfaction, and self-regulation and have correlated negatively with negative affect, neuroticism, and substance abuse as a means of coping with stress (Brown et al. 2011).

The MAAS-A is the only self-report measure that has been validated in a clinical population—mainly adolescents with anxiety- and mood-related disorders (Brown et al. 2011). It has been validated cross-culturally in the United States, the Netherlands, and China. The indirect assessment approach (i.e., negative wording) on the MAAS-A and similar measures has drawn some criticism related to the foggy mirror problem, or one's ability to make self-attributions about the frequency of not being mindful in everyday life (Grossman 2011). Like the CAMM, a single-factor solution was found for the MAAS-A, which limits its ability to ascertain subcomponents of mindfulness.

Mindful Attention Awareness Scale for Children

The Mindful Attention Awareness Scale for Children (MAAS-C; R. Benn, Modified Mindful Attention Awareness Scale, unpublished data, 2004) is an adapted version of the MAAS-A for children ages 9–13. The MAAS-C contains the same 14 items as the MAAS-A, but with more child-friendly language, and adds one additional item. As with the MAAS-A, all 15 items on the MAAS-C are negatively worded. However, the Likert scale on the MAAS-C is scored in the opposite direction (1=almost never; 6=almost always). Higher scores therefore reflect greater mindfulness.

The MAAS-C has been validated with the youngest sample of children. It therefore may be advantageous to practitioners working with elementary school–age children as young as fourth grade. Similar to the CAMM and MAAS-A, the MAAS-C has a single-factor construct of mindfulness. Its indirect assessment approach prompts the same validity concerns as the MAAS-A and similar measures (Grossman 2011). The MAAS-C has not yet been evaluated in clinical samples.

Comprehensive Inventory of Mindfulness Experiences-Adolescents

The Comprehensive Inventory of Mindfulness Experiences-Adolescents (CHIME-A) is a 25-item measure of trait mindfulness for adolescents (Johnson et al. 2017). It was adapted from the 37-item adult CHIME (Bergomi et al. 2014). Items on the CHIME-A are both positively and negatively worded. Responses are based on a 5-point scale (0=never true; 4=always true). The CHIME-A contains eight distinct mindfulness subscales: awareness of internal experiences, awareness of external experiences, acting with awareness, accepting and nonjudgmental orientation, decentering and nonreactivity, openness to experience, relativity of thoughts, and insightful understanding. CHIME-A scores have correlated positively with well-being and negatively with weight and body concerns, anxiety, depression, negative affect, emotion dysregulation, and perfectionism (Johnson et al. 2017).

The eight-factor structure of the CHIME-A benefits practitioners interested in more nuanced components of mindfulness. One drawback is that, to date, it has been evaluated only in 12- to 14-year-old youth, which is a limited range. The CHIME-A has not yet been tested in a clinical sample. Finally, the authors of the CHIME-A recommend using only the subscale scores, versus the total score, because of poor internal consistency of the total score during the initial validation studies (Johnson et al. 2017).

Mindful Thinking and Action Scale for Adolescents

The Mindful Thinking and Action Scale for Adolescents (MTASA) is a 32-item self-report measure of trait mindfulness for adolescents age 13–17 (A.M. West, T. Penix-Sbraga, and D.A. Poole, "Measuring mindfulness in youth: development of the mindful thinking and action scale for adolescents," unpublished manuscript, Central Michigan University, 2005). Items are both positively and negatively worded and based on a 5-point scale (1=never; 5=almost always). The MTASA has four subscales: healthy self-regulation, active attention, awareness and observation, and accepting experience. The MTASA has correlated positively with positive affect and life satisfaction and correlated negatively with negative affect. As with the CHIME-A, the four subscales on the MTASA benefit practitioners wishing to examine subcomponents of mindfulness. Its utility for younger children and clinical populations is unknown.

Adolescent and Adult Mindfulness Scale

The Adolescent and Adult Mindfulness Scale (AAMS) is a 19-item self-report measure of trait mindfulness. Before its publication by Droutman et al. (2018), the AAMS had been presented as the Mindfulness Scale for Pre-Teens, Teens, and Adults (MSPTA; Droutman 2015). The AAMS and MSPTA are the same instrument. The AAMS has been validated in adolescents ages 11–19 as well as adults. Items are both positively and negatively worded and rated on a 5-point scale (1 = never true; 5 = always true). The AAMS contains four subscales: focus on the present moment (i.e., paying attention to surroundings, thoughts, feelings, and emotions), being nonreactive, being nonjudgmental, and self-acceptance. AAMS scores have correlated with measures of self-compassion and emotion regulation (Droutman et al. 2018).

As with the CHIME-A and MTASA, the multifactor construct of mindfulness on the AAMS is beneficial in assessing separate components of mindfulness. In its initial validation, the AAMS captured changes in mindfulness following an 8-week mindfulness intervention for adolescents ages 11–18. It also demonstrated evidence of temporal stability and longitudinal invariance (Droutman et al. 2018). The AAMS has yet to be evaluated in a clinical sample.

Mindfulness School Questionnaire

The Mindfulness School Questionnaire (MSQ; Renshaw 2017) is a 15-item self-report measure of trait mindfulness for adolescents in grades 6–8. Items were designed to be relevant to mindfulness in a school setting (e.g., "When I am at school, I notice..."). All items are positively worded and rated on a 4-point scale (1 = almost never; 4 = almost always) such that higher scores reflect greater mindfulness. The MSQ contains three subscales: mindful attention, mindful acceptance, and approach and persistence. MSQ scores have correlated positively with aspects of subjective well-being, including joy of learning, school connectedness, educational purpose, academic efficiency, and academic achievement (Renshaw 2017).

Similar to the CHIME-A, MTASA, and MSPTA, the three subscales of the MSQ allow for a multifaceted assessment of mindfulness. Another benefit of the MSQ is its relevance for assessing mindfulness in school-specific settings. The validity of the MSQ has not yet been evaluated with elementary or high school students or with clinical populations.

Administering Self-Report Questionnaires to Children

Self-report questionnaires in any social or behavioral science, including the assessment of mindfulness, inherently include biases in self-perception, social desirability, and item interpretation. There are a few ways to help minimize these biases. For example, remind children that there are no "right" or "wrong" answers. Children may be eager to try to impress or manage the perceptions of teachers, clinicians, or others whom they respect or admire by responding in a way that they believe is desirable. It can be useful to read questions aloud and invite children to ask clarifying questions. Some questions can be confusing, even for adults, and it is important to ensure that children thoroughly understand them. In settings where the standardization of assessments is less important (i.e., outside of a research context), it might be helpful to expand on questionnaires and directly ask children or adolescents what mindfulness means to them or give examples of how they are mindful. If you are assessing before and after an intervention, children's self-perceptions will likely shift—often in the direction of becoming more aware of how their minds wander (i.e., being more mindful of not being mindful). Therefore, in addition to tracking a score on a self-report measure, it can be valuable to gather qualitative data about how cognitive or emotional responses might have changed. Asking supplemental questions about how mindfulness has been used in everyday life may minimize the problem that simply being exposed to mindfulness jargon (e.g., present-moment, attention, compassion) during an intervention provides children with clues to the "right" answer (Grossman 2011).

Assessing Mindfulness in the Clinic

Some readers may be working with youth in clinical settings. Although administering a self-report measure of mindfulness can be useful in this situation, it is not always necessary or beneficial. There are other methods of collecting information about a child or adolescent's degree of mindfulness. Rather than asking patients to report on the proclivities of their mind, we might assess mindfulness directly. This is akin to administering a memory (or other neurocognitive) task rather than asking, "How is your memory?" Because there are no validated measures for objectively assessing state mindfulness in youth, however, doing this requires some creativity. We offer a few suggestions for assessing mindfulness in clinics.

1. Invite the youth to count his or her breath cycles and raise his or her hand after five breaths (then start over).

- Count breath cycles by watching the rise and fall of the youth's chest or belly. Notice the patient's accuracy by matching your count to the hand raising. Inaccuracies are an indication that the mind has wandered.
- Repeat this same exercise with other objects of attention, such as ringing a bell and asking the youth to raise his or her hand when he or she no longer hears the sound.

2. Invite the youth to explore his or her thoughts, emotions, and body sensations for a few minutes. Then guide an inquiry into what he or she experienced.

- Assess whether the youth can distinguish between thoughts, feelings, and body sensations. Can he or she identify thoughts and emotions as being distinct from each other? How does he or she know the difference? Can he or she locate specific body sensations or locations in the body where those thoughts and emotions manifest? Can the youth use descriptive language (e.g., tingling, tightness, warmth) versus "judging" language (e.g., good, bad, hate it, love it)? Can he or she describe other qualities of experience (e.g., shape, color, texture, movement)? How long did those experiences last?
- If the youth is unable to come up with an answer, this is still interesting data in the sense that the mind may have been completely distracted, or the youth may have had difficulty identifying internal experiences. If the youth demonstrates resistance, hesitancy, or confusion about engaging in the exercise, consider using external objects of focus, especially those that elicit more buy-in, such as mindfully observing a food item. You can elicit descriptions of what the youth sees, smells, tastes, or touches and what internal responses he or she has to the object.

3. Assess how the youth relates to his or her own experiences, particularly those that feel "bad" or uncomfortable.

- In conversation, we can ascertain if the youth greets his or her internal experiences with aversion, self-criticism, automatic or impulsive reactions, or an underlying urge to "get rid of this experience." Alternatively, does the youth tend to relate to his or her experiences with curiosity, openness, kindness, and patience? Understanding this may also reveal useful targets for therapeutic interventions. This kind of assessment can be done naturally in the course of a therapy session by noticing language and inviting exploration of ways the youth tends to "work with" challenges or difficulties that arise in his or her life.

Clinicians might also consider assessing other qualities that are associated with mindfulness. Cognitive qualities might include thought suppression;

identification with thoughts (i.e., thoughts as representations of reality); psychological flexibility; or aspects of executive functioning such as concentration, working memory, or inhibition. Affective qualities might include empathy, self-compassion, or distress tolerance. Clinicians might also examine qualities associated with mindfulness that predict life satisfaction, for example, gratitude, perseverance, and empathic concern for others. The point to remember is that mindfulness exists within a matrix of other related constructs—many of which can provide clues to a patient's mindfulness and offer additional valuable information about his or her cognitions, emotions, personality, and behavior. An understanding of how mindfulness relates to other constructs adds nuance and depth to mindfulness assessments and interventions.

In assessing mindfulness in clinical populations, we must consider the interaction between mindfulness and psychopathology. Youth with anxiety, depression, trauma, or other emotional or behavioral difficulties may find it difficult to learn or practice mindfulness. Anxiety and depression are known to interfere with attention and emotion regulation and to promote experiential avoidance. A child with a trauma history, for example, not only may find it challenging to observe his or her thoughts and body sensations but also may experience great discomfort or distress when attempting to do so. Mindfulness interventions for youth with anxiety, mood, and trauma-related disorders is discussed in Part II, "Mindfulness Application to Specific Clinical Populations."

In assessing mindfulness in youth with psychopathology, we must also assess for reactions *to* mindfulness practice. Children who find these practices uncomfortable or are unwilling to explore their internal states might focus instead on developing a sense of safety, for example, or using mindfulness to explore external phenomena (e.g., sights, smells, sounds). Some experienced mindfulness teachers have suggested that the closer the attention is to the core of the body (stomach, chest, or head), the more likely it may be to elicit difficult emotions or uncomfortable body sensations. An assessment of mindfulness might invite the traumatized youth to explore sensations in his or her hands or feet or in the environment around him or her (Pollak et al. 2014, p. 11).

Assessing Mindfulness in the Classroom

Teachers, school psychologists, or counselors may be interested in assessing a child or adolescent's mindfulness at school. The MSQ may be a useful starting point. The activities suggested for therapists working in clinical settings are also relevant to therapists working in schools.

Mindfulness can also be inferred from examining other context-relevant constructs. A school psychologist might administer a test of executive functioning to infer attentional capacity in the classroom, whereas teachers might use academic performance or scales that assess socioemotional development. Parents can look beyond academic achievement or performance in the classroom for evidence of mindfulness-related qualities such as resiliency, perseverance, prosocial behaviors, and compassion toward oneself and others.

Researchers have examined socioemotional behavior in preschool-age children by using a sharing task whereby children are given a set of stickers and prompted to either keep as many as they would like or share as many as they like with other classmates (see Flook et al. 2015). Other examples include assessing the degree to which children or adolescents can describe their thoughts, feelings, and body sensations after an event (e.g., conflict on the playground) or inviting the child or adolescent to describe the emotional experiences from the other person's perspective.

Assessing Mindfulness in the Community

Parents or other adults working with youth in the community may also have an interest in assessing mindfulness. Parents might be curious about their child's lack of mindfulness (e.g., having a tendency to forget tasks), noting the frequency of absent-minded safety behaviors (e.g., crossing the street without looking) or evaluating the child's ability to recognize his or her emotional experiences. A parent might observe these behaviors directly or gather information from a teacher, sports coach, or other adult who interacts with the child in different settings. Self-report measures and some of the alternative assessment methods discussed in this chapter are other assessment options. As mindfulness retreats become more popular with youth, some readers might be interested in implementing mindfulness in nature in a family setting or with groups of youth. Fun activities related to assessment might include listening for sounds in nature, spotting items on a walk (e.g., scavenger hunt), or exercises involving deep listening and retelling of a partner's story. Adults working with youth in the community, classroom, or clinic should consider cultural factors when assessing and applying mindfulness. The meaning of mindfulness and objectives for practicing may differ across religious, ethnic, or other cultural backgrounds.

Developmental Adaptations

Because the construct of mindfulness is likely to be interpreted and demonstrated differently across the lifespan, assessment approaches need to differ as well. A toddler does not possess the cognitive capacity to observe his or her inner experience with metacognitive awareness, nor does a toddler have the language to describe his or her experiences. Preliminary research in children ages 4, 6, and 8 years old found that the capacity to mindfully observe the breath and to process knowledge about thoughts follows a predictable developmental progression; thus, assessments that focus on breath and thought awareness may be more appropriate for children ages 8 and older (Satlof-Bedrick and Johnson 2015).

Other behaviors in early childhood share overlapping neural networks with qualities of mindfulness and may be prerequisites to the development of state and trait mindfulness in adulthood. Mindfulness skills are closely related to networks involved in self-regulation, including emotion regulation and impulse control (Hölzel et al. 2011). In preschool- and kindergarten-age children, researchers often use "hot" and "cool" tasks to measure emotion regulation and attention. *Hot* tasks typically include an emotional component. Delay-of-gratification tasks are common (e.g., the Stanford marshmallow experiment in which children can either eat a marshmallow immediately or wait a short period for a larger reward [Mischel et al. 1972]). *Cool* tasks typically involve more top-down, attention- and/or motor-based assessments of executive function. Examples of cool tasks include go/no-go tasks, in which children either initiate or inhibit a response to competing stimuli (e.g., asking children to walk/stop or raise their hand/not raise their hand in response to green "go" or red "stop" signs), or other motor inhibition tasks (e.g., Simon Says). Stroop tasks (e.g., reading the names of colors that are printed in different color ink) is another example of a cool attention task.

It can sometimes be difficult to engage adolescents in mindfulness activities or to complete an assessment. Many of us have had trouble engaging high school–age students in anything—let alone an unfamiliar mindfulness activity. Using external objects of attention, such as focusing on sounds or mindfully tasting a food item, can initially elicit more buy-in. This might offer opportunities to explore the teen's ability to maintain focus on an object, use describing versus judging words, and notice any emotions or body sensations that might have been evoked (as reviewed in the section "Assessing Mindfulness in the Clinic"). The youth's language use offers other clues to inferring mindfulness. Notice if a teenager identifies with an experience or whether there is some separation of self from the experience. For example, the sentence "I *am* angry" is different from "I *feel* angry." The latter conveys less identification with the emotion and implies an understanding of temporality—I am experiencing anger in this moment, but anger is not who I am. Inviting youth to notice or feel the difference between "being" an emotion and "feeling" an emotion may suggest another target for intervention.

Alternative Assessment Methods

Mindfulness is a complex and challenging construct to assess. Self-report measures are currently the only validated tools for assessing mindfulness in youth. The examples provided previously in the sections on working with youth in the clinic, in the classroom, in the community, and across different age ranges offer several techniques that as of yet are not supported by empirical evidence. A few other promising alternative approaches are briefly described in this section.

Breath Counting Task

In the breath counting task, individuals press a button every breath cycle and a second button every ninth breath. This task has been validated in adults (Levinson et al. 2014), and it can easily be adapted to children. As noted in the section "Assessing Mindfulness in the Clinic," you can ask children simply to raise their hand or use another objective indicator as a means of measuring their attention to the breath.

Ecological Momentary Assessment

Ecological momentary assessment (EMA) enhances the ability to assess state mindfulness by sampling a child or adolescent's mindful state at different intervals throughout the day. For example, a teacher could pause every hour and ask students to notice whether their minds are wandering or whether they are on task. Researchers have used text messages and other technology (e.g., phone apps) to ask questions about the quality of a person's mind in a particular moment during a normal day. Although assessing mindfulness with EMA has been shown to be feasible in adults (Moore et al. 2016), no studies have yet implemented EMA with youth.

Physiological Data

Physiological correlates of mindfulness and self-regulation can be measured in children's natural environments using technology. For example, several devices are now on the market that discretely record respiration, heart rate, and other physiological data throughout the day. Although these data are not direct measures of mindfulness, they provide valuable information about health and stress resilience that may be associated with mindfulness. Heightened stress levels might inform professionals or parents of the need for a greater frequency of practice or the need for a particular type of practice (e.g., yoga, which more directly targets cardiovascular functioning) that may be most useful for an individual child or adolescent.

Qualitative Assessments

Children or adolescents can provide first-person descriptions of their experiences. Practitioners working directly with youth in clinics, schools, or the community may find a child's descriptions more helpful than fixed response choices from a questionnaire. Open-ended questions could evaluate the extent to which children are aware of their internal experiences, specific ways that they relate to their own thoughts and feelings, and how their understandings translate into emotional and behavioral responses.

Observer Reports

Instead of relying on child or adolescent self-reports of mindfulness, ratings can be obtained by observation. For example, a clinician may ask a teacher to complete a rating scale about a child's mindfulness in the classroom.

Conclusion

Seeing the nature of our minds clearly is a skill that is developed over the course of a lifetime, not only during childhood and adolescence. The assessment of mindfulness in youth presents unique challenges, but some of the background, techniques, and recommendations offered in this chapter may help orient and guide you toward practical methods of assessment. Understandings gained from your own mindfulness practice can be an essential guide—just as it will be when you begin putting mindfulness into practice. The more clearly you can see your own mind, the brighter the mirror you can hold up to the youth you are illuminating.

KEY POINTS

- Self-report measures are helpful assessment tools but are sometimes limited by the paradox that more mindfulness might be reported when we are less mindful and less mindfulness might be reported when we see our minds more clearly.
- Assessment approaches must be tailored to the setting and the child or adolescent's developmental level, mental and emotional health status, and cultural needs.
- Evidence-based assessment techniques can be enhanced by using measures of related constructs, in

conjunction with your own creativity and mindfulness practice.

Discussion Questions

1. What are some strengths and limitations to using self-report measures when assessing mindfulness in youth?
2. How might one's approach to assessing mindfulness differ across the developmental spectrum? What are the relevant cognitive differences between younger children and teenagers?
3. Given that mindfulness can be difficult to measure directly, name a few related constructs that can be measured instead of, or in addition to, mindfulness.
4. What are some alternative assessment approaches to using self-report?

Suggested Readings

Goodman MS, Madni LA, Semple RJ: Measuring mindfulness in youth: review of current assessments, challenges, and future directions. Mindfulness 8:1409–1420, 2017

Grossman P: Defining mindfulness by how poorly I think I pay attention during everyday awareness and other intractable problems for psychology's (re)invention of mindfulness: comment on Brown et al. (2011). Psychol Assess 23(4):1034–1040, discussion 1041–1046, 201122122674

Pallozzi R, Wertheim E, Paxton S, Ong B: Trait mindfulness measures for use with adolescents: A systematic review. Mindfulness 8:110–125, 2017

References

Bergomi C, Tschacher W, Kupper Z: Construction and initial validation of a questionnaire for the comprehensive investigation of mindfulness [in German]. Diagnostica 60:111–125, 2014

Brown KW, Ryan RM: The benefits of being present: mindfulness and its role in psychological well-being. J Pers Soc Psychol 84(4):822–848, 2003 12703651

Brown KW, West AM, Loverich TM, et al: Assessing adolescent mindfulness: validation of an adapted Mindful Attention Awareness Scale in adolescent normative and psychiatric populations. Psychol Assess 23(4):1023–1033, 2011 21319908

de Bruin EI, Zijlstra BJH, Bögels SM: The meaning of mindfulness in children and adolescents: further validation of the Child and Adolescent Mindfulness Measure (CAMM) in two independent samples from the Netherlands. Mindfulness 5:422–430, 2014

Droutman V: Mindfulness scale for pre-teens, teens and adults, in Clinical Applications of Mindfulness. Edited by Semple RJ. Research symposium conducted at the Bridging the Hearts and Minds of Youth: Mindfulness and Compassion in Clinical Practice, Education, and Research Conference, UC San Diego Center for Mindfulness, San Diego, CA, February 2015

Droutman V, Golub I, Oganesyan A, Read S: Development and initial validation of the Adolescent and Adult Mindfulness Scale (AAMS). Pers Individ Dif 123:34–43, 2018

Flook L, Goldberg SB, Pinger L, et al: Promoting prosocial behavior and self-regulatory skills in preschool children through a mindfulness-based kindness curriculum. Dev Psychol 51(1):44–51, 2015 25383689

Gogtay N, Giedd JN, Lusk L, et al: Dynamic mapping of human cortical development during childhood through early adulthood. Proc Natl Acad Sci U S A 101(21):8174–8179, 2004, 15148381

Goodman MS, Madni LA, Semple RJ: Measuring mindfulness in youth: Review of current assessments, challenges, and future directions. Mindfulness 8:1409–1420, 2017

Greco LA, Baer RA, Smith GT: Assessing mindfulness in children and adolescents: development and validation of the Child and Adolescent Mindfulness Measure (CAMM). Psychol Assess 23(3):606–614, 2011 21480722

Grossman P: Defining mindfulness by how poorly I think I pay attention during everyday awareness and other intractable problems for psychology's (re)invention of mindfulness: comment on Brown et al. (2011). Psychol Assess 23(4):1034–1040, discussion 1041–1046, 2011 22122674

Hölzel BK, Lazar SW, Gard T, et al: How does mindfulness meditation work? Proposing mechanisms of action from a conceptual and neural perspective. Perspect Psychol Sci 6(6):537–559, 2011 26168376

Johnson C, Burke C, Brinkman S, et al: Development and validation of a multifactor mindfulness scale in youth: the Comprehensive Inventory of Mindfulness Experiences-Adolescents (CHIME-A). Psychol Assess 29(3):264–281, 2017 27254018

Levinson DB, Stoll EL, Kindy SD, et al: A mind you can count on: validating breath counting as a behavioral measure of mindfulness. Front Psychol 5:1202, 2014 25386148

Mischel W, Ebbesen EB, Zeiss AR: Cognitive and attentional mechanisms in delay of gratification. J Pers Soc Psychol 21(2)204–218, 1972 5010404

Moore RC, Depp CA, Wetherell JL, Lenze EJ: Ecological momentary assessment versus standard assessment instruments for measuring mindfulness, depressed mood, and anxiety among older adults. J Psychiatr Res 75:116–123, 2016 26851494

Pollak SM, Pedulla T, Siegel RD: Sitting Together: Essential Skills for Mindfulness-Based Psychotherapy. New York, Guilford, 2014

Renshaw TL: Preliminary development and validation of the Mindful Student Questionnaire. Assess Eff Interv 42(3):168–175, 2017

Satlof-Bedrick E, Johnson CN: Children's metacognition and mindful awareness of breathing and thinking. Cogn Dev 36:83–92, 2015

Thompson BL, Waltz J: Everyday mindfulness and mindfulness meditation: overlapping constructs or not? Pers Individ Dif 43(7):1875–1885, 2007

Part II

Mindfulness Application to Specific Clinical Diagnoses

Chapter 5

Anxiety and Depression

Laila A. Madni, Psy.D.
Matthew S. Goodman, M.A.
Randye J. Semple, Ph.D.

The curious paradox is that when I accept myself just as I am, then I change.
—*Carl Rogers* (1995)

CHILDHOOD is a time to explore the world, whether by adventuring through a pillow fort or scrupulously evaluating all the ice cream flavors—before choosing vanilla (or maybe chocolate if it's been one of "those" days). Adolescents face increasing academic and social challenges as they move into middle or high school, such as making new friends or awkwardly navigating a first date. Our society often portrays youth as a carefree time filled with play and excitement, but for many children and adolescents, it can be a difficult time. This is particularly true for youth trying to cope with mood or anxiety disorders.

Anxiety is the most common disorder of childhood and adolescence, with estimates of more than 32% of youth ages 13–17 meeting criteria for lifetime prevalence of an anxiety disorder. Specific disorders range from approximately 2% for generalized anxiety disorder to 20% for specific phobias (Kessler et al. 2012). As many as 50% of adolescents experience anxiety symptoms by age 6 (Merikangas et al. 2010). Exacerbating the problem, the majority of youth with one anxiety disorder often have a co-occurring anxiety or depressive disorder (Costello et al. 2003).

Although anxiety disorders often begin in childhood, the common age of onset for mood disorders is adolescence (Merikangas et al. 2010). The lifetime prevalence of adolescent mood disorders is also high, with an estimated 14% of youth ages 13–18 meeting criteria for a mood disorder (Kessler et al. 2012). Unipolar depression affects the majority, with a lower rate of bipolar disorders. One concern is that mood disorders tend to increase with age; nearly twice as many 17- to 18-year-olds are affected than 13- to 14-year-olds (Merikangas et al. 2010). Another worrying trend is that the prevalence of adolescent mood disorders appears to be increasing over time (Mojtabai et al. 2016).

Evidence-Based Interventions

Although some youth benefit from pharmacological and psychotherapeutic interventions, many more either have no access to these treatments or find them to be not entirely effective. There continues to be a pressing need for additional interventions that are effective for treating anxiety and mood disorders and are readily accessible.

In this chapter, we review four evidence-based mindfulness interventions for youth with anxiety and mood disorders. We begin by providing an overview of dialectical behavior therapy for adolescents (DBT-A) and acceptance and commitment therapy (ACT), which are mindfulness-informed interventions that teach general concepts and a few mindfulness-based skills. We then discuss two mindfulness-based therapies that provide intensive training in formal and informal meditative practices: mindfulness-based stress reduction for teens (MBSR-T), which is followed by a more detailed description of another practice-based intervention, mindfulness-based cognitive therapy for children (MBCT-C). We discuss the theoretical foundations, core components, main interventions, and research support for these mindfulness-informed interventions and mindfulness-based interventions (MBIs). Table 5–1 summarizes the research findings for all four treatment models. We close by describing some clinical concerns to consider before implementing MBIs with youth and offer a few important take-home points. The treatment manuals or workbooks for each model are included in the Suggested Readings.

TABLE 5-1. Research support for treating child and adolescent mood and anxiety disorders with mindfulness

Study	Population	N	Setting	Research design	Control group	Main findings
Dialectical behavior therapy for adolescents (DBT-A)						
Del Conte et al. 2016	Adolescents with general psychiatric symptoms	48	Partial hospitalization program	Open trial	None	• Decreased anxiety • Decreased depression • Decreased general psychiatric symptoms • Decreased somatic complaints • Reduced interpersonal sensitivity and hostility • Decreased maladaptive coping • Increased emotion regulation • Increased mindfulness
Goldstein et al. 2007	Adolescents with bipolar disorder	10	Pediatric specialty clinic	Open trial	None	• Decreased suicidality • Decreased depressive symptoms • Decreased nonsuicidal self-injurious behavior • Reduced emotion dysregulation
Goldstein et al. 2015	Adolescents with bipolar disorder	20	Pediatric specialty clinic	Randomized clinical trial	Yes	• Decreased depressive symptoms ($p=0.05$) • Trend toward reduced suicidal ideation ($p=0.07$)

TABLE 5–1. Research support for treating child and adolescent mood and anxiety disorders with mindfulness *(continued)*

Study	Population	N	Setting	Research design	Control group	Main findings
Dialectical behavior therapy for adolescents (DBT-A) (continued)						
Mehlum et al. 2014	Adolescents with suicidal and self-harm behaviors	77	Psychiatric outpatient clinic	Randomized controlled trial	Yes	• Decreased depressive symptoms • Less suicidal ideation • Fewer self-harm behaviors
Acceptance and commitment therapy (ACT)						
Hancock et al. 2016	Children with anxiety disorders	157	Children's hospital, psychology department	Randomized clinical trial	Waitlist control and CBT	• Decreased anxiety • Increased quality of life
Hayes et al. 1999	Adolescents with depression	30	Psychiatric outpatient clinic	Randomized clinical trial	Yes	• Decreased depression
Mindfulness-based stress reduction for teens (MBSR-T)						
Biegel et al. 2009	Adolescent psychiatric outpatients	74	Outpatient psychiatric facility	Randomized clinical trial	Yes	• Decreased anxiety • Decreased depression • Decreased somatic distress • Increased self-esteem • Increased sleep quality

TABLE 5-1. Research support for treating child and adolescent mood and anxiety disorders with mindfulness *(continued)*

Study	Population	N	Setting	Research design	Control group	Main findings
Mindfulness–based cognitive therapy for children (MBCT-C)						
Ames et al. 2014	Adolescents with mood and/or anxiety disorders	6	Outpatient mood disorders clinic and hospital	Open trial	None	• Decreased depression • Decreased rumination • Decreased worry • Increased mindfulness • Increased perceived quality of life • Decreased emotional distress • Decreased symptom impact
Cotton et al. 2016	Children and adolescents at risk for bipolar disorder	10	Outpatient treatment facility	Open trial	None	• Increased mindfulness • Decreased emotional lability • Increased emotion regulation • Less clinician-rated anxiety • Less child-rated state anxiety • Less child-rated trait anxiety
Dehghani et al. 2014	Children with generalized anxiety disorder	14	Elementary school	Randomized clinical trial	Yes	• Decreased worry • Decreased anxiety

TABLE 5–1. Research support for treating child and adolescent mood and anxiety disorders with mindfulness (*continued*)

Study	Population	N	Setting	Research design	Control group	Main findings
Mindfulness-based cognitive therapy for children (MBCT-C) (*continued*)						
Esmailian et al. 2013	Children of divorced parents	30	Elementary school	Randomized controlled trial	Yes	• Decreased depressive symptoms • Increased acceptance and mindfulness
Lee et al. 2008	Children with academic problems	25	Psychiatric outpatient clinic	Open trial	None	• Decreased externalizing symptoms
Semple et al. 2010	Children with anxiety, attention, and academic problems	25	Psychiatric outpatient clinic	Randomized controlled trial	Waitlist control	• Reduction in attention and behavioral problems • Reductions in anxiety for children with clinically elevated anxiety
Strawn et al. 2016	Children and adolescents at risk for bipolar disorder	9	Outpatient treatment facility	Open trial	None	• fMRI examination found activation in insula and anterior cingulate structures associated with anxiety disorders and emotion regulation

Abbreviation. CBT=cognitive-behavioral therapy; fMRI=functional magnetic resonance imaging.

Dialectical Behavior Therapy for Adolescents

Background and Approach

DBT-A (Rathus and Miller 2002) was adapted from the adult dialectical behavior therapy program (Linehan 1993) and was originally focused on treating suicidal adolescents. DBT-A adopts a biopsychosocial model, which emphasizes that biological vulnerabilities combined with psychological and social factors result in emotion regulation difficulties. DBT-A primarily targets emotion dysregulation and incorporates cognitive and behavioral strategies to improve emotion regulation and distress tolerance, interpersonal relationships, communication skills, and mindfulness. In terms of mindfulness skills, DBT-A stresses learning to take a nonjudgmental stance as a way of shifting into "wise mind," which balances emotionality and rationality (Rathus and Miller 2002).

DBT-A takes a multimodal approach, combining individual therapy, a therapist consultation team, phone coaching with patients, and group skills training. Family interventions are incorporated as needed and may include family skills training and/or family therapy. Suggested treatment for adults is 6 months to 1 year, but for adolescents, this tends to be more flexible to accommodate teens' differing needs and situations. Although some programs do encourage participating in a yearlong program, a common variation includes a 16-week acute treatment phase, with an option to extend treatment as needed. The shorter duration may help gain "buy-in" from adolescents who are often wary of treatment. DBT-A uses simpler handouts than does the adult program and conducts skills training in multifamily groups. One module not included in DBT for adults (Walking the Middle Path) was added to the teen program to teach that there is more than one way to interpret a situation or solve a problem (Rathus and Miller 2015). The primary adaptations are age-appropriate language and handouts and the inclusion of families, who play a major role in adolescents' lives.

Main Interventions

DBT-A implements a treatment hierarchy that prioritizes the patient's most urgent needs. The first priority is always to address life-threatening behaviors, which include suicidality, self-harming behaviors (e.g., cutting, burning, bruising), and other dangerous or reckless behaviors (e.g., alcohol or substances, promiscuous sex, reckless driving). Once these behaviors are successfully managed, the second priority is to focus on therapy-interfering behaviors. These refer to actions by either patients or therapists that impede progress in treatment. If neither of these needs is present, issues related to the patient's quality of life are addressed. These include difficulties maintaining daily activities and use of maladaptive coping skills. One way treatment targets are assessed is by use of a daily diary card that is completed by the teen. This contains ratings of emotions, thoughts, and behaviors from each treatment target, as well as monitoring applications of acquired skills. The teens complete ratings each day, which are then reviewed with the therapist during the weekly individual sessions.

DBT-A includes five modules: mindfulness, interpersonal effectiveness, distress tolerance, emotion regulation, and walking the middle path. DBT-A is a mindfulness-informed intervention, and it includes a variety of mindfulness-based concepts as well as short activities and lessons. A major goal is to establish mindful awareness—balancing emotionality and rationality rather than relying exclusively on either. Mindfulness skills can help patients more effectively use the other skills modules, such as selecting and implementing distress tolerance skills, applying emotion regulation strategies, and building healthy relationships.

Research Support

Although DBT-A was initially intended to treat adolescent suicidality, several recent studies suggested that it may be helpful for adolescents with anxiety, depression, and bipolar disorders. Del Conte et al. (2016) conducted a 6-week program of DBT-A for adolescents with anxiety and mood disorders in a partial-hospitalization program. Following the intervention, they found a significant reduction in psychological symptoms, particularly anxiety and depression, but also in hostility and interpersonal sensitivity. They also found increased emotion regulation and use of mindfulness practices. Participants endorsed less dysfunctional ways of coping and reduced blaming of others. Goldstein et al. (2015) implemented DBT-A for adolescents with bipolar disorder over the span of a year. At the end of treatment, they found significant improvement in participants' suicidality, nonsuicidal self-injurious behavior, depressive symptoms, and emotional dysregulation. Following a 19-week DBT-A intervention, Mehlum et al. (2014) found reductions in depressive symptoms, self-harm behaviors, and suicidality in a group of adolescents with repeated suicidal and self-harm behaviors.

Acceptance and Commitment Therapy

Background and Approach

ACT (Hayes et al. 1999) is based on relational frame theory, an approach grounded in language and cognitive development (Coyne et al. 2011). ACT is used with both adults and youth. The primary goal of ACT is to increase psychological flexibility (e.g., the ability to think adaptively, consider more options, and choose from a broader range of behaviors). ACT can be used alone in an individual or group format or can be incorporated into other psychosocial treatments. ACT's metaphorical, sometimes paradoxical, and experiential approach may be better suited to older children and adolescents. Some concerns have arisen about the developmental appropriateness of ACT for young children—in particular, that they may have difficulty comprehending some of the more abstract terminology. In order to avoid this, therapists should select or modify the program to match the needs of the population with whom they are working.

Main Interventions

ACT is based on six core principles. The first is *acceptance*, which is a nonjudgmental attitude of noticing, accepting, and embracing one's experiences—even those that may be unpleasant or unwanted. One series of interventions is aimed at developing *cognitive defusion*, by which patients learn how not to take misleading, often problematic thoughts so seriously—to experience thoughts simply as words, not as binding realities. What may be unique to ACT is an emphasis on eliciting *core values* and then making *commitments* to behavior change that are consistent with those values. *Mindfulness* practices are encouraged to support patients connecting with present-moment experience. The sixth principle is recognizing that the *self in context* allows patients to develop multiple perspectives of themselves as beings who can observe their own moods and anxieties without becoming overly identified with them.

Research Support

Although research on ACT with youth is still in its early stages, several studies have found ACT (mindfulness-informed intervention) to be helpful for children with anxiety and adolescents with depression. Hancock et al. (2016) conducted a randomized clinical trial of ACT with anxious children. They found significant reductions in symptom severity at the end of treatment and at 3-month follow-up. Hayes et al. (2011) conducted a randomized clinical trial of ACT with depressed adolescents and found that at the end of treatment, adolescents who received ACT endorsed greater symptom improvement than those who received treatment as usual. Although limited follow-up data are available, there were indications that symptoms continued to improve 3 months later.

Mindfulness-Based Stress Reduction for Teens

Background and Approach

MBSR-T (Biegel et al. 2014) is intended for adolescents, ages 13–18, and can be implemented as a stand-alone program or to supplement other treatments.

One well-known MBSR-T program is Stressed Teens (Biegel 2009). The primary aim of this model is to increase teens' adaptability and improve their quality of life. This is done by teaching them mindfulness skills in both formal and informal practices. MBSR-T was adapted from the adult mindfulness-based stress reduction program (Kabat-Zinn 1994), with components adapted from mindfulness-based cognitive therapy (Segal et al. 2002).

Although variations of MBSR-T are offered (e.g., individual sessions, 12-week programs), an 8-week group format is most common. Teens initially attend a pretreatment orientation session followed by 90-minute sessions once weekly. However, MBSR-T is flexible in terms of how it is delivered (e.g., one 90-minute session vs. two 45-minute sessions), depending on treatment setting and availability of instructors. MBSR-T also provides suggested homework called "on-your-own practices" that relate to each week's topic.

MBSR-T offers guidelines for therapists to become effective teachers. A professional training program and certification are also available. MBSR-T teacher trainees are encouraged to participate in an MBSR course to experience the process of learning and practicing mindfulness in their daily lives. Teachers are expected to maintain a personal mindfulness practice and convey empathy while creating a safe space for teens to share experiences without feeling vulnerable. Other desirable qualities include authenticity, willingness to participate, respectfulness, compassion, and knowing how to maintain appropriate group boundaries. Furthermore, teachers should express interest in the teens' lives, particularly by asking clarifying questions, listening to what is important to them, and using examples that are relevant and meaningful to the teens. Therapists are reminded to be sensitive to teens' willingness to learn and practice new skills and to suggest that teens may be most receptive when MBSR is started with basic concepts before working up to more complex ones. However, therapists are also cautioned not to simplify too much because most teens are capable of learning the original MBSR program, with only slight changes to account for adolescent development.

Similar to MBSR, the teen program incorporates formal meditation practices, although they are generally 10–20 minutes rather than the 40-minute activities seen in the adult program. Initially, teens may not be comfortable or able to tolerate sitting for even short periods, so practices are initially very brief and gradually increase in length. MBSR-T adapts language from the adult program to which teens may not relate. For example, MBSR-T refers to maladaptive coping skills as *blocking*. The concept of blocking (e.g., via substance abuse, social isolation, denial) is more familiar to most teens than the concept of maladaptive coping. Therapists must engage teens or risk losing their attention to thoughts of that night's homework or who they plan to Skype with after the session. MBSR-T, therefore, focuses on teen-specific topics that include school-related stressors, social and peer demands, and self-harm behaviors. Mindfulness skills can be applied to teen problems as easily as to adult problems. The topics of discussion vary, but the aims and practices at the core of the teen and adult programs are similar.

Main Interventions

MBSR-T is based on three foundational skills: awareness of intentions, mindful breathing, and mindfulness across the five senses. A workbook that offers additional activities (Biegel 2017) is often provided to participants. Before most sessions, teens participate in mindful check-ins, during which they review previous topics and on-your-own-practices, identify their highs and lows since the last session, and discuss *mindful qualities* (e.g., foundations, components, or outcomes of mindful practice). These check-ins also give teens opportunities to connect with each other and identify current issues that may be discussed in that session.

The first two sessions introduce mindfulness and focus on defining and processing stress. Teens articulate their intentions for the program, define personal goals, and relate teen-specific stressors to the practices of MBSR-T. They also learn how stress affects their minds and bodies, in both helpful and harmful ways.

The middle sessions focus on cultivating awareness and acceptance. Specifically, teens engage in exercises to increase present-moment awareness of both positive and negative aspects of their lives. They practice noticing versus judging, responding versus reacting, and dealing with unpleasant experiences. Teens engage in self-care and learn to distinguish self-care from selfishness. They also learn the distinction between caring and worrying. They are then taught to use mindfulness skills (e.g., observing, describing, nonreacting) to enhance awareness and learn to use effective coping strategies. Teens discuss practical applications of stress management in school, at home, and in their social lives. The aim is to live with, rather than avoid, difficult experiences.

The closing sessions focus on generalizing mindfulness skills. Mindful resilience and mindful relationships include practicing mindful communications; cultivating forgiveness, compassion, and empathy; expressing trust and respect; and evaluating one's own strengths and weaknesses. Then, experiences of the program are discussed. The teacher facilitates discussion about forming intentions for the future, reviewing past intentions, and exploring ways that mindfulness may be integrated into the teens' daily lives.

Research Support

MBSR-T is a newer intervention. However, one study has shown promising results. Biegel et al. (2009) conducted a randomized clinical trial that evaluated

MBSR-T with teens ages 14–18 with heterogeneous psychiatric disorders. As compared with a treatment-as-usual control group (individual or group psychotherapy and medication included in routine clinical care), MBSR-T participants self-reported significantly reduced symptoms of anxiety, depression, and somatic distress and increased self-esteem and sleep quality. Additionally, existing literature describes a correlation between time spent engaging in formal mindfulness meditation and decreased anxiety, stress, and overall psychological well-being (Carmody and Baer 2008). Carmody and Baer's findings provide support for the inclusion of on-your-own-practices in MBSR-T.

Mindfulness-Based Cognitive Therapy for Children

Background and Approach

MBCT-C (Semple and Lee 2011) is a manualized intervention for children with anxiety disorders ages 8–12. It was developed as a downward adaptation from MBCT (initially used for adults with major depression) and MBSR (developed for use with adult chronic pain patients). MBCT-C has seven primary aims: 1) acceptance; 2) understanding obstacles to mindfulness practice; 3) developing personal motivations; 4) mindfulness of thoughts, feelings, and body sensations; 5) nonjudgmental awareness; 6) decentering; and 7) discovering choice points.

MBCT-C was developed as a group intervention. Groups consist of six to eight children and are facilitated by one or two therapists. Home practice activities are assigned at the end of each session. Children are expected to practice brief mindfulness activities (10–15 minutes per day) between sessions. The treatment manual offers additional guidelines for implementing MBCT-C in individual therapy, in which the therapist needs to take a more active participant role. Individual sessions may also be shortened from 90 minutes to 45–60 minutes.

For two important reasons, therapists are expected to establish and maintain a personal mindfulness practice. First, MBCT-C is an acceptance-based model, not directly change oriented. This can be unfamiliar territory for therapists who typically practice conventional therapies that focus on changing thoughts or behaviors. Facilitators embody present-moment awareness and express nonjudgmental acceptance of what is happening in the moment, both internally and externally. Every moment, however, changes—inviting us into a fluid, moment-by-moment awareness of thoughts, feelings, choices, speech, and behaviors.

Second, knowledge is not the same as understanding. MBCT-C teachers who understand the principles of mindfulness only intellectually by reading about present-moment awareness and nonjudgment or how to conduct mindfulness activities are unlikely to be effective. Semple and Lee (2011) make it clear that effective facilitators of MBCT-C embody mindfulness. To learn to play a violin, one must actually pick one up and practice. In order to embody mindfulness, therapists must actually practice bringing mindfulness into their own lives. This means that we must commit to developing a personal practice. There are no requirements specifying frequency, duration, or type of practice. The intent is to practice what we aim to teach. The therapist's own mindfulness practice can act as a container to help youth stay present with strong thoughts and emotions. Additionally, modeling mindfulness within the patient-therapist dyad may help children internalize these skills and more effectively self-regulate their internal experiences.

Developmental Adaptations

MBCT-C identifies three important developmental differences between adults and children. First, children are less able to express their thoughts and feelings than are most adults. Limited verbal fluency can sometimes make it difficult to communicate their feelings. Instead, they may express emotions through actions (e.g., hitting someone, giving a hug, isolating). MBCT and MBCT-C both focus on cultivating nonjudgmental observation of thoughts and feelings and use breath and body practices to develop mindfulness awareness. In addition, MBCT-C engages children in short, interactive activities that teach mindful awareness through touch, taste, sound, sight, smell, and movement.

Second, children have a shorter attention span and less tolerance for boredom. To address these issues, MBCT-C shortens the sessions from two-and-a-half-hour sessions conducted weekly for 8 weeks to 90-minute weekly sessions for 12 weeks. Moreover, MBCT-C groups have fewer children and a higher therapist-to-patient ratio than in adult groups, which allows for more individualized attention. MBCT-C incorporates a wider variety of short hands-on activities than does MBCT.

Third, addressing children's interrelatedness with parents or caregivers, MBCT-C makes a point of including caregivers in the program. Although the adult caregivers do not attend the child sessions, they are invited to attend a separate 2-hour group orientation session that introduces the program, allows opportunities for parents to experience some of the mindfulness activities, and invites questions. Therapists lead the parents through several practices that their children will participate in during the program and discuss how they can participate in and support their child's home-based activities. Children are also encouraged to share with their parents the written session summaries and home practice activities given out each week. Parents and therapists remain in open communication throughout the program. Finally, parents attend a group review session at the end of the program and explore ways to support and maintain their own and their child's ongoing mindfulness practice.

Main Interventions

Each session begins with an introduction, home practice review, and the aims of that session. Children are then asked to check in with their experience in the moment using a self-rated Feely Faces Scale (Semple et al. 2010, p. 267). Next, the children participate in session activities. Each session ends with the reading of a poem or story related to that week's topic, checking in with themselves with their Feely Faces Scale, and, finally, reviewing the assigned home practices for that week.

The first three sessions focus on introducing the children to mindfulness and teaching them specific ways to develop mindful awareness. They are introduced to the concept of *automatic pilot*, during which one's thoughts may be far away from the present moment. During several hands-on introductory mindfulness activities, children learn about turning off automatic pilot and explore how doing so may benefit them. They practice connecting with the breath as a way of bringing awareness to the present. Children begin to understand the challenges inherent in developing mindfulness practice, despite the simplicity of the activities. Mindfulness is explained as a different way of being present in one's life. The children learn that they can practice mindful awareness whenever they choose to do so and practice awareness of breath and body sensations. The concept of *decentering* from thoughts is introduced. Similar to defusion in ACT, decentering is the metacognitive ability to experience thoughts, feelings, and body sensations as internal experiences, not necessarily facts about reality. Children practice observing and describing their own thoughts, feelings, and body sensations with openness and nonjudgmental awareness. Insights gained from mindfulness practice include greater awareness of both internal and external events. This allows the children to gain a clearer understanding of their choices in any given moment. They practice this new way of being during mindfulness of the breath, body scans, visualization activities, and listening to the sounds of silence.

The middle sessions focus on cultivating mindfulness across the senses. First, children explore mindfulness through sense of taste. They compare eating with mindful awareness to how they may regularly eat. Children explore the idea that thoughts, feelings, and body sensations do not define who they are and may not align with situations or events in their lives. They learn that cultivating awareness of thoughts, feelings, and body sensations may help them make more skillful choices. Children are introduced to mindful hearing—gaining new perspectives on sounds in the environment and increasing awareness of the complexity of music. They explore thoughts, feelings, and body sensations associated with different sounds. Children take turns acting as a "conductor" and practice expressing sounds that convey emotions. They receive feedback on how the other children interpreted their composition, which is often different from what they intended. Children also discuss the importance of nonverbal expression as communication. They are introduced to mindful seeing and practice looking clearly (see Appendix, "Example MBCT-C Script," at the end of the chapter). The concept of subjectivity is introduced: children learn the difference between judging and noting (nonjudgmental observation) and examine how thoughts and feelings influence their felt experiences. They discuss how multiple factors influence visual experiences, which is a composite of what is actually seen, combined with their cognitive interpretations and emotional responses. Mindfulness-of-seeing activities further enhance attention and increase the ability to intentionally shift attention. Children practice perspective taking by focusing on different parts of their surroundings. They are introduced to *choice points*, which are defined as moments in which mindful choices can be made, as opposed to responding in emotionally reactive, often unhelpful ways. In particular, they are empowered to choose how to respond to their own thoughts and feelings. Mindfulness of touch and mindful smelling help demonstrate how judgments can influence perceptions.

The closing sessions focus on generalizing and maintaining mindful awareness skills. Children review ways in which mindfulness may be practiced in everyday life. The role of mindful awareness in managing or responding to strong emotions is explored. Children have opportunities to reflect on their personal understandings of mindfulness and express them through artwork. They plan a graduation party for session 12 to celebrate the MBCT-C shared journey. Therapists and children have a dialogue about how to remember to bring mindful awareness and skillful choices into their lives, brainstorm potential obstacles to continued practice, and identify ways to address those obstacles.

Research Support

At least seven studies have supported the use of MBCT-C for young patients with clinical levels of anxiety and depression (see Table 5–1). For example, Cotton et al. (2016) and Strawn et al. (2016) examined the impact of MBCT-C on children and adolescents at risk for bipolar disorder and found, among other benefits, increased emotion regulation. Other studies noted decreased symptoms for children with anxiety disorders and for anxious children with academic problems, reductions in attentional problems, and fewer externalizing behaviors following MBCT-C (see Table 5–1). Because anxious thoughts are often future focused and depressive thoughts are often past focused, it follows that cultivating the ability to maintain present-moment awareness may be useful in alleviating the impact of both types of unhelpful thought patterns. As with MBSR-T, Carmody and Baer's (2008) findings of the correlation between time spent engaging in formal meditation and decreased anxiety, stress, and overall psychological well-being provide support for the strong emphasis on home practice in MBCT-C.

Contraindications to Using Mindfulness-Based Interventions

In preparing to teach mindfulness-based interventions to youth with anxiety and mood disorders, it is important to remain vigilant for potential adverse reactions, particularly because emotion dysregulation and unstable moods are features of these disorders. As most experienced mindfulness facilitators know, some participants may initially experience increases in anxiety. Sitting down to meditate can be likened to stirring a glass of water with fine sand at the bottom: strong thoughts and emotions can arise and feel overwhelming to some youth who already have difficulties regulating their emotions. Although there is little research that focuses on potential adverse reactions in youth, Dobkin et al. (2012) highlight five contraindications to mindfulness practice for adults that child therapists might also consider. First, they emphasize the importance of screening patients for severe psychopathology, substance abuse, and posttraumatic distress. A child who is suicidal or psychotic is unlikely to benefit from mindfulness training, and the internally focused orientation of mindfulness could conceivably worsen these symptoms.

Second, if a patient is found to have significant psychiatric problems, the therapist should first determine whether the current treatment is sufficient and consider how mindfulness training might augment an existing treatment plan. An MBI may be combined with a current treatment or it may provide an alternative for youth who refuse or do not respond to medication. For example, although a child with attention-deficit/hyperactivity disorder may be doing well on stimulant medications, mindfulness training may bolster attentional skills and reduce the impulsivity associated with this disorder.

Third, particularly with patients who are highly reactive (emotionally or behaviorally), therapists should assess each child's expectations of the program, discuss potential challenges that may arise, and identify coping strategies before starting the program. For example, a teen with conduct problems may be noncompliant in a group, which may encourage other participants to be noncompliant. Bögels et al. (2008) suggested that adolescents with oppositional defiant disorder or conduct disorder might do better by beginning mindfulness training in individual settings.

Fourth, therapists should have the clinical skills and resources to support their patients if strong anxieties emerge or depression worsens and should have psychiatric referrals available if needed. Finally, Dobkin and colleagues (2012) suggest following each patient's lead regarding what they feel they can and cannot do on the basis of their individual needs. A child who has been sexually abused, for example, may not be prepared to engage in a body scan activity. No child should ever feel pressured to engage in a mindfulness activity with which he or she is uncomfortable and should be offered alternatives (e.g., sitting quietly) when these activities are done. Lustyk et al. (2009) also reviewed the research literature and suggested that mindfulness practices may be contraindicated for patients with severe posttraumatic stress disorder (potential retraumatization arising from intrusive memories or flashbacks with subsequent increases in dissociation); psychosis (increased hallucinations, disorientation, depersonalization, or derealization); suicidality; mania; and some medical concerns related to pain, extreme psychomotor agitation, and seizure disorders (possible reduction in an individual's seizure threshold). Although no formal guidelines have yet been developed, careful screening and mindful attention to changes in a patient's needs throughout the intervention should significantly reduce the potential for adverse effects.

Conclusion and Future Directions

There is clearly a need for further research into the efficacy of mindfulness-based and mindfulness-informed interventions for youth, but we now have preliminary evidence suggesting that mindfulness can be beneficial for youth with anxiety and mood disorders. DBT-A, MBSR-T, and MBCT-C are developmentally appropriate child or adolescent adaptations of evidence-based adult interventions. ACT, although not exclusively for youth, allows for flexibility and consideration of developmental appropriateness when selecting activities for younger patients. Overall, the future of mindfulness treatments for children and adolescents appears bright and can offer hope for our young patients who struggle to manage symptoms of anxiety and mood disturbances.

KEY POINTS

- We believe that the most effective way to teach mindfulness to others is to start by practicing it ourselves.
- When working with youth, we recommend including parents and families.

- Children and adolescents often do better with shorter-duration, dynamic, and participatory activities, with content that is tailored according to their developmental needs.

- Use caution when determining the appropriateness of mindfulness interventions for youth with severe psychopathology, those who may have experienced severe trauma, or those who are expressing extreme emotional or behavioral reactivity.

Discussion Questions

1. Identify obstacles to including parents and families in treatment. What are some potential strategies to increase familial involvement in MBIs for youth?

2. What aspects of facilitators' personal mindfulness practice are most influential when teaching mindfulness to youth?

3. What are some important factors to consider when teaching mindfulness to children with severe emotional dysregulation or trauma?

Suggested Readings

Biegel GM: The Stress Reduction Workbook for Teens: Mindfulness Skills to Help You Deal With Stress. Oakland, CA, New Harbinger, 2017

Hayes SC, Strosahl KD, Wilson KG: Acceptance and Commitment Therapy: An Experiential Approach to Behavior Change. New York, Guilford, 1999

Rathus JH, Miller AL: DBT Skills Manual for Adolescents. New York, Guilford, 2015

Semple RJ, Lee J: Mindfulness-Based Cognitive Therapy for Anxious Children: A Manual for Treating Childhood Anxiety. Oakland, CA, New Harbinger, 2011

References

Ames CS, Richardson J, Payne S, et al: Mindfulness-based cognitive therapy for depression in adolescents. Child Adolesc Ment Health 19(1):74–78, 2014

Biegel GM: The Stress Reduction Workbook for Teens: Mindfulness Skills to Help You Deal With Stress. Oakland, CA, New Harbinger, 2009

Biegel GM: The Stress Reduction Workbook for Teens: Mindfulness Skills to Help You Deal With Stress, 2nd Edition. Oakland, CA, New Harbinger, 2017

Biegel GM, Brown KW, Shapiro SL, et al: Mindfulness-based stress reduction for the treatment of adolescent psychiatric outpatients: a randomized clinical trial. J Consult Clin Psychol 77(5):855–866, 2009 19803566

Biegel GM, Chang K, Garrett A, et al: Mindfulness-based stress reduction for teens, in Mindfulness-Based Treatment Approaches: Clinician's Guide to Evidence Base and Applications. Edited by Baer R. San Diego, CA, Elsevier, 2014, pp 189–212

Bögels SM, Hoogstad B, van Dun L, et al: Mindfulness training for adolescents with externalizing disorders and their parents. Behav Cogn Psychother 36:193–209, 2008

Carmody J, Baer RA: Relationships between mindfulness practice and levels of mindfulness, medical and psychological symptoms and well-being in a mindfulness-based stress reduction program. J Behav Med 31(1):23–33, 2008 17899351

Costello EJ, Mustillo S, Erkanli A, et al: Prevalence and development of psychiatric disorders in childhood and adolescence. Arch Gen Psychiatry 60(8):837–844, 2003 12912767

Cotton S, Luberto CM, Sears RW, et al: Mindfulness-based cognitive therapy for youth with anxiety disorders at risk for bipolar disorder: a pilot trial. Early Interv Psychiatry 10(5):426–434, 2016 25582800

Coyne LW, McHugh L, Martinez ER: Acceptance and commitment therapy (ACT): advances and applications with children, adolescents, and families. Child Adolesc Psychiatr Clin N Am 20(2):379–399, 2011 21440862

Del Conte G, Lenz AS, Hollenbaugh KM: A pilot evaluation of dialectical behavior therapy for adolescents within a partial hospitalization treatment milieu. Journal of Child and Adolescent Counseling 2:16–32, 2016

Dehghani F, Amiri S, Molavi H, et al: Effectiveness of mindfulness based cognitive therapy on female elementary students with generalized anxiety disorder. Int J Psychol Behav Res 3:59–165, 2014

Dobkin PL, Irving JA, Amar S: For whom may participation in a mindfulness-based stress reduction program be contraindicated? Mindfulness 3:44–50, 2012

Esmailian N, Tahmasian K, Dehghani M, et al: Effectiveness of mindfulness-based cognitive therapy on depression symptoms in children with divorced parents. J Clin Psychol 3:47–57, 2013

Goldstein TR, Axelson DA, Birmaher B, et al: Dialectical behavior therapy for adolescents with bipolar disorder: a 1-year open trial. J Am Acad Child Adolesc Psychiatry 46(7):820–830, 2007 17581446

Goldstein TR, Fersch-Podrat RK, Rivera M, et al: Dialectical behavior therapy for adolescents with bipolar disorder: results from a pilot randomized trial. J Child Adolesc Psychopharmacol 25(2):140–149, 2015 25010702

Hancock KM, Swain J, Hainsworth CJ, et al: Acceptance and commitment therapy versus cognitive behavior therapy for children with anxiety: outcomes of a randomized controlled trial. J Clin Child Adolesc Psychol 47(2):296–311, 2016 26998803

Hayes L, Boyd CP, Sewell J: Acceptance and commitment therapy for the treatment of adolescent depression: A pilot study in a psychiatric outpatient setting. Mindfulness 2:86–94, 2011

Hayes SC, Strosahl KD, Wilson KG: Acceptance and Commitment Therapy: An Experiential Approach to Behavior Change. New York, Guilford, 1999

Kabat-Zinn J: Wherever You Go There You Are: Mindfulness Meditation for Everyday Life. New York, Hyperion, 1994

Kessler RC, Petukhova M, Sampson NA, et al: Twelve-month and lifetime prevalence and lifetime morbid risk of anxiety and mood disorders in the United States. Int J Methods Psychiatr Res 21(3):169–184, 2012 22865617

Lee J, Semple RJ, Rosa D, et al: Mindfulness-based cognitive therapy for children: results of a pilot study. J Cogn Psychother 22:15–28, 2008

Linehan M: Cognitive-Behavioral Treatment of Borderline Personality Disorder. New York, Guilford, 1993

Lustyk MK, Chawla N, Nolan RS, et al: Mindfulness meditation research: issues of participant screening, safety procedures, and researcher training. Adv Mind Body Med 24(1):20–30, 2009 20671334

Mehlum L, Tørmoen AJ, Ramberg M, et al: Dialectical behavior therapy for adolescents with repeated suicidal and self-harming behavior: a randomized trial. J Am Acad Child Adolesc Psychiatry 53(10):1082–1091, 2014 25245352

Merikangas KR, He JP, Burstein M, et al: Lifetime prevalence of mental disorders in U.S. adolescents: results from the National Comorbidity Survey Replication—Adolescent Supplement (NCS-A). J Am Acad Child Adolesc Psychiatry 49(10):980–989, 2010 20855043

Mojtabai R, Olfson M, Han B: National trends in the prevalence and treatment of depression in adolescents and young adults. Pediatrics 138(6):e20161878, 2016 27940701

Rathus JH, Miller AL: Dialectical behavior therapy adapted for suicidal adolescents. Suicide Life Threat Behav 32(2):146–157, 2002 12079031

Rathus JH, Miller AL: DBT® Skills Manual for Adolescents. New York, Guilford, 2015

Rogers CR: On Becoming a Person: A Therapist's View of Psychotherapy. Boston, MA, Houghton Mifflin Harcourt, 1995

Segal ZV, Williams JMG, Teasdale JD: Mindfulness-Based Cognitive Therapy for Depression: A New Approach to Relapse Prevention. New York, Guilford, 2002

Semple RJ, Lee J: Mindfulness-Based Cognitive Therapy for Anxious Children: A Manual for Treating Childhood Anxiety. Oakland, CA, New Harbinger, 2011

Semple RJ, Lee J, Rosa D, et al: A randomized trial of mindfulness-based cognitive therapy for children: Promoting mindful attention to enhance social-emotional resiliency in children. J Child Fam Stud 19:218–229, 2010

Strawn JR, Cotton S, Luberto CM, et al: Neural function before and after mindfulness-based cognitive therapy in anxious adolescents at risk for developing bipolar disorder. J Child Adolesc Psychopharmacol 26(4):372–379, 2016 26783833

Appendix

Example MBCT-C Script

Practice: Seeing Through Illusions

How often do we look closely and see clearly? We often miss small but important details, because our attention is focused on thoughts in our heads—anticipating the future, remembering the past, or not paying attention at all. When we choose to look with mindful awareness, we may discover a clearer, more focused way of seeing. Practicing mindful awareness, we simply observe what is, and so may develop greater acceptance of ourselves and our experiences.

Choice points are those moments in which we can make choices. When we look with mindful attention, we may see choices that we didn't know were there. We may see previously unnoticed things that help us make those choices. When we look very closely, we may see many choice points. But—we must look at the present, not the past or future. The present is the only moment in which choice points occur.

Today we continue to explore mindful seeing. Start by asking the children not to discuss what is seen, only to look with mindful attention and then quietly write down in their notebooks whatever they see. Then show the group the first optical illusion. Allow the children to observe the image for about thirty to sixty seconds while inviting them to write down what they saw. Then present the next illusion. After each image has been seen once and the children have written

Seeing Through Illusions is a mindfulness activity from session eight of the MBCT-C program. Republished with permission of New Harbinger Publications, from Semple RJ and Lee J: *Mindfulness-Based Cognitive Therapy for Anxious Children*, 2011, pp. 189–190. Copyright © 2011 by New Harbinger Publications, permission conveyed through Copyright Clearance Center, Inc.

down what was seen, show each illusion a second time and elicit verbal descriptions of what was observed. For example, one image that may be used is called "Duck and Rabbit." Some children initially will have seen the duck figure while others will have seen the rabbit. You can help each to see the other figure.

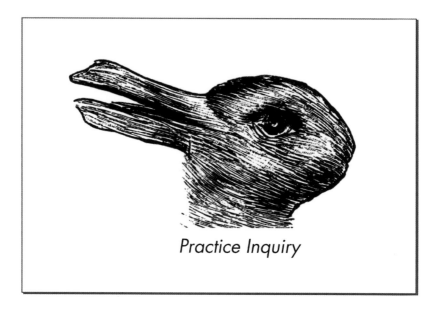

Practice Inquiry

When all children can see both figures, invite them to shift their attention back and forth—first to see one figure and then the other. Explore the experience of shifting attention at will. Invite the children to see both figures at the same time and explore how the effort to do so changes the quality of the experience. The children may learn that it is not possible to see both figures at the same time. They may learn that they can choose what they see simply by redirecting their attention.

Practice Inquiry

This inquiry is intended to draw out the understanding that shifting attention can change the quality or nature of the experience. During this discussion, elicit descriptions of the experience of willfully shifting attention and how this may change what is seen. What else might have contributed to different children initially seeing images in different ways? Explore how thoughts and feelings might influence what is seen.

Shifting attention to see different things may help a child learn that he has choices in how he relates to his experiences. He can choose to attend to different elements of his experiences or not to attend at all. He can develop conscious intentions to be more present. He can notice when he functions on "automatic pilot" and then choose to bring more awareness to the activities in the moment.

Chapter

6

Attention-Deficit/ Hyperactivity Disorder

Mari Kurahashi, M.D., M.P.H.

THE WORD *attention* stems from Middle English roots that translate into "apply[ing] the mind to something" through "a selective narrowing or focusing of consciousness and receptivity." (www.merriam-webster.com/dictionary/attention). The current zeitgeist of technological innovation, screen time, and overscheduled schedules can contribute to the constant stimulation and multitasking that overAt the same time, there has been a recent mindfulness boom that strengthens the tendency to fully attend to one's current experience, which may be a response to the current tendency of having one's attention frantically moving among competing stimuli in a mindless, automatic manner. The current demands and strain on the individual's and families' attention and lifestyle may be an importanload one's mind and energies and, therefore, one's ability to pay attention. t factor in the increasing rates of attention-deficit/hyperactivity disorder (ADHD), for which mindfulness-based interventions may be a helpful treatment.

ADHD is now the most commonly diagnosed childhood mental health disorder in the United States (Centers for Disease Control and Prevention

2013). According to the Centers for Disease Control and Prevention (CDC), approximately 11% of children (ages 4–17) have had an ADHD diagnosis (Centers for Disease Control and Prevention 2013). The rate of children with an ADHD diagnosis increased from 7.8% in 2003 to 9.5% in 2007 to 11% in 2011–2012. As the name implies, the core issues with ADHD are difficulties with sustained attention and hyperactivity, as well as impulsivity, all of which can significantly impair one's academic and social functioning (Box 6–1). Although hyperactivity tends to improve with age, the often chronic condition can continue to impair adults. The estimated prevalence of adult ADHD in the United States is 4.4% (Kessler et al. 2006). Adult ADHD can result in difficulty with paying attention and a tendency to make impulsive choices that then have significant repercussions on individuals' work performance and social relationships.

Box 6–1.   DSM-5 diagnostic criteria for attention-deficit/hyperactivity disorder

---

A. A persistent pattern of inattention and/or hyperactivity-impulsivity that interferes with functioning or development, as characterized by (1) and/or (2):

1. **Inattention:** Six (or more) of the following symptoms have persisted for at least 6 months to a degree that is inconsistent with developmental level and that negatively impacts directly on social and academic/occupational activities:

   Note: The symptoms are not solely a manifestation of oppositional behavior, defiance, hostility, or failure to understand tasks or instructions. For older adolescents and adults (age 17 and older), at least five symptoms are required.

   a. Often fails to give close attention to details or makes careless mistakes in schoolwork, at work, or during other activities (e.g., overlooks or misses details, work is inaccurate).

   b. Often has difficulty sustaining attention in tasks or play activities (e.g., has difficulty remaining focused during lectures, conversations, or lengthy reading).

   c. Often does not seem to listen when spoken to directly (e.g., mind seems elsewhere, even in the absence of any obvious distraction).

   d. Often does not follow through on instructions and fails to finish schoolwork, chores, or duties in the workplace (e.g., starts tasks but quickly loses focus and is easily sidetracked).

   e. Often has difficulty organizing tasks and activities (e.g., difficulty managing sequential tasks; difficulty keeping materials and belongings in order; messy, disorganized work; has poor time management; fails to meet deadlines).

   f. Often avoids, dislikes, or is reluctant to engage in tasks that require sustained mental effort (e.g., schoolwork or homework; for older adolescents and adults, preparing reports, completing forms, reviewing lengthy papers).

g. Often loses things necessary for tasks or activities (e.g., school materials, pencils, books, tools, wallets, keys, paperwork, eyeglasses, mobile telephones).

h. Is often easily distracted by extraneous stimuli (for older adolescents and adults, may include unrelated thoughts).

i. Is often forgetful in daily activities (e.g., doing chores, running errands; for older adolescents and adults, returning calls, paying bills, keeping appointments).

2. **Hyperactivity and impulsivity:** Six (or more) of the following symptoms have persisted for at least 6 months to a degree that is inconsistent with developmental level and that negatively impacts directly on social and academic/occupational activities:

Note: The symptoms are not solely a manifestation of oppositional behavior, defiance, hostility, or a failure to understand tasks or instructions. For older adolescents and adults (age 17 and older), at least five symptoms are required.

a. Often fidgets with or taps hands or feet or squirms in seat.

b. Often leaves seat in situations when remaining seated is expected (e.g., leaves his or her place in the classroom, in the office or other workplace, or in other situations that require remaining in place).

c. Often runs about or climbs in situations where it is inappropriate. (Note: In adolescents or adults, may be limited to feeling restless.)

d. Often unable to play or engage in leisure activities quietly.

e. Is often "on the go," acting as if "driven by a motor" (e.g., is unable to be or uncomfortable being still for extended time, as in restaurants, meetings; may be experienced by others as being restless or difficult to keep up with).

f. Often talks excessively.

g. Often blurts out an answer before a question has been completed (e.g., completes people's sentences; cannot wait for turn in conversation).

h. Often has difficulty waiting his or her turn (e.g., while waiting in line).

i. Often interrupts or intrudes on others (e.g., butts into conversations, games, or activities; may start using other people's things without asking or receiving permission; for adolescents and adults, may intrude into or take over what others are doing).

B. Several inattentive or hyperactive-impulsive symptoms were present prior to age 12 years.

C. Several inattentive or hyperactive-impulsive symptoms are present in two or more settings (e.g., at home, school, or work; with friends or relatives; in other activities).

D. There is clear evidence that the symptoms interfere with, or reduce the quality of, social, academic, or occupational functioning.

E. The symptoms do not occur exclusively during the course of schizophrenia or another psychotic disorder and are not better explained by another mental disorder (e.g., mood disorder, anxiety disorder, dissociative disorder, personality disorder, substance intoxication or withdrawal).

Specify whether:

314.01 (F90.2) Combined presentation: If both Criterion A1 (inattention) and Criterion A2 (hyperactivity-impulsivity) are met for the past 6 months.

314.00 (F90.0) Predominantly inattentive presentation: If Criterion A1 (inattention) is met but Criterion A2 (hyperactivity-impulsivity) is not met for the past 6 months.

314.01 (F90.1) Predominantly hyperactive/impulsive presentation: If Criterion A2 (hyperactivity-impulsivity) is met and Criterion A1 (inattention) is not met for the past 6 months.

Specify if:

In partial remission: When full criteria were previously met, fewer than the full criteria have been met for the past 6 months, and the symptoms still result in impairment in social, academic, or occupational functioning.

Specify current severity:

Mild: Few, if any, symptoms in excess of those required to make the diagnosis are present, and symptoms result in no more than minor impairments in social or occupational functioning.

Moderate: Symptoms or functional impairment between "mild" and "severe" are present.

Severe: Many symptoms in excess of those required to make the diagnosis, or several symptoms that are particularly severe, are present, or the symptoms result in marked impairment in social or occupational functioning.

This widely prevalent disorder puts people at a higher risk for adverse life outcomes, including significant impairments socially, academically, and professionally. People with ADHD are at higher risk of failed relationships, truancy, academic difficulties, substance use, incarceration, and other psychiatric disorders (Sciberra et al. 2009). Children with ADHD often cause significant parental stress that can then exacerbate the child's stress and thereby behavioral problems and result in worse functioning for both the child and the family (Bhide et al. 2016). Although there are established psychopharmacological and psychotherapeutic ADHD treatments, these treatments also have limitations.

Mindfulness-based treatment may be especially helpful for targeting the core ADHD symptoms of inattention and impulsivity and therefore may be a critical adjunct to the established treatments.

Current ADHD Treatment

Studies show that behavioral therapy with medication can have positive benefits for ADHD symptoms and that stimulants have a more effective impact on ADHD symptoms than behavioral therapy for children who are older than preschool age (MTA Cooperative Group 1999). The 14-month Multimodal Treatment of Attention Deficit Hyperactivity Disorder (MTA) study showed that combined behavior and medication treatment was not significantly more efficacious than medication alone for the core ADHD symptoms in children ages 7–9. However, the study did show that the combined behavior and medication treatment resulted in greater academic and conduct improvements if ADHD coexisted with anxiety and for children living in lower socioeconomic environments. Parents and teachers of children in the combined group also reported greater satisfaction with the treatment. In addition, the combined treatment allows for lower doses of medication, which may then decrease the risk of adverse effects. Furthermore, combined treatment also demonstrated advantages in secondary analysis of the MTA data (Hinshaw et al. 2015). For treatment guidelines for different age groups, see Table 6–1.

Studies indicate that both psychotherapy and pharmacotherapy can be effective for ADHD treatment in adults, with some studies finding similar effectiveness on symptoms for cognitive-behavioral therapy (CBT) and medications (Cherkasova et al. 2016; Young et al. 2015). However, because of the limitations on the psychotherapy studies, including shorter trials and a smaller number of studies, the current guideline for adult ADHD treatment is to start with medication. At the same time, psychotherapy is recognized as a helpful adjunct treatment, especially to help with executive function, impulse control, and interpersonal functioning. Some studies also indicate that combined medication and psychotherapy treatment results in greater ADHD symptom reduction than either treatment alone.

Limitations to Current ADHD Treatment

Although there is research to support the methodology of diagnosing ADHD and how to intervene after the diagnosis is made, how to effectively treat

TABLE 6–1.   Guidelines for treatment of ADHD

Age of child with ADHD	Treatment recommendations
Preschool age	• Begin with behavioral treatment administered by the parents and/or teacher. • Apply core behavioral principles of positive reinforcement, active ignoring, and time-out and provide psychoeducation on ADHD and child development and expectations. • If behavioral and parenting intervention is ineffective, then medication may be warranted.
School age	• Begin medication and/or behavioral therapy administered by parents and/or teacher, with a preference for combined treatment.
Adolescents	• Prescribe medication and potentially provide behavioral therapy, with preference for both.

Source.   Wolraich et al. 2011.

ADHD on a long-term basis remains unclear. The sentinel MTA study showed that by the 3-year follow-up, there were no longer any differences between the four treatment groups (optimal medication management, optimal behavioral management, combination of optimal medication and behavioral management, and community treatment) (Hinshaw et al. 2015). Although stimulant treatment of adult ADHD has been shown to have 70%–80% efficacy (Spencer et al. 2005) and CBT for adult ADHD is shown to be effective, there is no study looking at a 3-year or more follow-up on pharmacotherapy or psychotherapy interventions for adult ADHD.

The current limits on ADHD treatment may be where mindfulness-based therapy can be helpful. Mindfulness is attention training with an emphasis on observing without reactivity that could target and strengthen the core deficient attention and impulse-control skills for people with ADHD, as well as increase compassion and decrease self-judgment of their difficulties. Therefore, mindfulness-based therapy could be a significant adjunct to the currently established ADHD treatments, with potentially longer-term benefits. In addition, both children and adults can be wary of taking controlled substances for ADHD treatment and can experience adverse effects from ADHD medications, such as insomnia and decreased appetite. Effective nonpsychopharmacological interventions such as mindfulness practice may help in decreasing the dosage of required medication and thus help with side effects.

Mindfulness-Based Intervention for Children and Adolescents With ADHD

MYMind Protocol

Some of the studies of mindfulness-based interventions for children with ADHD used the mindfulness training for youth (MYmind) protocol called Mindfulness Training for Youngsters With ADHD and Their Parents (Bögels et al. 2008). The MYmind protocol follows an 8-week manualized group treatment based on mindfulness-based cognitive therapy (MBCT) for depression (Segal et al. 2002) that has been modified to address the different developmental needs of children, adolescents, and parents, with a focus on ADHD (Bögels et al. 2008). The purpose of this training is to cultivate mindfulness through exercises and then bring this mindful awareness into the daily lives of youth and their parents to help with ADHD symptoms, overall stress, relationships, and difficult emotions. Similar to MBCT, the MYmind protocol combines mindfulness, CBT, and psychoeducation. The mindfulness concepts emphasized include awareness, nonjudging, acceptance, letting go, beginner's mind, and being present in the moment (Shecter 2013).

Both the child or adolescent and parent groups meet in parallel sessions for 1.5 hours. They are mostly separate, other than parts of a few sessions that bring together both groups and provide opportunities for youth and parents to share their experiences. Each session begins with a mindfulness exercise, with a gradual build-up in the types and duration of mindfulness exercises. For example, participants begin with mindful walking, body scan, mindfulness of sound, and routine activities, then proceed to sitting meditation. For an example of a breath awareness exercise adapted for individuals with ADHD, refer to Audio 2 (available online at www.appi.org/Carrion).

 Audio 2: Breath Awareness Practice for Individuals With Attention-Deficit/Hyperactivity Disorder (5:39)

Developmental Considerations

MINDFULNESS-BASED INTERVENTION FOR CHILDREN

Because children, especially those with ADHD, have shorter attention spans, the mindfulness exercises in MYmind were modified to be shorter; have more variety; and be more task-oriented, with such tasks as mindful walking, mindful eating, and mindful listening (Bögels et al. 2008). The personal challenging experiences of the children's everyday lives were addressed as well (Bögels et al. 2008). During sitting meditation, children share a difficult experience, such as being excluded or teased. Children then are guided to notice their emotional, cognitive, and physical reactions and welcome and accept whatever arises. They are encouraged to say to themselves, "It's OK. Whatever it is, let me feel it." Then, they return to noticing their breath and total physical body.

Children also engage in role-playing a difficult situation they experienced. One child describes the difficult experience, and the other children help role-play while the child is guided to be mindful of thoughts, feelings, and physical sensations that arise. Then, all of the children take a 3-minute breathing space, during which the children first bring mindful awareness to whatever they are currently experiencing, next, bring focused attention to their breath in the body, and then bring awareness to their entire body. The same difficult situation is then replayed, with the child being encouraged to answer rather than react. Other children are also encouraged to share their reactions to the situation and offer alternative perspectives.

To increase motivation and compliance, children are rewarded for their attendance and participation and for completing their home practice (Bögels et al. 2008). The children earn points that can be traded in for rewards from their parents.

Child Case Example: Tom

Tom is an 8-year-old boy in third grade who was recently diagnosed with ADHD, combined presentation. He is smart and active and plays soccer. However, some of his friendships are strained because of his impulsive comments and difficulty with respecting personal space. At school, he is frequently reprimanded by his teacher for talking in class, being out of his seat, or forgetting to complete or turn in his work. He has a younger brother without ADHD who excels in school and in his social interactions. Tom's parents had become increasingly frustrated with his impulsivity and hyperactivity and made an appointment for a psychiatric assessment. Tom was diagnosed with ADHD, and his parents were reluctant to try a medication. They wanted to try another intervention first and signed up Tom for a mindfulness-based group for ADHD.

The mindfulness exercises were very challenging for Tom because it is difficult for him to sit still and focus, and he preferred the more active mindfulness exercises, such as walking meditation. However, over the weeks, the instructor noted that Tom was able to stay in his seat more and more. By the end of the group, Tom was much more familiar with what mindfulness means and how to be in touch with it. When he became stressed, he used some of the mindfulness exercises and found them helpful. It was difficult for him to assess any change in his ADHD symptoms because he did not appear to be aware of the ADHD symptoms he was exhibiting. However, he did note that relationships with his peers were going more smoothly and that he was having more playdates. Going to a group also allowed Tom the opportunity to see peers with similar issues. This was an incredibly powerful experience because he experienced significant shame at potentially requiring medication and therapy for being "out of control." His parents took a parenting mindfulness course simultaneously, and Tom noticed that they seemed less frustrated with him all the time, which helped his mood and anxiety.

The MYmind themes for children with ADHD are presented in Table 6–2 (Meppelink et al. 2016).

TABLE 6–2.   Content of the MYmind protocol for children with ADHD

Week	Theme
1	Beginner's mind
2	Home in our body
3	The breath
4	Distractors
5	Stress
6	High way, walking away
7	Acceptance and autonomy
8	The future
Follow-up	Beginning anew

MINDFULNESS-BASED INTERVENTION FOR ADOLESCENTS

The first four sessions of MYmind for adolescents also focus on ADHD psychoeducation, with an emphasis on awareness and acceptance (Shecter 2013). Discussion topics include ADHD symptoms, positive aspects of ADHD, challenges that teens face because of ADHD, the impact of ADHD on daily life, and how mindfulness applies to ADHD. The last four sessions focus on mindfulness in relationships and interactions with others. Adolescents learn to be more mindfully aware of their reactivity, how to have more choice in how they respond, how to regulate their emotions mindfully, and how to respond with empathy and decrease judgment overall.

Adolescent Case Example: Doug

Doug is a 15-year-old sophomore in high school with diagnoses of ADHD, combined presentation, and unspecified depressive disorder. He has also been increasing his marijuana consumption because of peer pressure and academic stress. He has refused to take his ADHD medication for the past few months because, as he states, "I don't feel like myself" when he takes it. He was reluctant to join the mindfulness-based intervention group for ADHD because it would take time away from hanging out with his friends, but his parents told him they would not pressure him to take the medication if he attended the group. They also told Doug that if he completed the program, they would buy him a pair of sneakers he had been asking for.

When he joined the group, Doug was open to what it had to offer but felt uncomfortable talking about himself in a group. He found the exercises challenging at times because of his difficulty concentrating, but he also thought they were interesting and different from his regular experience and felt hopeful about learning another way to address his ADHD other than with medication. Doug also really enjoyed the ADHD psychoeducation components. He had not had the experience of talking about ADHD with a group of other teens who also had ADHD. He had not realized how much self-judgment he experienced and felt supported by the group, which improved his mood and decreased his anxiety. He also practiced mindfulness exercises, such as mindful eating (which he learned from the raisin exercise) and increasing awareness during difficult moments with less reactivity by taking a breathing space (which he practiced and tracked with a difficult moment–breathing space–answering calendar). Through practicing mindfulness exercises, Doug noticed that he was becoming more aware of his thoughts, emotions, and physical experience and was less reactive to situations and even had more self-compassion, which helped his self-image and mood. He was more motivated to try to take charge of his own life and was better able to focus on school.

The MYmind themes for adolescents with ADHD are presented in Table 6–3 (Bögels et al. 2008).

Mindfulness-Based Intervention for Parents of Youth With ADHD

The MYmind protocol was also adapted for the parent role (Bögels et al. 2008). Additional mindfulness exercises that focus on mindfully interacting with their child are emphasized. Parents are also encouraged to be mindful and nonjudgmental in their observations of and when listening to their child. They learn to become more aware of when they are responding automatically to their child's behavior on the basis of their own personal upbringing and previous experiences with their child. Instead, they learn to start to pay full attention to the child in the present moment and have more awareness in how they answer their child. Parents also receive psychoeducation on their child's diagnosis, with an emphasis on cultivating acceptance of certain aspects of their child and the impact of ADHD on the family.

Daily mindfulness practice is strongly encouraged for parents (Bögels et al. 2008). Parents are important role models for their child, and children can be motivated and encouraged to maintain their own individual practice if they see their parents dedicated to their own. Parents also can better support their child's

TABLE 6–3. Content of the MYmind protocol for adolescents with ADHD

Week	Theme	Exercises
1	Man from Mars	Raisin exercise, mindful walking, mindfulness of routine activities, mindful listening, mindful eating, rewards
2	Home in my body	Body scan, mindful walking, pleasant events, mindfulness of routine activities
3	Breath	Mindful breathing, 3-minute breathing space, unpleasant events
4	Answering	Mindfulness of sounds and thoughts, impulsivity, difficult moment–breathing space–answering calendar
5	Judging	Yoga, acceptance, difficult moment-breathing space-answering calendar
6	Who am I?	Yoga, shame, listing everything you are, intuition calendar
7	Me and the others	Trust, role-play, vulnerable moment-breathing space-honest response
8	On my own	Mindfulness, planning, processing, stone meditation

mindfulness practice if the parents have real mindfulness experiences themselves. In addition, the daily practice, with an emphasis on self-care, helps decrease parent stress and therefore could lead to less stress on the family. In addition, there is a strong genetic ADHD predisposition, and therefore, mindfulness may help parents who might also have similar struggles as their child.

Each parent session begins with a progressively longer meditation and ends with a shorter meditation (Shecter 2013). Each meditation is followed by a group reflection during which parents can discuss their experiences. In addition to focusing on mindfulness, the parent sessions also focus on the role of parents and especially the challenges of raising an adolescent with ADHD and how to bring mindfulness into their relationship with their child.

For the last session in the eighth week, the children and parents make an action plan for how to maintain their mindfulness practices for the 8 weeks after treatment prior to the follow-up meeting (Bögels et al. 2008). They write down their action plan and share it with the rest of the group. During the follow-up booster session, participants review how they are making progress in their goals and what barriers they are experiencing and receive feedback (Shecter 2013).

Parent Case Example: Alice and Bruce

Tom's parents, Alice and Bruce, attended the mindful parenting group for parents of children with ADHD. Alice was dealing with a lot of stress and anxiety about Tom's challenges. Bruce had become more and more easily frustrated by Tom's behaviors and was angry with Tom's hyperactivity, limited attention span, and impulsivity. Alice and Bruce also disagreed on how to respond to Tom's difficult behaviors, which led to more conflict and stress in the family. Both parents benefited from the ADHD psychoeducation component of the mindfulness program because they felt that their challenges with their son were validated, supported, and normalized by the group. Through the mindfulness exercises, Alice was better able to observe her anxiety and respond with compassion, which then decreased some of her anxiety and resulted in fewer anxious and reactive behaviors, especially in relation to Tom. Bruce was better able to tolerate his anger and frustration and developed more compassion for himself and for Tom in their challenges. After speaking with other parents in the group and experiencing less complicated emotions about their son's ADHD, Alice and Bruce decided to see a psychiatrist about potential ADHD medications for Tom after the group ended.

The MYmind themes for parent training of children and adolescents with ADHD are presented in Table 6–4. (Bögels et al. 2008).

Mindfulness-Based Intervention for Adults With ADHD

A specific treatment approach for adults with ADHD is called the Mindful Awareness Practices (MAPs) for ADHD Program (Mitchell et al. 2015). The MAPs for ADHD Program was created by Lydia Zylowska, M.D., and her colleagues in 2008 initially for a group-based treatment and is now also available as a self-help book that clinicians can use to help individuals with ADHD (Zylowska, 2012).

Similar to the MYmind protocol, the MAPS for ADHD Program also consists of eight weekly group sessions (Mitchell et al. 2015). Each session lasts for 2.5 hours, similar to mindfulness-based stress reduction (MBSR) and MBCT for adults. The sessions begin with a mindfulness exercise, then proceed to a review of the previous week and the assigned home practice, introduction of new material with experiential exercises, assignment of home practice, and a meditation (Mitchell et al. 2015; Zylowska 2012). Participants are encouraged to participate in discussion of the topics and in the mindfulness meditation practices. The weekly content of the MAPS for ADHD Program is shown in Table 6–5 (Mitchell et al. 2015; Zylowska 2012).

The MAPs for ADHD Program follows some of the overall framework used by MBSR and MBCT protocols, with modifications to meet the needs of

TABLE 6–4. Content of the MYmind protocol for parents of youth with ADHD

Week	Theme	Exercises
1	Being attentive	Raisin exercise, mindful walking, mindfulness of routine activities, child observation, rewards
2	Home in your body	Body scan, mindful walking, pleasant events, child observation, mindfulness of routine activities
3	Breath	Mindful breathing, 3-minute breathing space, unpleasant events
4	Answering	Mindfulness of sounds and thoughts, difficult moment–breathing space–answering
5	Acceptance	Yoga, sitting with "it is OK," what can(not) be changed about child, action plan
6	Identity	Yoga, Who am I?/Who is my child?, allowing growth of child's autonomy
7	Mindful communication	Open and authentic communication with child, vulnerable moment-breathing space-honest response calendar, life goals
8	The future	Mindfulness, planning, processing, stone meditation

adults with ADHD (Mitchell et al. 2015; Zylowska 2012). For example, the first two sessions focus on ADHD psychoeducation, with an emphasis on ADHD being a neurobiological disorder on the more severe end of a spectrum of functioning. There is also an emphasis on sitting with one's ADHD symptoms in a nonjudgmental manner. The meditation practices are shorter and range from 5 to 15 minutes rather than 45 minutes to accommodate the shorter attention spans of people with ADHD, with a gradual increase in the duration of the sitting meditation exercises. To further accommodate the limited attention span of people with ADHD, participants can substitute walking meditation for sitting meditation. There is also an emphasis on informal meditation—bringing mindful awareness to the daily activities one typically does such as brushing teeth or washing hands—in contrast to formal meditation, in which time is set aside from daily activity to focus on the breath, sounds, and body sensations. In addition, lovingkindness meditation occurs in every session, starting with the second week, to cultivate compassion toward self and others and to potentially

TABLE 6–5. Content of the MAPs for ADHD Program

Week	Topics	Exercises
1: Introduction to ADHD and mindfulness; re-framing of ADHD	ADHD psychoeducation, mindfulness definition, individual ADHD experiences, awareness and experience quality, sitting meditation	Mindful eating, mindfulness of breath
2: Mindful awareness of ADHD patterns	Common difficulties of meditation and overlap with ADHD symptoms, dialectic of acceptance and change, modifications for formal practice, mindfulness of movement	Mindfulness of breath, mindful walking, lovingkindness
3: Mindful awareness of breath, body, and sound	Shifts in attention, breath as anchor, attention check-in	Three-minute breath space; mindfulness of music; mindfulness of sound; mindfulness of movement; mindfulness of breath, body, and sound; lovingkindness
4: Mindful awareness of body sensations	Being present in the body, body movement and ADHD, physical pain vs. suffering, ADHD and "automatic pilot"	Mindfulness of breath, body scan, mindfulness of physical pain, mindfulness of putting on shoes, lovingkindness
5: Mindful awareness of thoughts	Metaphors, noticing thoughts, ADHD and self-esteem	Mindfulness of breath, mindfulness of thoughts, mindful walking, lovingkindness
6: Mindful awareness of emotions	Awareness of emotions, RAIN mnemonic, cultivating positive emotions	Mindfulness of breath, mindfulness of emotions, mindful walking, mindful presence, lovingkindness
7: Mindful awareness of interactions	Open awareness, interpersonal interactions, mindful communication	Mindfulness of breath, mindful presence, mindful walking, mindful listening (dyads), lovingkindness
8: Review and wrap-up	Mindfulness as part of daily life, how to continue practice, beyond MAPs, resources	Mindfulness of breath, mindful presence, mindful walking, lovingkindness

Abbreviations. MAPs=Mindful Awareness Practices; RAIN=recognize, accept, investigate, not-identify.

counter the negative thinking and depression that can occur with ADHD. Finally, CBT aspects are discussed in the last session to help participants continue their mindfulness practice.

Zylowska made further adaptations to the MAPs for ADHD Program in her book (Mitchell et al. 2015; Zylowska 2012). These adaptations include a focus on values, similar to the focus of acceptance and commitment therapy (ACT), and the dialectic of acceptance and change, similar to ideas from dialectical behavior therapy (DBT). Other adaptations include applications of imagery for negative emotional states and body posture for assertiveness and engagement. Another adaptation is the use of the mnemonic STOP from MBSR for informal mindfulness practice. The letters stand for stop, take a breath, observe in the present moment, and proceed. There is also a focus on willingness to change behaviors and using the reward of being fully aware of the experience of completing tasks and thereby potentially reinforcing subsequent behaviors. The final adaptation is use of a mindfulness buddy to help support each other's ongoing mindfulness practice.

Adult Case Example: Julia

Julia is a 35-year-old white single woman without children who has a history of generalized anxiety disorder and who was recently diagnosed with ADHD, predominantly inattentive presentation. She works as a nurse in the emergency department and enjoys her job, although she is often forgetful about things she needs to do and often stays late to complete her charting. As a child, she was an introvert who did not have any behavioral problems but often daydreamed and struggled with focusing on the teacher and on her schoolwork. She was usually an average student with low motivation to excel in school.

Julia's recent diagnosis and participation in a mindfulness group for ADHD helped her better understand her lifelong struggles in a more compassionate and less critical manner. She felt supported by being with others with similar experiences. She found the mindfulness exercises difficult because she quickly became distracted and then self-critical and self-judgmental. Over time, although Julia continued to be distracted during mindfulness exercises, her self-judgmental reaction softened. Overall, her tendency to be self-critical and self-judgmental decreased, and her general anxiety decreased as well. She found many of the mindfulness exercises helpful at work as well in keeping her grounded in the present moment and on task.

Research Support for Mindfulness-Based ADHD Treatment

Mindfulness-based activities are widely practiced, with popularity in schools and in work environments to help with overall well-being. Parents, teachers, colleagues, and health care providers of various levels of training and experience are leading and teaching a wide range of mindfulness-based activities, such as yoga and various forms of meditation. There have been two recent reviews to assess the efficacy of mindfulness-based interventions specific for ADHD: one for children and the other for adults.

Research Support for Mindfulness-Based ADHD Treatment for Children

Evans and colleagues (2018) recently conducted a much-needed systemic review of meditation-based interventions for children with ADHD. Their main objectives were to determine the validity of the following assertions:

- Meditation-based interventions may decrease core ADHD symptoms, increase child well-being, and decrease internalizing and externalizing problems.
- Meditation-based interventions for parents of children with ADHD improve the parent-child relationship and parent functioning.
- Combined meditation-based interventions that include both parents and children are more effective than interventions that include only the parents or the children.

Evans and colleagues found a high risk of bias in the studies they reviewed. The biases were the result of uncontrolled, single-arm studies; use of self-report and nonvalidated measures; small sample sizes; and analytical methodologies that did not control for covariates or missing data. These studies did not comment on adverse effects, and it is unclear if there was a protocol to measure them if they did occur.

In their attempts to address their main objectives, Evans et al. (2018) found the following:

- Overall, meditation-based interventions decreased ADHD symptoms in the majority of the studies. However, there was significant concern regarding the high risk of bias, and two of the three controlled studies did not find positive impact from the meditation-based intervention.
- Parents reported an improvement in child self-esteem and social functioning, but there was no indication of improvement in child-reported self-esteem and social functioning. Child-reported happiness was also decreased in one study. Some results indicated a positive benefit for academic functioning from the meditation-based intervention.
- There was very limited support for decreased internalizing and externalizing symptoms associated with ADHD.

- There was also limited and inconsistent support for improving parent functioning.
- There was moderate improvement of the parent-child relationship without improvement in the children's well-being, such as their self-esteem, social functioning, happiness, and internalizing or externalizing symptoms.
- The child-only interventions largely showed a decrease in ADHD symptoms, but there were significant limitations to the studies, and two studies indicated an increase in ADHD symptoms after yoga and mindful martial arts.
- The combined intervention (parent and child) may be more helpful than medications alone; including parents in the treatment resulted in larger effect sizes, fewer negative outcomes, and positive impact on adults, which may then result in benefits for their children.

Ultimately, Evans et al. (2018) found that they could not make a definitive conclusion on the effectiveness of meditation-based interventions for children with ADHD and/or their parents because of the poor quality of methodological quality of the studies. There was only one RCT for mindfulness-based intervention for children with ADHD. Evans and colleagues (2018, p. 24) also used a broad definition of meditation or mindfulness-based intervention as "any treatment that involved the cultivation of attention with the goals of increased awareness, presence and an integrated sense of self." Therefore, they included studies that used yoga, martial arts, or mindful walking as well as more formal sitting meditation. The instructors in the studies also had a broad range of experience, from high school volunteers with brief training to an instructor with 40 years of personal meditation practice. Evans and colleagues commented that the general intuitive recommendation is that instructors receive training in and maintain their own personal meditation practice, but they also commented that it is not yet established that the instructor's expertise directly impacts the outcome of the studies.

Research Support for Mindfulness-Based ADHD Treatment for Adults

Cairncross and Miller (2016) conducted a meta-analytic review on whether mindfulness-based therapies for ADHD were effective for adults. They hypothesized that mindfulness-based treatments would be more effective in decreasing ADHD symptoms in adults than in children because inattentive symptoms are more common with adult ADHD and mindfulness is more helpful for improving attention. They concluded that preliminary findings supported mindfulness-based treatments for decreasing ADHD symptoms. There were many limitations to this study, including the use of a small number of studies, limited information on what the mindfulness intervention consisted of, and small sample size. In addition, many of the same studies that were part of the systematic review conducted by Evans et al. (2018) were included in the Cairncross and Miller (2016) meta-analysis, but there was much less emphasis on the poor methodology that precluded Evans et al. from being able to conclude that mindfulness-based interventions were effective for childhood ADHD.

Strengths

Most of the mindfulness-based interventions that showed preliminary efficacy for decreasing ADHD symptoms follow manualized protocols that help to streamline the treatment. Manualized treatments also help with training instructors for the specific intervention. In addition, most of the participants in these studies reported a positive experience, regardless of how much impact there was on their ADHD symptoms. Overall, adverse effects from the mindfulness-based interventions were not reported, although it is not clear that all of the studies were designed to include ways to monitor for potential adverse effects.

Areas for Development

There continues to be an increase in studies looking at the efficacy of mindfulness-based intervention and, more recently, with a focus on mindfulness-based interventions for specific mental health issues, including ADHD in children, adolescents, and adults. Although studies continue to show preliminary indications for potential efficacy, the main area for further development remains the same as for most of the mindfulness-based intervention studies: the need for better methodology. The other common issue is the heterogeneity of what is considered *mindfulness-based intervention*. The commonly used definitions for mindfulness are broad enough that many types of interventions can fit under this category. At the same time, each of those approaches also has significant differences that can potentially have different effects; therefore, these differences and their potential impacts also need to be further studied.

Conclusion and Future Directions

ADHD is a widely prevalent disorder that continues to increase in prevalence. It is unclear if the increasing prevalence is due to more awareness of the disorder, overdiagnosis, and/or the unique time we live in. Although there are evidence-based treatments for ADHD, there continue to be limits to the well-established treatments, such as pharmacology and behavioral therapy. Therefore, there remains a significant need for additional treatment modalities. Mindfulness-based interventions may be especially suited for treatment of ADHD, as well as being especially challenging for individuals with ADHD, given that ADHD is largely a problem of attention and mindfulness is largely attention training.

Although the research shows preliminary indications that mindfulness-based interventions may be helpful for ADHD, more methodologically sound studies are critical to better establish mindfulness as an effective treatment for ADHD. This issue has been an ongoing challenge for mindfulness research in general.

The current third wave of behavioral therapy, such as DBT, ACT, and MBCT, is characterized by incorporation of mindfulness into the therapy. This third wave of behavioral therapy addresses the individual's relationship to thought and emotion, in addition to the content of those thoughts and emotions (Hayes and Hofmann 2017). Many of the mindfulness-based interventions for ADHD appear to be based on the MBCT structure, with significant adaptions to address the challenges faced by individuals with ADHD. Further adaptations to meet the specific needs of persons with ADHD may be warranted for greater efficacy. For example, given that many of the meditation exercises are shorter to accommodate the shorter attention span of persons with ADHD, it may be important to consider a longer duration of treatment. Also, for individuals with more significant ADHD symptoms for whom mindfulness exercises may be especially difficult, discussion of the potentially important role of medication for ADHD may also be warranted to decrease stigma and normalize the role of medication. This is especially important because medication is the first-line treatment for ADHD, with the exception of preschool-age children. It may be helpful to have a mindful space to discuss the experience of taking psychotropic medication as well, given that there is significant variability in people's experiences.

In addition, similar to the adult MAPs for ADHD Program, the protocols for children and adolescents may benefit from an emphasis on lovingkindness and/or compassion cultivation. Many people with ADHD struggle with a negative self-concept, given the academic and social challenges that they internalize rather than attribute to their ADHD. This negative self-concept can result in other comorbidities and poorer functioning overall. Zylowska's additional adaptations to the MAPs for ADHD Program, including discussion of values, the dialectic of acceptance and change, and the buddy system, may also be helpful for adolescents. The mindfulness discussed in MBSR and MBCT stems from Eastern Buddhist traditions, and some other adaptations of lovingkindness and compassion cultivation, such as living by a code of values and intentions, the dialectic of acceptance and change, and the connection to others to help support one's mindfulness practice, are also important features of this tradition.

Another consideration is the idea of a third wave of therapy supporting parenting. There is evidence of benefits from parent behavioral therapy, as well as some preliminary indication of mindful parenting practices, for ADHD treatment. Combining these modalities, similar to incorporating mindfulness into CBT, in which parent behavioral strategies remain a significant portion of the treatment, may have even greater impact. The balance of specific strategies based on effective principles of behaviorism, combined with staying present with less reactivity and more compassion, may have even greater efficacy overall for parents and their children.

KEY POINTS

- The key limitations to current ADHD treatment include the use of strong medications from a young age, limited and variable benefits from current psychotherapeutic modalities, and the lack of clear long-term benefit.

- Mindfulness, as a way to compassionately train attention, may be helpful in the prevention of and early intervention for ADHD as well as a helpful adjunct for standard ADHD treatment.

- The key components of current mindfulness-based interventions for ADHD include increasing attention and compassion while decreasing reactivity.

- Research is showing preliminary indications for mindfulness-based interventions for ADHD, although methodologically sound studies are critical to better establish these interventions.

Discussion Questions

1. How might mindfulness be helpful for and challenging for persons with ADHD?
2. What are important adaptations to keep in mind when incorporating mindfulness in treating ADHD?
3. Given that medication can be an important part of ADHD treatment, should medications be integrated into the mindfulness-based intervention? And if so, how?

Suggested Readings

Evans S, Ling M, Hill B, et al: Systematic review of meditation-based interventions for children with ADHD. Eur Child Adolesc Psychiatry 27(1):9–27, 2017 28547119

Mitchell JT, Zylowska L, Kollins SH: Mindfulness meditation training for attention-deficit/hyperactivity disorder in adulthood: current empirical support, treatment overview, and future directions. Con Behav Pract 22(2):172–101, 2015 25908900

Zylowska L: The Mindfulness Prescription for Adult ADHD. Boulder, CO, Trumpeter Books, 2012

References

American Psychiatric Association: Attention-deficit/hyperactivity disorder, in Diagnostic and Statistical Manual of Mental Disorders, 5th Edition. Arlington, VA, American Psychiatric Association, 2013, p 59

Bhide S, Sciberras E, Anderson V, et al: Association between parenting style and socioemotional and academic functioning in children with and without ADHD: a community-based study. J Atten Disord July 28, 2016 [Epub ahead of print] 27474160

Bögels S, Hoogstad B, Schutter S, et al: Mindfulness training for adolescents with externalizing disorders and their parents. Behav Cogn Psychother 36:193–209, 2008

Cairncross M, Miller CJ: The effectiveness of mindfulness-based therapies for ADHD: a meta-analytic review. J Atten Disord February 2, 2016 [Epub ahead of print] 26838555

Centers for Disease Control and Prevention: Mental health surveillance among children—United States, 2005–2011. Morbidity and Mortality Weekly Report. Atlanta, GA, Centers for Disease Control and Prevention, 2013. Available at: www.cdc.gov/ncbddd/adhd/data.html. Accessed May 16, 2018.

Cherkasova MV, French LR, Syer CA, et al: Efficacy of cognitive behavioral therapy with and without medication for adults with ADHD. J Atten Disord October 1, 2016 [Epub ahead of print] 28413900

Evans S, Ling M, Hill B, et al: Systematic review of meditation-based interventions for children with ADHD. Eur Child Adolesc Psychiatry 27(1):9–27, 2018 28547119

Hayes SC, Hofmann SG: The third wave of cognitive behavioral therapy and the rise of process-based care. World Psychiatry 16(3):245–246, 2017 28941087

Hinshaw SP, Arnold LE; For the MTA Cooperative Group: ADHD, multimodal treatment, and longitudinal outcome: evidence, paradox, and challenge. Wiley Interdiscip Rev Cogn Sci 6(1):39–52, 2015 25558298

Kessler RC, Adler L, Barkley R, et al: The prevalence and correlates of adult ADHD in the United States: results from the National Comorbidity Survey Replication. Am J Psychiatry 163(4):716–723, 2006 16585449

Meppelink R, de Bruin EI, Bögels SM: Meditation or medication? Mindfulness training versus medication in the treatment of childhood ADHD: a randomized controlled trial. BMC Psychiatry 16:267, 2016 27460004

Mitchell JT, Zylowska L, Kollins SH: Mindfulness meditation training for attention-
deficit/hyperactivity disorder in adulthood: current empirical support, treatment
overview, and future directions. Cognit Behav Pract 22(2):172–191, 2015 25908900

MTA Cooperative Group: Multimodal Treatment Study of Children with ADHD: a
14-month randomized clinical trial of treatment strategies for attention-deficit/
hyperactivity disorder. Arch Gen Psychiatry 56(12):1073–1086, 1999 10591283

Sciberra E, Roos LE, Efron D: Review of prospective longitudinal studies of children
with ADHD: mental health, educational, and social outcomes. Curr Atten Disord
Rep 1:171–177, 2009

Segal ZV, Williams JMG, Teasdale JD: Mindfulness-Based Cognitive Therapy for Depression. New York, Guilford, 2002

Shecter C: Mindfulness training for adolescents with ADHD and their families: a time-
series evaluation. Doctor of philosophy thesis, University of Toronto, Toronto,
Canada, 2013. Available at: https://tspace.library.utoronto.ca/bitstream/1807/
43718/1/Shecter_Carly_M_201311_PhD_thesis.pdf. Accessed on May 16, 2018.

Spencer T, Biederman J, Wilens T, et al: A large, double-blind, randomized clinical trial of methylphenidate in the treatment of adults with attention-deficit/hyperactiv-
ity disorder. Biol Psychiatry 57(5):456–463, 2005 15737659

Wolraich M, Brown L, Brown RT, et al; Subcommittee on Attention-Deficit/Hyper-
activity Disorder; Steering Committee on Quality Improvement and Management: ADHD: clinical practice guideline for the diagnosis, evaluation, and
treatment of attention-deficit/hyperactivity disorder in children and adolescents.
Pediatrics 128(5):1007–1022, 2011 22003063

Young S, Khondoker M, Emilsson B, et al: Cognitive-behavioural therapy in medica-
tion-treated adults with attention-deficit/hyperactivity disorder and co-morbid
psychopathology: a randomized controlled trial using multi-level analysis. Psychol
Med 45(13):2793–2804, 2015 26022103

Zylowska L: The Mindfulness Prescription for Adult ADHD. Boulder, CO, Trumpeter
Books, 2012

Chapter

7

Grief and Loss

Susan Delaney, Psy.D.

No one ever told me that grief felt so like fear.
—*C. S. Lewis (1968, p. 5)*

If we practice mindfulness, we always have a place to be when we are
afraid.
—*Thich Nhat Hanh (1992)*

THERE is no hierarchy of grief, but the death of a child brings a profound loss that sets it aside from any other loss. Children carry our DNA, our future, and when a child dies, the dreams of the parents die too; their assumptive world is shattered. A parent burying a child goes against the natural order of things, the cycle of life. One hundred years ago, we did not expect to raise all our offspring to adulthood, but with improvements in health care, nutrition, and medical intervention, delivering healthy children and having them remain healthy throughout their lifetime is expected. We no longer wait until a child is born to invest all our hopes in him or her. In utero, we already connect to this fantasy

121

child. Fathers routinely attend scans, and we often know the gender of the child before birth. We pick names, paint the nursery, and make plans. Being a parent becomes central to how we define ourselves. A parent's grief is very difficult to bear, whether it is the result of a miscarriage, a stillbirth, a childhood accident, or illness. But this grief is also very difficult to witness. In this chapter I consider how we as practitioners can use mindfulness practices to support bereaved families on their journey of grief.

Bereavement work, by definition, is a shared experience. There is no place to hide; we are all the bereaved. Bereavement challenges us as practitioners, and it activates our own death anxiety. The loss can remind us of our own loss if we are bereaved parents or can trigger our own worst fears if we have living children. As Nicholas Wolterstorff (1987, p. 34) so beautifully described in a piece he wrote after the death of his son:

> If you think your task as comforter is to tell me that really, all things considered, it's not so bad, you do not sit with me in my grief but place yourself off in the distance from me. Over there, you are of no help. What I need to hear from you is that you recognize how painful it is. I need to hear from you that you are with me in my desperation. To comfort me, you have to come close. Come sit beside me on my mourning bench.

We can agree that therapeutic presence and the ability to develop and maintain a therapeutic connection with clients is key to any good counseling practice. In bereavement counseling, however, practitioners are additionally asked to remain present while managing their own death anxiety and can easily feel overwhelmed when faced with a grief-stricken parent filled with hopelessness and helplessness. As practitioners, we are asked to sit and bear witness to grief without trying to make it better.

Factors to Consider When Using Mindfulness With Bereaved Families

The first factor to consider when using mindfulness as therapy for bereaved families is that the death of a child is a risk factor for developing complicated grief (Kersting et al. 2011). *Complicated grief* (CG; also known as prolonged grief disorder or persistent complex bereavement disorder) occurs in approximately 10% of the bereaved population, and its hallmark is unrelenting grief that fails to integrate and continues to impact daily functioning. Not all bereaved parents will develop CG, but bereaved parents have the highest prevalence of CG (reported as 23.6% in a study by Kersting and Wagner 2012). Although mindfulness techniques may still be a useful support, it is recognized that bereaved parents who meet criteria for CG may well need additional intervention. The work of Kathy Shear, Director of the Center for Complicated Grief at Columbia University, is an excellent resource for further information on evidence-based treatment of CG (see https://complicatedgrief.columbia.edu).

Second, mindfulness and meditation practices may not be suitable for all bereaved clients. Sitting with strong feelings of grief may trigger anxiety, unleash repressed feelings, and trigger flooding in vulnerable people, particularly bereaved clients experiencing acute grief. Therefore, practitioners should carefully assess whether particular clients have the emotional capacity to manage the strong emotions that may emerge when they sit with their feelings and sensations.

Finally, and very importantly, before we engage bereaved people in mindfulness practices, it is crucial to have an established practice ourselves. A number of researchers have suggested that mindfulness practices can foster therapeutic presence (Bruce et al. 2010), and Campbell and Christopher (2012) concluded that training counselors in mindfulness-based interventions can help them realize and embody the personal characteristics that foster therapeutic presence. I came to mindfulness through hospice work. It is what sustains me in that work and helps me to stay present to the deep sorrow and pain that I encounter. Bereavement work asks of us that we show up in a different way, that we meet clients first as fellow human beings living with our own losses and griefs, that we can "sit beside them on their mourning bench." We must expect to be challenged, to be rocked out of our comfort zone, and to meet our own grief in the process.

Mindfulness in Grief Work: What We Know From Research

Joanne Cacciatore (2011) proposed a mindfulness-based bereavement care model known as the ATTEND model. The acronym stands for attunement, trust, therapeutic touch, egalitarianism, nuance, and death education. This ATTEND model has been adopted as a means to improve psychosocial care during both acute and chronic states of bereavement. This is a tripartite model that encourages practitioners first to engage in their own mindfulness practice to foster attunement to clients, second, to integrate aspects of the model into their client work, and finally to introduce clients to formal and informal mindfulness practices. The utility of the model has been endorsed by several researchers (Cacciatore and Flint 2012; Thieleman and Cacciatore 2014), with reports of a reduction in trauma and depressive and anxious symptoms in traumatically bereaved people (Rando 1985; Thieleman and Cacciatore 2014). Neimeyer and Young-Eisendrath (2015) developed and assessed a Buddhist intervention for bereaved clients that incorporated mindfulness practice, creative arts, and meaning making and reported significant decreases in grief-related suffering and increases in meaning making and personal growth across the course of a workshop experience.

Mindfulness-based cognitive therapy (MBCT; see Chapter 5, "Anxiety and Depression") has been established as an effective treatment for depression relapse prevention. It aims to equip clients with tools to notice, and thereby avoid, the escalation of negative thoughts into ruminative loops and emotional avoidance. Grief differs from depression, but there are overlapping features. Susan O'Flanagan in her unpublished thesis (O'Flanagan 2013) examined the efficacy of using MBCT to reduce the symptoms of prolonged grief disorder in a sample of Irish clients. Her findings suggested that MBCT is a promising treatment approach for CG. In particular, she notes, "Considering the fundamental role of rumination and avoidance in maintaining and exacerbating prolonged grief reactions, developing an understanding of mindfulness may well prove a worthy pursuit for those suffering from intense and unremitting grief" (O'Flanagan 2013, p. 83). Heather Stang (2014) has written extensively on the topic and provides online training on grief and loss to guide people through their grief, using meditation to calm the mind and restore a sense of hope. For further information, see her website, http://mindfulnessandgrief.com.

The research on the benefits of mindfulness practices in grief work is both recent and limited. Practitioners working in the field have both clinical and anecdotal evidence of its efficacy, but much of what we know is extrapolated from findings on the efficacy of mindfulness-based stress reduction and MBCT. There is an increasing need for researchers and practitioners to consider the place of mindfulness in grief work and to publish and share their research and clinical findings. We must also correct misunderstandings. Many people, and certainly many bereaved people, get much of their information via the Internet and social media. A recent piece doing the rounds on Facebook suggested that mindfulness was not appropriate in grief work because it urged bereaved people to change their thoughts and accept that everything is just as it should be. This is the complete opposite of mindfulness teaching. Mindfulness encourages a noticing of thoughts, of feelings, and of body sensations, without judgment, and certainly without any expectation of changing or getting rid of them. As we notice what is already present, we pause, and rather than engage in habitual reactivity, mindfulness provides the opportunity to respond in a more skillful and compassionate way.

Grieving Parents

Each parent's grief is unique, but all grief has some commonalities. In acute grief, most people experience a myriad of intense feelings, including sadness, anger, guilt, relief, irritability, and self-recrimination. Some days, grief can feel manageable; other days, it can bring us to our knees. Sometimes we feel we are managing, only to wake up the next day feeling quite ambushed by grief and totally overwhelmed by the experience. We can struggle with facing feelings of grief or finding ways to take breaks from our grief. This is sometimes called *dosing our grief.* Of course, no parent ever gets over the death of a child. The grief is transformative and becomes part of who that person is in the world. But over time grief changes; it reshapes. For bereaved parents, grieving can be described as the oscillation between engaging with the heartache of losing a child and adapting to life without that child. The course of grief will vary for each family member, but the overall trajectory is forward as the grief slowly begins to integrate. Our job as practitioners is to facilitate this natural process, to witness and honor the grief while allowing resilience and the psychological immune system to bring about healing.

The grief journey for bereaved parents is both similar to and different from other grief journeys. Its course will differ depending on such factors as the timing and circumstances of the death and the psychological makeup of the bereaved parent. It is beyond the scope of this chapter to consider the many ways parents can grieve and the impact of a child's death on their psychological functioning. Readers who are interested in this topic can refer to the work of Therese Rando (1985) and Denis Klass (1999).

Below are some of the ways a bereaved parent might present. As you read them, notice the sensations you are experiencing and imagine how you respond to this bereaved parent.

> **Emotion dysregulation:** "I try not to think about her at all because I simply go to pieces and I can't cope." "If I wake up thinking about him, I know that the whole day is shot and I just stay in bed."
> **Recrimination:** "How could I have let him die? Dads are supposed to keep their children safe. I should have taken him to the doctor sooner."
> **Loss of sense of self:** "I only ever wanted to be a mother; now I am nothing. I am only a shadow of myself."
> **Guilt:** "I didn't really want this child." "This was my favorite child."
> **Shame:** "I am a monster. I prayed for her pain to end. This is my punishment for having an abortion when I was younger."
> **Self-loathing:** "I don't deserve to be happy. I punish myself every day for not noticing she was sick."
> **Counterfactual thinking:** "It was my fault she died."
> **Hopelessness:** "I will never have a moment's peace. I wish I could die too."
> **Unimaginable sadness:** "I know I will never be happy again. My life now is just existing until I see my child again. There is nothing that you can do to help me."

How did it feel to read those sentences? Did you notice your body reacting? Where were you aware of it in your body? What was your breathing like? As practitioners we are called on to witness grief and to create a space where bereaved parents can say the unsayable. To do this well, we must anchor ourselves in our body and acknowledge the impact of grief on ourselves before we attend to our clients' grief.

Using Mindfulness to Support Grieving Parents

Bereaved parents don't wish to get over their grief because their grief connects them to their child. As therapists, we emphasize that we are not going to ask them to give up their grief. We offer the possibility of finding a way to remember their child with love rather than with pain. We help them learn gentle ways to turn toward difficult feelings such as shame, guilt, isolation, and sorrow while also learning to redirect attention if the feeling becomes too intense. At this point, oscillation—the ability to move toward grief and move away from grief— begins to occur. Emotion regulation is slowly reestablished. Parents notice that they can tolerate strong emotion, that thoughts are just mental events, not truths. Importantly, they are introduced to the concept of self-compassion, which is an integral part of mindfulness practice. They are reminded that pain is inevitable, but suffering is eased in a landscape of compassion. They learn how to come to a moment and notice that it is a moment of suffering, a moment that calls for self-kindness and patience. Offering themselves simple words of comfort and small acts of self-care through this time of turbulence opens up possibilities of self-compassion.

We can work with bereaved parents on finding new ways of imagining grief. We remind them that they don't need to wait for their grief to change; they can change their relationship with their grief. It is possible to grow around grief. As grief begins to heal, they are no longer simply the parents whose child died. That may well continue to be a defining part of how they see themselves, but it does not define every part of them. We allow for posttraumatic growth. We allow for the possibility of finding purpose and moments of joy again. There is a laminated sign in my office, a favorite quote from Thich Nhat Hanh (1992), that reads "Although the seed of suffering in you may be strong, don't wait until you have no more suffering before allowing yourself to be happy." It's a challenging concept. In grief, parents can lose the ability to experience joy in life and truly come to believe that after the death of a child, they will never experience happy moments again. However, this is not true, and, indeed, an inability to feel any joy or find purpose in life should raise a red flag to the presence of CG. Through mindful practice, we encourage bereaved parents to come out of autopilot and into awareness and acceptance of grief while also noticing how grief reshapes and changes and allows space for other experiences as well. Although it is true that after the death of a special person even the happiest of days will be tinged with sadness, it is also true that even on the saddest of days there can be moments of joy or contentment if we are awake to them.

Suggestions for Incorporating Simple Mindfulness Practices Into Your Work With Bereaved Parents

Bereaved parents have the freedom to attend to their grief when practitioners are able to bear witness to their pain right in the moment, nonjudgmentally and with full acceptance of emotional, social, and existential states. Our job as practitioners is to hold a space where bereaved parents can be met with kindness, understanding, and compassion. As practitioners, we model a state of mindfulness and allow bereaved parents to find their own way to presence, to tolerance for what is, and this also allows for the possibility of growth. Learning how to pause and use the breath as an anchor allows some sense of control over grief, a noticing that grief is not solid, that it changes as we interact with it, and a noticing that we all have the ability to move up close to grief and to move back from grief.

MINDFUL BREATHING

One of the most powerful tools can be the introduction of mindful breathing. Because grief can feel so much like fear, many bereaved people feel as if they are under threat. The simple act of noticing the breath and taking a pause to breathe and allow the body to settle can be both calming and reassuring.

At the start of each meeting, sit with the bereaved parent in companionable silence. We become aware of what is present for us as practitioners and attune to the other, the client. Allow the body and the mind to settle. Guide the client in the following breathing exercise (it can be useful to keep a jar of muddy water as a visual aid):

> Use the breath, at whatever point you are most aware of it, to connect you to the body and whatever sensations are present there. Just breathing now, perhaps imagining a jar of muddy water and what happens when we shake it and then when we hold it still; the silt sinks to the bottom and the water becomes clearer. Noticing what's arising, what is present, but just like the clear water, the part of us that sees the difficulty is separate from the difficulty, and we can work from there.

Mindful breathing can facilitate the activation of the parasympathetic nervous system, which allows clients to remain present, to know that they have survived the death of their child and that this is a grief experience and there is nothing to fear. They can begin to look at how and where they hold grief in their body, where they are most aware of their grief, and how the sensations of grief can change. This allows bereaved clients to feel some control over their grief and to notice how their relationship with grief can change, can wax and wane—such is the nature of grief.

THE POWER OF PAUSE

It is important to pause regularly in the conversation: to ask clients to take a moment, to become aware of their breathing, and to notice what is arising for them. The phrase "stop, drop, and roll" can sometimes be useful. For example, the practitioner might say, "Let's stop here for a moment" or "Let's drop into the body and roll with whatever is arising for you." The three-step breathing practice described in th following subsection can be used during a pause.

THREE-STEP BREATHING SPACE PRACTICE

This is a useful practice when the client feels overwhelmed by grief. It takes approximately 3 minutes and can help clients feel less overwhelmed by the emotions and feelings that accompany grief. Encourage clients to visualize an hourglass as they narrow and expand their field of focus. Coming to the breath allows for a pause and the possibility to see grief rising and falling and our ability to breathe through the difficult times. Coming to the breath simply means noticing the breath as it enters and leaves the body. Just focus on where you most readily feel the breath—it might be at the nostrils, the chest, or the tummy. There are three steps to this practice:

First step: awareness. When you become aware of strong grief feelings during the day, pause, close your eyes if possible, and ask yourself, "What am I experiencing right now? What sensations are in my body? What feelings are present? What thoughts am I aware of relating to my grief?" Acknowledge and register the experience, even if it is unpleasant or unwanted.

Second step: gathering. Narrow the field of attention to a single, pointed focus on the breath in the body. Attention is redirected, and the breath functions as an anchor, allowing present-moment awareness and a moment of stillness and pause.

Third step: expanding. Widen attention again to include the body as a whole and any sensations that are present.

HOME PRACTICE

Engaging mindfully with grief. Encourage clients to engage mindfully with their grief every day for short periods of time. This can help with the integration of their grief. Encourage clients to attend to specific practices each day and also to keep a reflective journal in which they can jot down any notes, insights, or questions that arise for them. For example, you might suggest the following home practice.

Until we next meet:
1. During the day, take time to pause and notice how you are feeling in your grief. It helps to have a reminder, such as drinking coffee, brushing your teeth, stopping at red traffic lights—anything that you do on a daily basis— to remind you to stop and notice. Just be curious and open to the changing experience that is grief.
2. Once a day, take the time to do the lovingkindness practice (see below).
3. At least once a day, engage in self-compassion. Very consciously, remind yourself that grieving can be exhausting. Take a nap, take a leisurely walk, listen to soothing music. It can also help to say quietly to yourself, "This is a time of suffering; may I be kind to myself."
4. Continue to use the three-step breathing exercise any time you feel over-whelmed by grief.
5. Continue to write in your reflective journal, without judgment or editing. You might like to comment on the above practices or just note down your grief feelings or thoughts.

Lovingkindness practice.
Self-kindness and self-compassion are core elements in mindfulness practice. Bereaved parents can sometimes be hard on themselves, and this practice can help them develop a kinder disposition to themselves, serve as a reminder that suffering is part of life, and provide a sense of connection to others. Guide the client in the following practice:

Find a comfortable position where you can be relaxed and alert. Place your hands on the tummy and notice the rise and fall of the tummy as you breathe [*pause*]. Now move your awareness up toward the chest and the heart region, the areas where we hold love and grief. Allow an image of [child's name] to form in your mind's eye, making it as clear as suits you today [*pause*]. Allow a half smile to form as you feel that connection to your beloved child. Now whisper or say the following silently to yourself:
> *May you be safe.*
> *May you feel the love we share.*
> *May you be at peace.*

Then allow the image of [child's name] to fade, just for now, allowing an image of yourself to form in your mind's eye. Keep breathing and perhaps gently massage the chest or heart area. Offer the same comforting words to yourself:
> *May I be safe.*
> *May I feel the love we shared.*
> *May I be at peace.*

Case Example

Mary opened with "It should have been me." She presented with unrelenting grief over the death of her daughter, Sarah, who died in a car crash at age 10. Mary described going to see a "lovely counselor" previously but reported that in three sessions they never spoke of her daughter even though she really wanted to talk about Sarah. Finally, Mary just gave up going to the sessions.

Mary was very much caught in ruminations, and although one might expect the ruminations to be around the death of her child, the real sticky point for Mary was obsessive and intrusive thoughts that she should have given up her baby for adoption and that if she had not been so selfish, her little girl would still be alive. Mary was housebound, unable to tolerate seeing other mothers out with their daughters or to allow people to sympathize with her. She was barely sleeping or eating. When I inquired about this, she answered, "How could I possibly ever sleep well or enjoy food again when my baby is gone?" Mary experienced relief from this unrelenting thought by practicing *thought watching*, in which she noticed the ruminations when they occurred. I gave her a copy of the saying "Thoughts are not truths," and she developed her own reminder system: she noticed that this thought arose whenever she made a pot of coffee, and this allowed her to focus on letting it go, like a puff of smoke, rather than lapsing into rumination.

Mary used simple mindful movement practices to engage with her body and get out of her head, and we noticed together that as her body moved, the grief also moved. Mary believed that she was responsible for Sarah's death because she chose to bring her up as a single parent. With no challenge to this counterfactual belief, it had taken root. Mary's growing ability to sit with whatever thoughts and feelings arose around her grief served her well. She learned that although the grief felt overwhelming, she could use her breath as an anchor and move toward or away from her grief at will. She was able to remind herself how she loved her daughter to the best of her ability, to remember good times she had shared with Sarah, and to recognize that she was always a good enough parent and occasionally a spectacularly good one. She learned to stop punishing herself and to start taking care of herself. She continued to engage in lovingkindness offerings to Sarah as a way of staying connected while letting go of the past and opening up to her future.

Mary continued her mindful movement and began taking a yoga class. She also attended a drop-in mindfulness class in her neighborhood. Both of these activities helped her to connect with other people as well as stay connected to her body. Mary learned that the tie to Sarah would never be severed and that by engaging again in her life, she was doing exactly what Sarah would have wanted. Does she still have difficult days, days when she feels crushed by the unfairness of it all? Absolutely. The difference now is that Mary is not afraid of the strong grief feelings; she knows how to manage them and knows that they will abate, and she engages in regular home practice.

Children and Grief

We often refer to children as forgotten mourners. In bygone times, children grew up with death: a stillbirth at home, the death of a grandparent who lived within the home. They knew death as part of life. In Ireland, young girls accompanied their mothers to the laying out of bodies, which was considered women's work. Then, somewhere along the line, we decided that children should be protected from death and grief. We outsourced death and stopped including children in death rituals. Now we are trying to reintroduce the reality of death to children and recognize that we cannot protect them from it. Our job as practitioners is to find age-appropriate ways to help children understand their grief, learn ways to manage strong feelings, and experience resilience first hand, learning that just as we heal from physical hurts, we also heal from psychological hurts.

The tiniest of children will have a response to loss, and by 5 or 6 years, most children will have some understanding of the finality of death. Although children's grief will be mediated by their cognitive and emotional development, they feel much the same grief feelings as adults. Their grief tends to occur in shorter bursts; in fact, children quite naturally oscillate from grief to everyday life activities. As I was explaining to my own children that a child in their school had died unexpectedly, my daughter, then 6 years old, replied, "That's very sad, Mom, but can we go watch TV now?" Children need to reestablish routine, to feel safe and secure following the death of someone in their life. They need help to understand what they are feeling and a safe place to express their grief. Bereaved siblings may harbor thoughts that what happened was their fault because secretly they wished their brother or sister would die. They may think that perhaps their parents preferred the sibling who died. They may feel guilty for still being alive and worry about dying themselves. They may feel scared, unsafe, vulnerable, different from peers, unsure of the future.

Extending Mindfulness Practices to Bereaved Children

Cacciatore's ATTEND model can possibly be extended to a quadripartite model. Even if you work only with bereaved parents, take the opportunity to pass on some simple mindfulness techniques that your client can use at home with bereaved children, nieces, nephews, or friends of the deceased child. For many children, this will be their first encounter with death, and it presents an opportunity to introduce children to simple ways of managing the strong emotions that can accompany grief and a way for families to connect in their shared grief.

Children are naturally mindful; they live in the present and are often more connected to their bodies than are adults. My 7-year-old nephew was able to tell me that he knew he was anxious about going back to school because he had butterflies in his bottom. Children can often locate body sensations better than we can.

Simple Mindfulness Techniques to Use With Bereaved Children

All bereaved children need accurate, age-appropriate information about the family member who died. Children are also entitled to their grief and to be part of family and community rituals marking the death. A small number of children will benefit from more targeted bereavement counseling, but most bereaved children can navigate their way through grief with the help of supportive adults in their lives, adults who will answer their questions honestly and respect their need to grieve and the need to intersperse their grief with the business of being a child. Simple mindfulness techniques can be useful in providing children with the skills to meet their grief in a safe way and to develop the capacity to tolerate the strong emotions and thoughts that accompany grief. Most important, through mindfulness, bereaved children can learn to self-soothe and to self-regulate, which makes the grief path a little less scary.

One example of using mindfulness with bereaved children is the use of mindful breathing as an anchor. The following techniques can be useful.

1. Ask children to lie down with a stuffed toy on their chest and simply watch it rise and fall. Older children or teens may prefer to use a book or a mobile phone. This exercise can be used to help children calm down or when there are strong emotions present.
2. Teach children to notice thoughts arising about the person who died and help them understand that thoughts are just thoughts. They come and they go, just like feelings.
3. Encourage children to locate their grief feelings in their body. Ask questions such as "Where do you feel the sadness in your body?" "How do you know that you feel mad?" "Can you describe that guilty feeling in your tummy?" "If your sadness had a face, what would it look like?" "If mad was a color, what would it be?" "Does it feel hot or cold? Hard or soft?" Most children can relate to questions like these, but you may need to adjust the nature of the inquiry depending on the child you are working with.
4. Encourage bereaved children to observe the grief from the safety of their breath and to notice what happens when they breathe right into that place in their body that holds the grief.

Unless you are a trained mindfulness teacher, it is important to keep the practices general and simple. Any practices will, of course, need to fit the emotional and cognitive developmental level of the child. These simple practices can be very powerful; they are an opportunity for children to learn that the only way through grief is through grief. Children can easily learn to use their breath as their anchor as they move up close to their grief feelings, and they can learn that when they need a break from these feelings they can shift their attention away from the strong emotion and back to the breath. Consider using practices to help children notice how grief is held in the body, how they can choose where they place their attention, and how feelings begin to change as we pay attention to them.

KEY POINTS

- Service providers are encouraged to develop their own mindfulness practice as a way of managing death anxiety when working with grieving families.
- Mindfulness practices can be a useful support to bereaved families on their grief journey.
- Bereaved children can be introduced to simple mindfulness practices to help them understand and cope with their grief.

Discussion Questions

1. Review your own practice. Are there ways you might begin, or deepen, your own mindfulness practice to support your work with bereaved families?

2. Review the mindfulness techniques you already incorporate into your grief work. Which mindfulness practices might benefit someone you are currently supporting through bereavement?

3. What benefits do you notice in your clients when you include mindfulness in your bereavement work?

Suggested Readings

Cacciatore J, Flint M: ATTEND: toward a mindfulness-based bereavement care model. Death Stud 36(1):61–82, 201224567995

Campbell J, Christopher J: Teaching mindfulness to create effective counselors. J Ment Health Couns 34(3):213–226, 2012

Stang H: Mindfulness and Grief. London, CICO Books, 2014

References

Bruce N, Shapiro SL, Constantino MJ, et al: Psychotherapist mindfulness and the psychotherapy process. Psychotherapy (Chic) 47(1):83–97, 2010 22402003

Cacciatore J: ATTEND: Towards a patient-centred model of psycho-social care, in Still Birth: Prediction, Prevention, and Management. Edited by Spong C. West Sussex, UK, Wiley Blackwell, 2011, pp 203–228

Cacciatore J, Flint M: ATTEND: toward a mindfulness-based bereavement care model. Death Stud 36(1):61–82, 2012 24567995

Campbell J, Christopher J: Teaching mindfulness to create effective counselors. J Ment Health Couns 34(3):213–226, 2012

Kersting A, Wagner B: Complicated grief after perinatal loss. Dialogues Clin Neurosci 14(2):187–194, 2012 22754291

Kersting A, Brähler E, Glaesmer H, et al: Prevalence of complicated grief in a representative population-based sample. J Affect Disord 131(1):339–343, 2011 21216470

Klass D: The Spiritual Lives of Bereaved Parents. Philadelphia, PA, Taylor & Francis, 1999

Lewis CS: A Grief Observed. London, Faber & Faber, 1968

Neimeyer RA, Young-Eisendrath P: Assessing a Buddhist treatment for bereavement and loss: the mustard seed project. Death Stud 39(1–5):263–273, 2015 25365540

O'Flanagan S: Moving mindfully with grief: testing the efficacy of a mindfulness-based cognitive therapy intervention for prolonged grief disorder. Unpublished MLitt thesis, Irish Hospice Foundation Library, Dublin, 2013

Rando TA: Bereaved parents: particular difficulties, unique factors, and treatment issues. Soc Work 30(1):19–23, 1985 10270480

Stang H: Mindfulness and Grief. London, CICO Books, 2014

Thich Nhat Hanh: Peace Is Every Step: The Path of Mindfulness in Everyday Life. New York, Bantam Books, 1992

Thieleman K, Cacciatore J: Witness to suffering: mindfulness and compassion fatigue among traumatic bereavement volunteers and professionals. Soc Work 59(1):34–41, 2014 24640229

Wolterstorff N: Lament for a Son. Grand Rapids, MI, Williamm B Eerdmans, 1987

Chapter 8

Substance Abuse

Sam Himelstein, Ph.D.
Alejandro Nunez, B.A.

AS EXEMPLIFIED in the wide range of topics covered in this book, it is clear that mindfulness offers value to a diverse set of populations for a wide array of psychological concerns. Alongside the advancements in research, the first author, S.H., has taught mindfulness to substance-abusing teenagers for more than 10 years. This experience has given S.H. the opportunity to offer a number of anecdotes that will be discussed in this chapter along with original research. As mindfulness has grown in popularity, it has also grown with niche interests (e.g., use of mindfulness as an effective intervention with young people who abuse drugs and alcohol). In this chapter we provide foundational knowledge for how mindfulness can be an effective treatment tool and review the therapeutic process and core ways in which mindfulness can be used with adolescents.

Mindfulness With Addiction Populations: A Brief Review of the Literature

Preliminary results from studies researching mindfulness with addiction populations are promising. Bowen et al. (2006) conducted a meditation study with prisoners in a correctional setting in the Pacific Northwest. A total of 305 adult inmates volunteered to participate in a 10-day Vipassana course. Of these participants, 173 completed posttest measures. Multiple scales were used to assess daily drinking and drug use, impulse control, thought suppression, psychiatric symptoms, and optimism prior to the course. Follow-up assessments were also conducted at 3 and 6 months after completion of the course. Results showed a decrease in the use of alcohol, marijuana, and crack cocaine at the 3-month follow-up assessment ($P<0.05$). Furthermore, decreases in psychiatric symptoms and increases in optimism and internal locus of control related to alcohol were also significant ($P<0.05$). In a similar study, Simpson et al. (2007) measured daily alcohol and drug use, impulse control, and posttraumatic stress disorder symptoms prior to the course and at 3-month follow-up. As in the study by Bowen and colleagues, participants demonstrated significant differences that did not manifest for the control groups. The decrease in alcohol and drug use ($P<0.001$) 3 months after completion of the course suggested that the meditation course may have been beneficial in reducing substance use in prison populations (Simpson et al. 2007).

Bowen et al. (2011) developed the mindfulness-based relapse prevention (MBRP) program, an 8-week intervention modeled after Kabat-Zinn's (1996, 2013) mindfulness-based stress reduction, Segal et al.'s (2013) mindfulness-based cognitive therapy, and Marlatt's relapse prevention (Marlatt and Gordon 1985). Research examining MBRP has been promising. Bowen et al. (2009) conducted a randomized control trial with 168 participants who had recently completed intensive inpatient or outpatient treatment for alcohol and drug use disorders. Participants were randomly assigned to either an 8-week MBRP course or a standard aftercare group. Substance use measures were administered before and after treatment and at 2- and 4-month follow-ups. Participants in the MBRP group demonstrated significantly greater decreases in drug cravings than did those in the control group. MBRP group participants also demonstrated significantly fewer days using substances than did the control groups.

Mindfulness-based interventions also have been the subject of pilot studies with youth dealing with substance use disorders (Himelstein 2011; Himelstein et al. 2014, 2015). Himelstein (2011) conducted a study investigating the impact of a mindfulness-based intervention on self-regulation, attitudes toward drugs, and impulsiveness in 60 incarcerated male youth. Results showed that impulsiveness decreased significantly, and perceived risk of drugs significantly increased from pretest to posttest. Additionally, Himelstein et al. (2014) conducted a grounded theory study in order to develop teaching methods for effective mindfulness instruction to adolescents. Ten participants were taught various mindfulness meditations over a 10-week period. At the end of the 10-week period, participants' self-report measures reflected improved self-regulation and problem solving and a decrease in substance use as a result of the mindfulness practice. Furthermore, in a pilot randomized clinical trial conducted by Himelstein et al. (2015), 44 participants recruited from a juvenile detention camp received mindfulness training for 10–12 weeks. Test results suggested that both problem solving and self-esteem significantly improved at the end of the mindfulness training period. Most notably, self-esteem scores increased at significantly higher rates in the mindfulness training group than in the control group. These studies demonstrated the feasibility of using mindfulness as an intervention with substance-abusing youth.

Therapy Process

As noted in the aforementioned research, mindfulness is promising as an intervention for youth struggling with substance abuse. This is in part because of the impact mindfulness can have on many comorbid issues (e.g., depression, anxiety, impulsiveness) that arise with substance abuse and in part because the practice of mindfulness targets critical aspects of relapse prevention: awareness of and response to cravings and general life insights. See the other chapters in Part II for examples of working with youth with various clinical diagnoses.

Mindfulness practice enhances awareness of craving for a substance in the moment and enhances the ability to consciously choose an action in response to the craving (i.e., self-regulation), and sustained practice may offer insight into or perspective on why substances were sought in the first place. As in standard substance abuse treatment with adolescents, assessment, therapist and patient expectations, and core treatment goals are vital to a positive outcome.

Use of Assessment

In most psychotherapeutic interventions, assessment determines specific treatment objectives and goals. Working with substance-abusing adolescents is no different. Although standard substance abuse assessment information is critical, detailed discussion of assessment tools is beyond the scope of this chapter (for a comprehensive review of substance abuse assessment, see Juhnke 2017). Instead, we focus on how and when mindfulness may be indicated as an appropriate intervention for substance-abusing adolescents. It is crucial to understand that mindfulness is absolutely not appropriate for all youth, let alone all those who abuse substances. Youth who are experiencing active psychotic symptoms, are severely depressed, and/or have high levels of trauma should be approached with caution. For example, youth who have active psychotic symptoms and are severely depressed may find practicing mindfulness meditation particularly decompensating. Recent research has shown that meditative experiences can lead to depersonalization and other negative experiences (Lindahl et al. 2017). Youth who have been victims of extreme trauma may find it difficult to follow cognitive-based directions and may feel a sense of inner regulation when closing their eyes. They can even become hyperaroused because of past traumatic experiences, traumatic triggers, mistrust, discomfort, and/or physical or mental experiences that arise from the meditation practice. Further, mindfulness may prove difficult to use with resistant youth. These youth may simply not want to engage. Attempting to force or manipulate youth to practice mindfulness will only lead to impasse. Therefore, the above situations should trigger caution among clinicians who wish to teach mindfulness, and clinical judgment and intuition should be leveraged as necessary.

Mindfulness meditation is simply one aspect of mindfulness practice, and many other informal mindfulness techniques can be implemented that do not necessarily have the same contraindications as above. Although most mindfulness interventions incorporate both forms of mindfulness (formal meditation and informal activities), it is unclear if both lead to positive outcomes from a research standpoint. I (S.H.) can say with full confidence from my anecdotal experience with patients that both mindfulness meditation and informal mindfulness techniques can be very powerful, and sometimes, informal mindfulness techniques can be a gateway to helping patients who are resistant or for whom meditation may be contraindicated be more open to and ready for (from an emotion regulation standpoint) formal meditation.

Therapeutic Frame

Mindfulness-based substance abuse treatment with adolescents can be lengthy. Mindfulness-based substance abuse treatment (MBSAT; Himelstein and Saul 2016) is a 12-session 1.5-hour weekly program, mostly by circumstance. Most group-based substance abuse interventions are between 8 and 16 sessions because it is difficult to maintain program participation beyond that timeline. Ideally, individual youth and their families would be assessed via a comprehensive clinical interview to determine treatment needs, which may include a program such as MBSAT along with individual and family counseling for anywhere between 4 months to a year of treatment. Although a detailed summary is beyond the scope of this chapter, some of the best outcome research for substance-abusing adolescents comes from family-based interventions.

Expectations for the Therapist

In our view, it is highly probable that the most important factor in teaching mindfulness to substance-abusing youth is the clinician. In psychotherapy, it seems to be a truth that in general, patients who view the therapist as caring and genuinely wanting to help and who perceive the therapy relationship or alliance to be strong tend to have a higher likelihood of achieving a better outcome. This is arguably more crucial when working with young people. Therapist qualities and practices that enhance outcome with youth include but are not limited to authenticity, skillful self-disclosure, and an alternative stance on behavioral change. We will review each in brief and refer the reader to Himelstein (2013) and Himelstein and Saul (2016) for a more in-depth analysis.

AUTHENTICITY

Working with teenagers, let alone substance-abusing teens, requires a commitment to authenticity if a goal of patient receptiveness is desired. Adolescents are in the process of developing their identity, and youth who struggle with both trust issues and extreme trauma need guidance from caring adults who are consistent in authenticity. Trying to "fit in" with youth often leads to the opposite effect than intended: a decrease in a sense of safety rather than an increase. Frankly put: be yourself. Do not try to adopt slang or mannerisms of the youth you work with if they aren't part of your already established authentic way of being. Youth will sense the inauthenticity, and it will be extremely difficult to develop trust. It is possible to be your authentic self, establish rapport, and maintain a sense of professionalism.

SKILLFUL SELF-DISCLOSURE

Inevitably, when working with young people, you will get asked about yourself. How you respond sets the tone for the type of relationship you develop with your patients. If you opt to not say anything about your own life history, preferences, or values, it's not that you cannot work with young people, it's just that you may encounter more impasses than if you skillfully and appropriately self-disclose.

What is skillful self-disclosure? It's always asking oneself prior to disclosing, "is this in the best interest of the patient?" You may not always be right, but asking that question leads to a better chance of being skillful. For example, the most common question that arises when I (S.H.) facilitate trainings on the topic is how to respond when a young person asks if you have used or currently use drugs and/or alcohol. There is no simple answer. Sometimes sharing that you have used or haven't used drugs is indicated; other times it is not. Disclosing that you have not used has its own set of advantages and disadvantages. The critical aspect is asking oneself how, if at all, disclosure is in the best interest of the patient. It could be, for example, that a youth is looking for connection and is feeling isolated in his or her experience, in which case offering your experience could provide hope. Other times, it may prompt more resistance or even colluding with a patient. The more you practice skillful self-disclosure (or contemplating it via case conceptualization), the better you will get at discerning when it is indicated.

ALTERNATIVE STANCE ON BEHAVIORAL CHANGE

The last of the therapist qualities discussed here is to not force change—in this case, demanding that a youth stop using drugs. There are many people in the youth's lives who can and do have the right to do so (e.g., parents, probation officers, judges), but if you pass harsh judgment on youth for using and try to manipulate them to get clean, they will often push back, and an impasse will occur (unless they have an explicit goal to get clean). This doesn't mean that a clinician should give up or not be concerned about risky behaviors such as drug use and delinquency. Rather, the path to addressing such issues is not direct confrontation but the building of the authentic relationship—trust, connection, alliance—so the clinician can leverage the relationship to discuss behavior. This mainly applies to youth who do not want to change (e.g., stop using drugs) and are resistant in treatment. In this situation, focus treatment goals on developing self-awareness and building the therapeutic relationship. Often, when I (S.H.) first meet a young person in substance abuse treatment, I state that I am not there to tell him or her what to do or judge him or her. I indicate that I simply have an intention to be authentic, to build a relationship, and to help the patient build self-awareness. The sighs of relief I get from young people in that first session after hearing that brief spiel are evident of the constant pressuring and "demands" they get from adults. Such demands do not work and often create resistance.

Core Treatment Goals

Treatment objectives and goals are heavily related to both therapist and patient expectations. Treatment plans should be uniquely tailored to the needs of the youth; however, a couple of general goals related specifically to this mindfulness-based approach are indicated:

Develop an authentic relationship. This goal is met by the objectives of building rapport (i.e., initial comfort and trust in the beginning stages of treatment), developing a clear alliance (i.e., being on the same page about what you're doing in treatment), and intentionally strengthening the therapeutic relationship over time as appropriate.

Increase self-awareness. This goal is met by the objectives of practicing self-awareness exercises (i.e., mindfulness) to increase general emotional awareness and self-knowledge and by increasing insight into substance use.

Other treatment goals may be agreed on depending on circumstances. For example, some youth do in fact want to decrease or quit drug use all together. For those youth, setting an explicit goal to stop use can be appropriate. For other youth who may be resistant to quitting use, a goal might be developed around "not needing" the substance and practicing tapering off of it (i.e., a harm reduction approach) and learning to deal with an underlying issue that influences and causes use (e.g., social anxiety). Other goals related to family and peer relationships and other external variables such as school or delinquency should be tailored to the unique needs and strengths of the patient.

Core Therapy Interventions and Techniques

The following core therapy interventions and techniques are an aggregate of practices from the MBSAT 12-session curriculum for youth and my (S.H.) more than 10 years of providing mindfulness-based intervention with substance-abusing youth. For emphasis, it is reiterated here that to be effective, all interventions and techniques depend on the quality of the therapy relationship.

Mindfulness Meditation Techniques

The mindfulness meditation practices offered in the MBSAT curriculum are obviously neither new nor invented by myself. However, in our research (see Himelstein et al. 2014), we found that it is worth considering how those standard mindfulness meditation practices are delivered and implemented with teenagers. We suggest a progression of mindfulness meditation techniques from tactile, easy-to-follow instructions with the potential for immediate positive outcome (i.e., feeling relaxed) to more abstract and difficult techniques (Himelstein et al. 2014). For example, both body scan meditation and mindfulness of deep breathing were rated highest among youth for techniques to teach first because of their simple, easy-to-follow instructions and the sometimes immediate physiological relaxation response (Himelstein et al. 2014). Thus, the progression of mindfulness meditation techniques in the MBSAT curriculum is as follows.

1. **Mindfulness of deep breathing.** In this technique, you specifically instruct youth to take slow, protracted deep breaths in and deep breaths out, with an option of placing theirs hands on the belly.

2. **Mindfulness of the breath.** In this technique, you instruct youth to keep their breath in awareness by focusing on the touch of the breath on the nostrils, belly, or chest. When the mind wanders, youth should nonjudgmentally bring their attention back to the breath. This is often the standard meditation taught to beginners in Western society; however, we found it too abstract for youth. It is therefore taught after a number of sessions of mindfulness of deep breathing, which is easier for young people to start with.

3. **Body scan.** In this technique, you instruct youth to systematically scan sensations in their body from head to toes or toes to head. Youth are encouraged to notice sensations and not judge them over time.

4. **Nonmoving body scan.** This technique is similar to the body scan, but you instruct youth not to move or readjust at all during the meditation. Youth often view this as a challenge and will compete at it with each other.

5. **Compassion practices.** We offer a number of compassion-based meditations that send compassion to family members, loved ones, the self, and so on. These are good practices to use when some form of concentration and mindfulness has been established through practice and youth have bought into the idea of mindfulness somewhat.

Informal Mindfulness Techniques

The MBSAT curriculum also has a number of informal mindfulness techniques that can be taught without having youth close their eyes and engage in meditation. These techniques do not require the facilitator to even mention the words *mindfulness* or *meditation*. The following techniques are also not new; rather, they are versions of psychotherapeutic practices adapted specifically for substance-abusing adolescents.

1. **Mindful check-in.** This technique can also be called just a *check-in*. The premise is that the youth should take a deep breath and pause before checking in on his or her mental, emotional, and/or physical state. Articulate words are encouraged, and such words as "fine," "cool," "OK," and other nondescriptors are discouraged.

2. **STIC cognitive acronym.** Similar to other mindfulness-based cognitive acronyms, STIC is an acronym that fosters mindfulness and choice. STIC stands for stop, take a breath, imagine the future consequences, and choose. This technique can be taught individually or in groups and can be turned into such activities as role-plays or visualizations.

3. **Mindful eating.** This is an ancient technique; what's innovative is that we use it in the curriculum to highlight the urge often associated with food as a way to highlight urges and cravings related to drug use and other risky behaviors in order to help youth learn to recognize and forestall these urges.

4. **Mindful stretching.** Although not formally incorporated into the MBSAT curriculum, mindful stretching and movement are a great way to practice embodiment with young people, especially those with heightened arousal symptoms from trauma. Mindful stretching is distinct from traditional stretching exercises in that the connection of movement to breath is emphasized. I (S.H.) have used mindful stretching and movement with young people extensively as a centering exercise and as a core intervention. Mindful stretching is quite useful, especially for youth who have trouble meditating.

Insight-Oriented Interventions

Along with formal and informal mindfulness practices, insight is also a critical component of effective mindfulness-based substance abuse treatment with teenagers. Whereas the conceptual framework for the mindfulness techniques per se is to develop awareness and self-regulatory capacities for distress tolerance and craving control, insight-oriented interventions help young people understand the etiology of their substance use (and other behaviors) and contemplate future choices, meaning, and purpose. Insight-oriented interventions include but are not limited to identification of the following.

1. **Personal pros and cons of drug use.** We use the *decisional T* for getting youth to think about why they use drugs in the first place. The decisional T is the traditional method of creating two columns, with pros on one side and cons on the other side. In the MBSAT curriculum, it is implemented after a debate about the general pros and cons of drug use (to get the group thinking generally) and within the context of the question "How well do you know yourself?"
2. **Personal values.** This intervention can be implemented in individual and/or group settings. Youth are instructed to look at a number of nouns (e.g., trust, loyalty, family, self-awareness) either on a piece of paper in front of them or on Post-It notes on a wall and to pick their top two or three most important values and discuss why they chose them. This activity builds and solidifies self-knowledge and information gathered by the clinician used to highlight any discrepancies between the ideal presented values and the youths' actions (i.e., motivational interviewing).
3. **Personal triggers.** Important in substance abuse treatment is understanding one's triggers, and working with youth in this way is no different. In the MBSAT curriculum, youth are taught how to identify and categorize their triggers, along with techniques to regulate them as they arise. This is done via psychoeducation, process activities, and mindfulness practices.
4. **Knowledge of peers, family, and community.** Finally, youth are taught to contemplate the major relationships in their lives (family and peers) and how to

navigate the sometimes tumultuous territory associated with being an adolescent and how drugs sometimes mitigate those experiences. Youth are taught to identify who among their peers actually has their best interest at heart and how to start a dialogue with unhealthy accomplices and those who at times may pose as true friends in order to alter these relationships. Youth are also invited to think about their family and community context and how that has, if at all, influenced their drug use and other behaviors. Mindfulness and other contemplative activities are used to meet these objectives.

Psychoeducation on fatal drug combinations and how drugs impact the central nervous system are also helpful interventions. Table 8–1 lists the table of contents from the MBSAT 12-session curriculum to offer the reader some perspective on how the above core interventions are incorporated sequentially. This program was originally developed for groups of youth; however, it can be adapted for individual psychotherapy and some aspects of family psychotherapy.

Cultural and Other Individual Adaptations

If you plan on facilitating the MBSAT curriculum or using mindfulness with youth of diverse ethnic and gender backgrounds, it is extremely important to consider the diversity issues that may arise. You own cultural competence will be of extreme importance. Substance abuse and addiction are heavily interrelated with some of the socioeconomic issues related to marginalized communities, and it is important to understand these conjunctions (e.g., understanding the complexity and oppressive policies in the war on drugs and how those policies affect certain communities).

As discussed previously, another key aspect of working with young people from ethnically diverse backgrounds is authenticity. It is important to have a real, genuine, and honest approach to the challenges that at-risk youth face on a daily basis. Considering that communities of color experience vastly disproportionate mental health problems and are hindered by a lack of resources, we   as clinicians must be authentic in our approach to provide help and services to individuals who have been historically marginalized. Acknowledging our own place of privilege is an important step toward developing authenticity. Additionally, considering the cultural differences that can arise, it is important to use culturally relevant metaphors and examples when working with ethnically diverse groups. Cultural barriers are bound to arise, but in being authentic and honest in our interactions and being willing to be humble, accepting, and understanding of our own privilege, we can find ways to improve the therapeutic dynamic and reach our therapeutic goals.

TABLE 8–1. Mindfulness-based substance abuse treatment 12-session curriculum

Session	Title	Session agenda
1	Introduction to the program	• Informal greeting • Program overview • Group agreements • Defining mindfulness • Mindfulness of deep breathing • Group poll[a]
2	Mindfulness of drugs and their health effects	• Mindful check-in • Drug classifications • Fatal combinations • Mindfulness of deep breathing
3	Reacting vs. responding	• Role-play • Definitions of reacting and responding • STIC contemplation • STIC role-plays • Mindfulness of the breath • Mindful check-in
4	Mindfulness of delusion	• Shel Silverstein poem "The Perfect High"[b] • Mindful check-in • Pros and cons debate • Personal pros and cons of drug use • Body scan meditation
5	Emotional awareness	• Emotional categories • Emotional expression and gender norms • "Stand if" activity[c] • Deep disclosure • Game: Concentration[d]
6	The brain and drugs	• Mindful check-in • Brain presentation I • Meditation break • Brain presentation II • Body scan
7	Mindfulness of craving	• Mindful check-in • Mindful eating • Role of craving in drug use • Nonmoving body scan • Worksheet: roots of craving
8	Mindfulness of triggers	• Mindful check-in • Mindfulness of triggers • Three levels of influence • Noting awareness meditation

TABLE 8–1. Mindfulness-based substance abuse treatment 12-session curriculum *(continued)*

Session	Title	Session agenda
9	The family system and drugs	• "My children" contemplation[e] • Effects of drug use on family relationships • Addiction and intergenerational trauma • Compassion for family meditation
10	Mindfulness of the peer system	• Peer pressure role play • Discussion: friends vs. accomplices • Mindful check-in with prompt • Mindful communication • Youth-developed peer pressure skits • Meditation: compassion for friends and accomplices
11	Mindfulness of the external environment	• Mindful check-in • Mindfulness of the external environment • Transforming systems of influence • Meditation: compassion toward community
12	Closing ceremony	• Final meditation practice • Mindful check-in • Focus group • Group appreciations • Food celebration • Certificate of completion • Closing ceremony

[a]The final activity of the session is to take a brief poll on what the youth may want to learn during the course of the curriculum. This can help the clinician better understand the needs of the youth in regard to the idea of recovery and drug use.

[b]In "The Perfect High," a boy embarks on a search to find a guru who supposedly knows how to obtain the perfect high but is severely disappointed when he hears that the high is "inside oneself." The poem is a great teaching tool to highlight the role of delusion in drug use.

[c]The "Stand if" activity involves the reading of approximately 10 statements. Youth are instructed to stand up if the experience from the statement has been true for them. After everyone has sat back down, youth then take a few deep breaths and notice what thoughts, feelings, and images arose during the activity.

[d]The game "Concentration" is a built-in deescalator activity designed to help youth move from ruminating on the potentially tough experiences that arise from previous activities. Participants stand in a circle, a category is chosen, and on a clapping rhythm and beat, each participant has to say a specific thing from the category without hesitating or repeating words.

[e]The "My children" contemplation guides youth to think about the impact their decisions have had on their parents or caregivers. Youth are led to imagine what it would be like to have children who engaged in behaviors they have engaged in themselves (e.g., drug use, violence, illegal activities).

Abbreviation. STIC = stop, take a breath, imagine the future consequences, choose.

Source. Adapted from Himelstein and Saul 2016.

Evaluation of the Approach

Research conducted on the MBSAT curriculum thus far has focused primarily on feasibility and process, with one randomized controlled outcome study. In the first study of the curriculum, we investigated the effects of an adapted, 8-week version of the program on a sample of 60 male youth incarcerated at a juvenile detention camp (Himelstein 2011). Self-reported impulsivity, perceived drug risk, and healthy self-regulation assessments were administered before and after the 8-week program, with a total of $N=48$ participants completing both pretest and posttest measures. Paired t tests revealed a significant decrease in impulsiveness at posttest ($P<0.01$) and a significant increase in perceived drug risk ($P<0.05$). There were no significant differences found regarding healthy self-regulation at posttest. Although this study had important research method limitations (e.g., no control groups), it points toward the feasibility of using mindfulness as an intervention for adolescents dealing with substance abuse issues and lends credence to the idea that mindfulness coupled with substance abuse treatment could have the potential to increase participants' degree of perceived risk associated with drug use.

As the curriculum has been further developed, we have gathered data from participants regarding the efficacy of the meditations used in the curriculum. From these results, it was found that when starting out in the program, adolescents tend to prefer meditations or techniques that are tangible and easy to follow and remember (e.g., deep breathing, body scan). In a larger grounded theory study, we investigated the experiences and opinions of 40 incarcerated adolescents (Himelstein et al. 2014). Participants were asked about their experiences and preferences specifically regarding their receptiveness to the overall intervention, drug education, and relapse prevention strategies (not including mindfulness meditation). For this study, Corbin and Strauss's (1990) grounded theory approach was used to develop a theory for how to effectively facilitate group-based substance abuse interventions with adolescents. Results revealed that participants felt open to learning drug education information and to actually attempt relapse strategies when facilitators fostered authentic relationships and weren't overly concerned with forcing behavioral change (i.e., reducing drug use). Adoption of a harm reduction approach as opposed to an abstinence-only approach was found to facilitate a more open and positive atmosphere, including freedom of expression. These results are primarily concerned with the process of implementing this intervention rather than the outcomes among participants. From our results, it is clear that some of the relapse prevention mindfulness strategies used in this curriculum can have benefit (Himelstein et al. 2014). One youth who was interviewed described his ability to use the STIC acronym to abstain from drug use while on a home pass from a juvenile detention camp. He encountered a close friend for the first time since his friend had become wheelchair bound as a result of gun violence:

> I ain't gonna lie. I was supposed to not come back to camp, and I was supposed to hit the blunt [marijuana] when I was in the house. 'Cause my boy, when we got back to the house, he was out there rolling a blunt. I ain't gonna lie, once I seen him in the wheelchair, I already knew I was gonna do something: drink or something.... I used STIC. I kinda looked at him...and I took a deep breath and just calmed down, sat down, and I was like, "Damn man, it's good to see you." But at the same time I was really thinkin' about the blunt. He was like, "You gonna smoke?" I was like, "Nah, I'm good." He was like, "Fool, what the fuck? Since when do you say no?" I felt more me, doing me. I'm like, "Nah, I'm good"...you feel me? (Himelstein et al. 2014, pp. 566–567)

Last, in a pilot randomized clinical trial (Himelstein et al. 2015), 44 participants recruited from a juvenile detention camp were randomly assigned to either a treatment-as-usual group without incorporating mindfulness meditation or a treatment condition group that received mindfulness training as part of the psychotherapy. Treatment lasted 10–12 weeks, and participants were assessed preintervention and postintervention for locus of control, attitude toward drugs, self-esteem, decision making, and mindfulness. Self-report test results for both treatment and control groups showed that both decision making ($P<0.01$) and self-esteem ($P<0.05$) significantly increased from pretest to posttest. All other measures were found to be insignificant but moved in the expected direction. Interestingly, change scores for self-esteem increased at a significantly higher rate for the treatment group than for the control group ($P<0.05$), suggesting that mindfulness meditation coupled with psychotherapy may help foster self-esteem at a greater rate than psychotherapy alone.

Strengths

Although the studies mentioned in the previous subsection are limited in many ways, they do suggest the feasibility of using mindfulness as an intervention with adolescents dealing with substance abuse issues. As summarized in the evaluation of the approach, a number of key aspects of the intervention results suggest why mindfulness can be beneficial as a treatment intervention for adolescents dealing with substance abuse issues. These include, but are not limited to, an increased ability to manage strong emotions, reduced impulsiveness, reduced stress, decreased cravings to use drugs, ability to observe drug cravings without reaction, decreased stress, increased overall well-being, perception of increased risk in drug use, and, ultimately, decreased drug use. All in all, these stated benefits are critical skills for adolescents attempting to reduce the frequency of substance use or other unhealthy behaviors.

Areas for Development

Although the results in the previous subsection are promising, much more research is needed. More advanced randomized clinical designs, study of dependent variables such as trauma and recidivism, and qualitative data to further highlight the experience of young people are needed. However, such designs can be challenging to implement within a community-based participatory research model. It is very difficult to conduct randomized clinical trials in community or correctional settings because most organizations do not want to deal with the constraints of random assignment. As I (S.H.) have been told many times by collaborative gatekeepers, "We already know who needs the treatment." Balancing the importance of advanced-design research with the importance of helping the youth being served is critical to developing and maintaining community partnerships.

Conclusion

In this chapter we have reviewed a mindfulness-based approach to engaging substance-abusing adolescents and have discussed the therapy process, therapist expectations, and core interventions and techniques. Although promising advancements have taken place, further research is needed to develop the field. For clinicians looking to implement mindfulness into substance abuse work with young people, it is important to focus on building authentic relationships with patients. Start with easy-to-follow instructions and techniques that often result in immediate outcome (e.g., deep breathing, body scan) and remember to use informal mindfulness activities to facilitate mindfulness.

In addition, having your own practice is critical to being successful at facilitating mindfulness with youth. As a practitioner, you should develop and sustain a regular meditation practice, practice mindfulness in daily life, and have an overarching commitment to broadly defined self-awareness. This will ensure a constant strengthening of awareness around your practice and the limits of your practices, and overall, this will be a service to your patients.

KEY POINTS

- Focus on building authentic relationships with your patients.
- When introducing mindfulness meditation, start with easy-to-follow instructions and techniques that often result in immediate outcome (e.g., deep breathing, body scan).

- Do not rely solely on mindfulness meditation. Use informal mindfulness activities to facilitate mindfulness.
- Do not force someone who is extremely opposed to mindfulness to practice meditation or mindfulness. This kind of imposition of mindfulness will only lead to impasse.

Discussion Questions

1. What are some challenges therapists encounter when building authentic relationships with patients?

2. What are some instances in which using informal meditation practices may be a better alternative to using formal mindfulness activities with substance-abusing teens?

3. Considering the lack of resources in underserved at-risk communities, what are some ways that core components of an evidence-based mindfulness practices can be integrated into daily lives and across communities at large?

Suggested Readings

Himelstein S: A Mindfulness-Based Approach to Working With High-Risk Adolescents, Vol 35. New York, Routledge, 2013

Himelstein S, Saul S: Mindfulness-Based Substance Abuse Treatment for Adolescents: 12-Session Curriculum. New York, Routledge, 2016

Himelstein S, Saul S, Garcia-Romeu A: Does mindfulness meditation increase effectiveness of substance abuse treatment with incarcerated youth? A pilot randomized controlled trial. Mindfulness 6:1472–1480, 2015

References

Bowen S, Witkiewitz K, Dillworth TM, et al: Mindfulness meditation and substance use in an incarcerated population. Psychol Addict Behav 20(3):343–347, 2006 16938074

Bowen S, Chawla N, Collins SE, et al: Mindfulness-based relapse prevention for substance use disorders: a pilot efficacy trial. Subst Abus 30(4):295–305, 2009 19904665

Bowen S, Chawla N, Marlatt GA: Mindfulness-Based Relapse Prevention for Addictive Behaviors: A Clinician's Guide, Vol 1. New York, Guilford, 2011

Corbin J, Strauss A: Grounded theory research: procedures, canons, and evaluative criteria. Qual Sociol 13(1):3–21, 1990

Himelstein S: Mindfulness-based substance abuse treatment for incarcerated youth: a mixed-methods study. International Journal of Transpersonal Studies 30:1–30, 2011

Himelstein S: A Mindfulness-Based Approach to Working With High-Risk Adolescents, Vol 35. New York, Routledge, 2013

Himelstein S, Saul S: Mindfulness-Based Substance Abuse Treatment for Adolescents: A 12-Session Curriculum. New York, Routledge, 2016

Himelstein S, Saul S, Garcia-Romeu A, et al: Mindfulness training as an intervention for substance user incarcerated adolescents: a pilot grounded theory study. Subst Use Misuse 49(5):560–570, 2014 24611851

Himelstein S, Saul S, Garcia-Romeu A: Does mindfulness meditation increase effectiveness of substance abuse treatment with incarcerated youth? A pilot randomized controlled trial. Mindfulness 6:1472–1480, 2015

Juhnke GA: Substance Abuse Assessment and Diagnosis: A Comprehensive Guide for Counselors and Helping Professionals. New York, Routledge, 2017

Kabat-Zinn J: Full Catastrophe Living: How to Cope With Stress, Pain, and Illness Using Mindfulness Meditation. New York, Dell, 1996

Kabat-Zinn J: Full Catastrophe Living: Using the Wisdom of Your Body and Mind to Face Stress, Pain, and Illness. New York, Bantam, 2013

Lindahl JR, Fisher NE, Cooper DJ, et al: The varieties of contemplative experience: a mixed-methods study of meditation-related challenges in Western Buddhists. PLoS One 12(5):e0176239, 2017 28542181

Marlatt GA, Gordon JR: Relapse and Prevention: Maintenance Strategies in the Treatment of Addictive Behaviors. New York, Guilford, 1985

Segal ZV, Williams JMG, Teasedale JD: Mindfulness-based Cognitive Therapy for Depression, 2nd Edition, New York, NY, Guilford, 2013

Simpson TL, Kaysen D, Bowen S, et al: PTSD symptoms, substance use, and Vipassana meditation among incarcerated individuals. J Trauma Stress 20(3):239–249, 2007 17597132

Chapter 9

Autism Spectrum Disorders

Allison Morgan, M.A., OTR, E-RYT
Erik Jacobson, Ph.D.

SAM sits in the back of the classroom, with his aide keeping a watchful eye. The teacher is leading the class in a new math lesson. The overhead lights are dimmed while the students focus their visual attention on the colorfully illuminated, interactive smart board. Several students in this third-grade class are moving about the room to get a drink of water, go to the bathroom, or sharpen a pencil. A peer seated next to Sam drops his pencil, and it rolls under Sam's desk. A voice comes over the intercom to announce that recess will be held outside. The classroom erupts in excitement. The volume of the teacher's voice increases tenfold to quickly regain control and the attention of her students. Some semblance of silence resumes within the open space until the vibrating hum of a lawn mower begins to seep through the windows.

Sam is a student with autism spectrum disorder. His ability to take in, process, and respond to the multitude of pieces of information coming from the surrounding environment is compromised. For Sam, each of these minute, momentary events and subtle interactions are an immense distraction that has the potential to wreak havoc within his body and mind. Each individual sensory, communication, and cognitive challenge can be perceived as a threat to his nervous system, diverting his attention from learning to preserving his own sense of internal safety. Protecting a highly sensitive and easily overwhelmed nervous system is paramount for individuals with autism.

Sam begins to tighten his fists and rise up onto his toes. He squints his eyes, purses his lips, and begins to rock his torso back and forth. Sam's aide has learned that these behaviors are his quickest form of communication when he can't find the words to verbally express how he feels and what he needs. He uses his body to deliver the message "I am overwhelmed." His aide grabs a chair and sits beside Sam so as to not cause a distraction in the classroom. She begins to breathe deeply into her belly, a mindful breathing tool called *center breath* from a yoga and mindfulness program used in Sam's classroom called Educate 2B, a curriculum to support educators and therapists in sharing breathing, movement, and mindfulness activities with elementary-age students. Sam's school therapists, teacher, and aide attended a 1-day workshop provided by Zensational Kids to learn how to infuse these activities into the natural setting of the classroom.

Sam's aide then points to a picture card taped to Sam's desk that provides an illustration of a boy touching the fingertips of one hand to the fingertips of the other hand. This is the starting position for another Educate 2B mindful breathing tool, the *energy ball* (for directions for this tool, see the Appendix, "Educate 2B Exercises," at the end of the chapter). Sam knows exactly what to do to complete this breathing technique because he has practiced it in his class every day for the past 2 months. His teacher leads the entire class in short breaks throughout the day, practicing mindful breathing, movement, and guided visualizations. Sam follows the visual direction of the card on his desk and brings his fingertips together at the center of his body. He takes several deep breaths, expanding the energy ball as he draws his hands apart, filling his belly with breath and imagining a ball of energy between his hands. He exhales, bringing his fingertips together to touch again, focusing on containing the energy and getting his fingertips to reconnect.

After Sam completes several rounds of the energy ball quietly at his desk, his heels regain contact with the floor. His shoulders no longer flank his ears. His face relaxes. His body stills. Although he has missed part of the lesson while taking a few minutes to ground himself, he is able to refocus his attention and engage in learning again.

Prior to beginning the Educate 2B program, Sam would have needed to be excused from the classroom. His episodes of being overwhelmed typically escalated into rage, possibly due to his heightened level of anxiety. In his distressed state, he would begin to write on his paper and then erase incessantly until the paper ripped. Pencils would then be broken in half. Desk and chair might be toppled to the ground. The disarray of Sam's internal state would become a mirror to what would quickly ensue in the rest of the classroom. Heads would turn and eyes widen as the rest of the class observed his behavior, compounding Sam's social isolation from his peers.

In this chapter, we share our journeys as we discovered mindfulness through our personal and professional experiences. Having worked with a diverse set of special needs youth populations for a combined 50 years, we share a tremendous desire to help children with autism spectrum disorder (ASD) develop the necessary skills to thrive while maintaining a deep appreciation for their unique differences and abilities. Allison Morgan provides practical experience of adapting mindfulness-based approaches to the needs of children with ASD through her therapeutic practice as an occupational therapist and the formation of her approach of Zensational Kids and its classroom program, Educate 2B. Educate 2B teaches simple breathing, movement, and mindfulness exercises to help children develop inner resources of self-regulation, focused attention, and resilience. The program was designed to be integrated into traditional therapeutic approaches as well as a classroom setting. Erik Jacobson provides invaluable insight and evaluation into the approach and program from both an academic perspective and his own practical experience working as the chief psychologist at Upstate Cerebral Palsy Tradewinds Education Center, a residential treatment and education program in the state of New York serving children with the most complex developmental disabilities.

Through our combined professional experiences, we hope to help readers determine effective mindfulness methods that can be used universally to meet the needs of unique individuals, their community, and their therapists with ease, confidence, and reliable results. First, we introduce the effectiveness of mindfulness-based therapeutic programs for youth through review of the research. We briefly discuss the background medical history of ASD and analyze typical areas addressed in therapeutic interventions through the lens of adopting a mindfulness-based approach. We then introduce a model for sharing these practices with this population. Adaptations to the model are also suggested to allow the practices to become more accessible to varying learning styles and abilities. Specific meditation exercises are provided for you to use in initiating your own mindful practice as well as with the children and community you serve.

Literature Review of Autism Spectrum Disorder and Mindfulness

ASD is the fastest-growing developmental disorder in the United States. National statistics identify that 1 in 68 children in the United States are diagnosed with ASD, among which there is a significant increase in the diagnosis of boys (Christensen et al. 2016). ASD is a complex neurobiological developmental disorder. Individuals with ASD demonstrate a wide range of challenges, abilities, and gifts. Diagnostic symptoms include deficits in social communication, social interaction patterns, and restrictive and repetitive behavioral patterns.

Children with ASD are at an increased risk of experiencing mood dysregulation and deficits with self-regulation. Approximately 40% of children with ASD have at least one comorbid diagnosed anxiety disorder (van Steensel et al. 2011). Additional co-occurring symptoms in individuals with ASD include attention-deficit/hyperactivity disorder and depressive disorders (Belardinelli et al. 2016). Given the breadth of comorbidities experienced by children on the spectrum, it is common for children with ASD to face a variety of behavioral challenges, ranging from internalizing problems, such as self-injurious and highly repetitive behaviors, to external behaviors, such as tantrums and aggression toward others. Children with ASD often attempt to escape or avoid challenging situations, which is particularly difficult in the school setting. Reduction in interfering behaviors is one of the key areas addressed in treatment because it directly affects the everyday life of the child with ASD, as well as his or her caregivers, peers, teachers, and community.

Research With Youth

Over the past decade, there has been a growing body of evidence demonstrating the many benefits mindful practices can bring to neurotypical youth. Many of the findings confirm what we had anecdotally discovered. Initial results point to several benefits that may significantly assist children with ASD, such as increased active engagement and enhanced sense of well-being, self-awareness, and emotional control (Cook-Cottone 2017). Several studies also noted improved listening skills, reduction in stress-related symptoms, improved attention and concentration, and improved ability to manage emotions (Butzer et al. 2016, as cited in Cook-Cottone 2017). Youth participation in a mindful awareness practices program has been found to improve behavioral regulation, metacognition, and overall executive function. Flook and others found improvement in children's abilities to attend to their breath (initiating), focus on the breath and notice whether their attention has wandered (monitoring), and bring their attention back to the breath when the mind wanders (shifting) when mindful practices are taught (Flook et al. 2010, as cited in Cook-Cottone 2017).

Mindful practices such as breath awareness also help with developing self-regulation, an essential skill for coping with difficult life situations (Cook-Cottone 2017). Self-regulatory skills include the ability to manage emotions, engage, and interact in positive ways with others and the ability to establish appropriate behaviors based on the demands of a task or situation (Bronson 2000). Such skills are essential for children with ASD like Sam to develop so they may learn to proactively manage and become resilient to stressful situations within any environment that may be perceived as a threat or hindrance.

Foundational Research Inspiring the Use of Mindfulness for Autism Spectrum Disorder

Research on the application of mindfulness practices in the treatment of children with ASD is in its infancy. When Allison began this journey through developing Zensational Kids in 2008, research with this population was almost nonexistent. Because she was working in a school and often teaching these techniques to teachers and parents, the need for "proof" of her newfound modality was becoming more and more essential. Her education colleagues were accustomed to seeing scooter boards, swings, therabands, and weighted vests, typical equipment and materials used in therapy programs for students challenged with processing sensory information. The teachers were accustomed to using these types of external tools to facilitate inner states of being calm and focused; getting them to recognize that one's own breath, body, and mind are powerful tools as well was a bit of a challenge.

One of the most transformative aspects of using mindful practices as a treatment modality is that the tools for implementation are within us all the time. Mindful practices use our breath, our body, and our mind—things within us—to create change and balance within the nervous system. When students are able to access tools as they are needed in the moment, they become the facilitator of their own calm, focused, attentive, or peaceful states.

Although the teachers all noticed the positive changes within their students following our sessions, they were skeptical. At that time, the greatest evidence-based ally for mindfulness-based therapeutic interventions was the research of Dr. Herbert Benson, professor, author, cardiologist, Director Emeritus of the Benson-Henry Institute, and Mind Body Medicine Professor of Medicine at Harvard Medical School. His studies in the 1960s and 1970s demonstrated how a stress response can be deactivated, calming down the fight-flight-freeze centers of the brain. Benson found that a relaxation response can be elicited through visualization, breathing techniques, progressive muscle relaxation, and other mind-body practices (Benson and Klipper 1975).

In 1995, Stephen Porges introduced the polyvagal theory, providing a new perspective on the relationship between autonomic functioning and behavior (Porges 1995, as cited in Loizzo et al. 2017). Since that time, extensive research has been done to further explain the parasympathetic nervous system's role in not only calming the mind and body but also supporting social engagement behaviors and relieving anxiety (Hanson and Mendius 2009).

The research that examined the physiological changes that were occurring through mindfulness practices explained how the relaxation response was being activated, thereby helping students to achieve a calmer, more relaxed state, reducing the effects of anxiety and stress. We observed students becoming more engaged and less reactive in the classroom, long after our therapy session had ended. Their overall functioning during classroom activities was improving and their maladaptive and often disruptive behaviors were decreasing, all without explicitly addressing functional skills within the classroom such as handwriting, attention, and behavior.

Current Research for Therapeutic Use of Mindfulness for Autism Spectrum Disorder

Recent ASD research has found similar results as those studies performed with typically developing youth, such as improvements in attention, concentration, imitation skills, and self-regulation (Radhakrishna et al. 2010; Rosenblatt et al. 2011). Several research studies have also found a reduction in depression, anxiety, and rumination in intervention groups of adults and adolescents with ASD with a mindfulness-based therapy (MSD) that was modified for individuals with ASD (MBT-AS; de Bruin et al. 2014, as cited in Keenan-Mount et al. 2016; Spek et al. 2013).

Koenig et al. (2012) investigated the use of a 15- to 20-minute yoga video from the Get Ready to Learn program in self-contained classrooms with children with ASD. The video led the students and faculty through breathing techniques, mindful rhythmic movement, relaxation, and singing. Results showed decreases in maladaptive behavior and hyperactivity.

Singh et al. (2011) developed Soles of the Feet, a mindfulness-based technique to manage anger and aggression in youth with ASD. In the study, three male adolescents learned to maintain a meditative position while seated upright in a chair, hands resting on their laps, feet grounded on the floor. Using their breath as an anchor, they developed awareness of the present moment and became aware of negative thoughts that preceded an aggressive outburst. When negative thoughts occurred, they learned to shift their attention to a neutral object—the soles of their feet. Although the study employed a sample size of only three participants, results showed significant reduction in aggressive and injurious behaviors toward themselves and family members. General compliance also improved.

Although most of the studies within the ASD population had very small sample sizes (from as few as 3 participants to as many as 70 participants), results suggest that mindfulness practices not only can be taught to this population but also can elicit very beneficial results (for key details of significant current studies, refer to Table 9–1). It is also important to note that several of the studies were conducted in India, where familiarity with these practices may bring a level of acceptance and ease to implementing the activities, thus contributing to their positive results. A therapeutic approach that integrates mindfulness focuses on the development of inner awareness rather than explicitly addressing outward behaviors. When individuals learn to manage their internal state, the external behaviors tend to become more adaptive and appropriate as a natural consequence, leading us to believe that a therapeutic approach that integrates practices of mindfulness within its routinely instructed interventions may steadily provide children with ASD the tools to develop lifetime skills needed to succeed in their daily societal interactions and commitments, especially, but not limited to, within the classroom.

Core Benefits of Integrating a Mindful Practice for Children With Autism Spectrum Disorder

Mindfulness offers a holistic complement to many other models of therapeutic interventions. Therapies that address physical, cognitive, sensory, behavioral, and communicative challenges of ASD can benefit from the integration of mindfulness. The main goals of mindfulness for children with ASD, which can be applied in most therapeutic models, are as follows:

- Recognize internal states of dysregulation
- Develop an understanding of internal and external triggers that ignite the fight-flight-freeze response
- Identify emotions and notice how they manifest in the body and are communicated through behavior
- Use specific tools with greater independence to create ease within the nervous system
- Foster compassion for self and lovingkindness toward self and others

Principles to Guide You in Integrating Mindful Practices

Each of the above goals can be addressed through developing an awareness of breath, body, and mind. We may think of mindfulness practices as quiet, contemplative moments, seated upright on a cushion with legs crossed and spine straight. However, to help you understand how to share mindfulness with children with ASD, let's throw that picture out the window. These children are as unique as an individual's fingerprint. Their learning styles vary more greatly than those of their neurotypical counterparts, and these various learning styles must be considered when designing mindful practices that suit the children's variability and individuality. There are a few principles that we follow to guide us in sharing and developing accessible practices for students with all functional levels.

1. Mindfulness is a powerful practice for connecting you to the wisdom that is already inside you. This reservoir of inner knowledge is available to everyone—neurodiverse and neurotypical. It is nondiscriminatory. It awakens our capacity to see potential and possibilities where other people may see problems and deficits. As more therapeutic interventions begin to view

TABLE 9–1. Review of yoga and mindfulness therapeutic interventions for autism spectrum disorder

Author, design, and location	Participants	Content and facilitator	Duration	Data	Findings
de Bruin et al. 2014; pretest/posttest; Netherlands	23 adolescents (ages 11–23) and 29 parents	MyMind (mindfulness training tailored to adolescents with ASD) plus mindfulness parenting training; 2 mental health care professionals	1.5-hour weekly sessions for 9 weeks; 9-month follow-up joint booster session for parents and adolescents	Adolescent self-report on core symptoms, mindful awareness, quality of life, rumination, and worrying; parents reported effects on ASD core symptoms and social responsiveness	1. Improved quality of life 2. Decreased rumination
Koenig et al. 2012; pretest/posttest (between subject);[a] United States	48 students (ages 5–12)	Get Ready to Learn Yoga program; classroom teachers[b]	15- to 20-minute daily sessions for 16 weeks	ABC-Community to assess challenging behavior; VABS-II (parent interview) to assess independence and proficiency across several domains	1. Reduced maladaptive classroom behavior (specifically irritability, agitation, and crying) 2. Cumulative ABC scores also significantly reduced

TABLE 9–1. Review of yoga and mindfulness therapeutic interventions for autism spectrum disorder *(continued)*

Author, design, and location	Participants	Content and facilitator	Duration	Data	Findings
Radhakrishna et al. 2010; pretest/midtest/posttest (matched);[a] India	12 children (ages 8–14): 6 with intervention, 6 without intervention	Integrated approach to yoga therapy (IAYT): warm-up, strengthening, loosening, and calming asanas; yogic breathing practices; and chanting module along with ABA (control was ABA only); elementary teachers	15-hour ABA-based training and 5-hour IAYT training for two 10-month academic years with a 2-month summer holiday gap	Special educators assessed subjects on ASD's nine core targeted behaviors using the Autism Research Institute's form E-2 checklist to assess subjects on nine core targeted behaviors; Imitation Test Battery to measure imitating behavior; and Repetitive Stereotyped Behavior Test Battery to measure stereotyped, self-injurious, repetitive, restricted, and sameness behavior	1. By midsession: improved eye-to-eye gaze, sitting tolerance, body posture, receptive skills to verbal commands, imitation skills, self-stimulation, and self-injurious behavior 2. Increased alertness immediately following sessions 3. Postintervention: improved connection with therapist during yoga sessions; increased oral-facial movement imitation skills; improved communication, language, play, and joint attention, as well as eye contact 4. Parents reported improved ability to interact with other children and family members

TABLE 9-1. Review of yoga and mindfulness therapeutic interventions for autism spectrum disorder *(continued)*

Author, design, and location	Participants	Content and facilitator	Duration	Data	Findings
Rosenblatt et al. 2011; pretest/posttest (within subject); United States	24 children (ages 3–16)	Relaxation-response based yoga (dance, yoga, and music); licensed clinician with certification in dance and yoga[b]	45-minute sessions once a week for 8 weeks	ABC to assess challenging behavior); Behavioral Assessment System for Children to assess symptoms	1. Effective treatment of behavioral symptoms (especially irritability) 2. Effective treatment of some ASD core symptoms (especially on the atypicality scale) 3. Results most prominent for latency-age children (ages 5–12)
Singh et al. 2006; multiple baseline; United States	3 mothers of young children (ages 4–6)	Mindfulness training; senior investigator	2 hours per session weekly for 12 sessions plus 52 weeks of personal practice	Mothers observed their children on three target behaviors: aggression, noncompliance, and self-injury; fathers provided interrater agreement data; parents used self-report measures of mindfulness and satisfaction with both parenting and interactions	1. Significant decreases in all target behaviors for the children (aggression, noncompliance, and self-injury) 2. Increases in all parent self-report outcomes (mindfulness, parenting satisfaction, and interaction satisfaction)

TABLE 9–1. Review of yoga and mindfulness therapeutic interventions for autism spectrum disorder *(continued)*

Author, design, and location	Participants	Content and facilitator	Duration	Data	Findings
Singh et al. 2011; multiple baseline; United States	3 adolescents (ages 15, 13, and 18)	Meditation on the Soles of the Feet (mindfulness intervention involving attention from aggression-triggering event to neutral body part); mothers	15-minute sessions led by parents during training, then twice a day with mother plus any time the adolescent felt anger for 17–24 weeks (intervention concluded after 3 consecutive weeks without aggressive behavior)	Recorded incidents of physical aggression through parent and sibling reports and self-reports	1. Starting with moderate rates of aggression at baseline, incidents decreased during the mindfulness intervention for each participant, ending the intervention with 3 weeks without incident 2. No episodes occurred during 4-year follow-up

TABLE 9–1. Review of yoga and mindfulness therapeutic interventions for autism spectrum disorder (*continued*)

Author, design, and location	Participants	Content and facilitator	Duration	Data	Findings
Spek et al. 2013; pretest/posttest (waitlist);[a] Netherlands	42 high-functioning adults: 21 with experimental condition, 21 control	Mindfulness-based therapy modified for individuals with autism (MBT-AS); 2 trained and experienced therapists (psychologist and clinical psychologist)	Weekly 2.5-hour sessions for 9 weeks plus 40–60 minutes of meditation practice 6 days per week	Self-report: Symptom Checklist 90–Revised, Rumination-Reflection Questionnaire, and Dutch Global Mood Scale	1. Significant reduction in depression, anxiety, and rumination in intervention group as opposed to control group 2. Increase in positive affects for intervention but not for control

[a]Study included a control group.

[b]Study was performed as a group intervention.

Abbreviations. ABA=applied behavior analysis; ABC =Aberrant Behavior Checklist; ASD=autism spectrum disorder; VABS-II=Vineland Adaptive Behavior Scale, Second Edition.

ASD through a strength-based lens, mindful practices help us to open our sight toward these strengths rather than the multitude of challenges that may exist.

2. When teaching a new practice or tool, it is best to present it as an offering, as if the child is "trying it on." Then observe how it "fits." Without becoming attached to any postulated expected outcome, gently observe how the individual receives and communicates the effects of that tool. This can be done verbally by asking participants how they feel after a practice or by simply observing their behavior. This reduces our own professional propensity toward goal-driven expectations and allows for a more natural unfolding and integration of therapeutic mindful practices.

Where to Begin

Teaching mindfulness tools—sitting and following the breath or noticing thoughts—to children with ASD can be a challenge. Begin in the body through movement practices, such as *qigong* or yoga, to release anxiety and unbalanced energy. Movement assists in relieving physical and emotional tension, which often accompanies stress and anxiety. Exploring the breath to activate the parasympathetic nervous system is much more accessible when beginning with movement activities. We have found that students are able to relax, settle, and notice the mind (thoughts) and emotions (sensations) with greater ease by following the sequence of body, breath, and then stillness. In the following subsections, we describe some examples of how you can use the guiding principles of mindfulness and this sequence with your students.

BODY

Laura, a third grader, often flaps her hands whenever she is excited, a very typical repetitive pattern completed by individuals with ASD. Rather than cuing her to stop and rewarding her when she complies, we began using this movement to help her gain awareness of her body. Hand flapping becomes "earthquake": The facilitator encourages Laura to continue to shake her hands, then her arms, torso, legs, and head, and her entire body becomes the earthquake. The facilitator slowly counts to 10 while shaking her body as well. The movement ends with a big breath in as they stretch their arms toward the ceiling, then exhale slowly as they lower their arms back to their sides. This is a very enjoyable movement pattern for most of the children we have worked with. It is not often that they are encouraged to move in patterns that are intuitive and easy for them. As noted previously in the first principle of sharing mindfulness with this population, we honor their wisdom. We must consider that the patterns they prefer, although foreign to neurotypical individuals like us, holds something essential for their well-being. Why change or discard something that has the potential to help them gain awareness? Laura was pleased to be able to move in a way that innately felt good to her. Following this moment of vigorously shaking her entire body, she was able to relax. Her breath automatically became deeper and slower, supporting her awareness of her ability to change the flow of her breath. She was then able to attend to and notice the subtle sensations of her belly, ribcage, and chest moving as air filled and released from her lungs.

For many children with ASD, following their lead in terms of how they move their body provides a window into their nervous system. What feels good to them is not necessarily what we would choose for our body. Because these children's sensory systems are interpreting what they feel and how they move differently from their neurotypical counterparts, we must assume that what feels good to them, what helps them to settle, may vary from what feels good to us. With Laura, we followed her lead and inner wisdom, becoming a student, learning from her what was needed to release her body and organize her nervous system.

BREATH

Belly breath is a common mindful practice that is taught to adults and children. It is powerful and effective in activating a relaxation response through the parasympathetic nervous system. This exercise is typically explored by placing your hands on your abdomen, inhaling to feel your belly grow, then exhaling to allow your belly and body to relax. Like many individuals with ASD, Paul, an eighth grader, has very poor awareness of his body in space. He bumps into things often and has difficulty recognizing his personal space and realizing when he is invading someone else's. Precise, controlled gross and fine motor movements are challenging. To assist a child like Paul in recognizing the subtle movements of belly breathing, which involves awareness of the abdomen expanding and contracting, the use of props is helpful. The most effective adaptation is to provide resistance against the abdominal muscles as the belly expands with the breath. One means of achieving this is by placing a weighted lap pad or weighted bean bag (try making your own with rice or beans in a resealable plastic bag) on top of the abdomen while the youth is lying on his or her back. Another option is having the youth lie on his or her stomach, thereby positioning the abdomen to press against the floor as it expands with each breath.

STILLNESS

Owen is a second-grade student who always communicated his sense of being overwhelmed through states of rage. Since first grade, he would mutter under his breath, "I am so dumb. I am a mad boy." This seemed to become his mantra and inner dialogue. Owen needed healing and acceptance from not only others but also himself. The meditative exercise of *floating balloon* became Owen's bridge to internal awareness and compassion for himself. Try it with your own patients to see if it can become a bridge to greater self-esteem and motivation: Close your eyes and imagine using your breath to fill a huge balloon. Each breath contains positive, healing energy or something that you wish for yourself. It may help to have the youth create a list of things they would like to place in the balloon (e.g., happiness, peace, calm, strength, focus). Use your voice to guide them on each inhale. "Take a big breath in and fill your balloon with [*insert an appropriate affirmative word*]." Let them exhale on their own. With each exhale you can state, "You are [*insert whatever word you just stated during the inhale*]." Continue with each affirmative word. Once the balloon is filled, tell participants that they have this balloon of good feelings within them all the time. They can even share it with a friend.

When Owen began using the floating balloon meditation, he was tense and resistant and often looked at the facilitator as if she were crazy for even suggesting words of self-acceptance, kindness, and compassion. She told him that he didn't have to believe each word but just to repeat them after her as he used his breath to fill the balloon. What we noticed from the first breath to the tenth breath was that Owen's body began to relax and soften. His fisted hands naturally opened, and a smile began to form on his face. We were amazed. The next session, Owen had a new word to add to our list of affirmations. He stated, "I am awesome." He kept his list of affirmations on his desk with a picture of a balloon. His aide reported that he would often use this meditation at his desk to calm himself when he felt himself becoming agitated.

REFLECTION

In small-group sessions or individual treatment, we use the *feelings worksheet* (Figure 9–1) after introducing mindfulness practices. This provides an opportunity for youth to "try on" a practice and then observe and reflect on how they feel following each exercise. When used in a group setting, the feelings worksheet provides an opportunity for youth to compare sensations and emotions and notice that they are experienced differently with each practice and for each individual. After participants identify how they feel following a practice, we also discuss when they might choose to try it again on their own, such as when they feel bombarded by sensory input, become annoyed or overwhelmed by a situation, or feel anxious in a particular environment. Students have given us very specific examples such as "when I am going to lunch and I start smelling the foods that I hate," "when I am trying to fall asleep and I can't," or "when I get really confused in class." As with most youth, when they determine for themselves when they want to do something, it is more likely they will follow through, as opposed to when we (the adult) tell them to do something.

Your feelings	Dragon breath	Energy ball	Down dog pose	Center (belly) breathing	Drifting clouds	Melting butter
Happy						
Calm						
Relaxed						
Energized						
Silly/Wiggly						
Frustrated						
Anxious						
Worried						
Angry						

FIGURE 9–1. Your feelings worksheet.

Your feelings	Dragon breath	Energy ball	Down dog pose	Center (belly) breathing	Drifting clouds	Melting butter
Scared						
Sad						

Dragon breath: Inhale through the nose and exhale through the open mouth while sticking out your tongue.

Energy ball: Bring the fingertips of one hand to touch the respective fingertips of your other hand, making the shape of a ball with your hands. Imagine there is a glowing ball of energy in the center of the ball you just formed with your hands. Use your breath to grow that energy. Take a deep breath in, imagining the ball of energy getting bigger and bigger. As the energy grows, gradually separate your hands to create room for the energy. As you exhale, imagine you are containing that energy. Bring your fingertips back to meet. Continue using your breath to inhale and grow the energy and then exhale to contain the energy. Your breath and movement should happen at the same time.

Down dog: With hands and feet on the floor, press your bottom to the sky and form an upside-down "v." Hold this pose for 10 breaths.

Center breath: Sit with spine long or lie on the floor. Place your hands on your belly and feel the rise and fall of your abdomen as you inhale and exhale.

Drifting clouds: Imagine that you are lying on your back in a field of soft green grass. Feel the cool grass on your back. In your imagination, look up at the sky and notice the various shapes and sizes of the clouds against the deep blue color of the sky. Notice if there are thoughts that are making their way into your mind. As each thought comes in, imagine that you are placing it gently into one of the clouds, and allow it to drift away in the breeze without attaching to the thought. Thoughts come and go, just like these clouds. Let them come and let them go.

Melting butter: Imagine that you are a cold piece of frozen butter. Inhale and make every part of your body tight and tense as if it is a frozen block and hold that frozen form for a count of 5. As you slowly exhale, imagine that you were just placed on top of a warm piece of toast. Melt into all the nooks and crannies of the toast, filling up all the open spaces as your body begins to relax, soften, and gently glide over the toast. Inhale again and become that frozen piece of butter, tightening each part of your body to freeze it in place. Exhale and melt. Repeat 4–5 times.

After each practice, allow students to check off how they felt. Notice the changes and differences with each practice.

FIGURE 9–1. Your feelings worksheet. *(continued)*

We have also adapted the feelings worksheet for students with varied abilities and understanding of emotions. Replacing the words of emotions with pictures is helpful for students who cannot read. Reducing the number of emotions, even if only two are used, such as calm and excited, is also an option.

Practitioner's Mindfulness Practice and the Regulatory State of Youth

What we have learned throughout our years of mindful practice is that there is a direct correlation between our personal mindfulness practice and our regulatory state. And consequently, what we have learned throughout our numerous years of working with children with ASD is that there is also a direct correlation between our regulatory state and the regulatory state of our students. Our states of being tend to mirror each other through our innate, neurobiological capacity to coregulate. One thing we have noticed with many of our students with various developmental challenges is that they are quite astute at reading and picking up on the emotional states of those around them. This can produce both positive and negative interactions with youth. For instance, when we are lax with our personal practice, we have the tendency to mirror the state of children with ASD, which leans toward dysregulation. Dysregulation does not look or feel good on us and, unfortunately, dysregulation perpetuates the state within the youth we are treating. When we give ourselves the space and time to sit with our breath, to become present with our emotions and thoughts, we are able to carry a grounded, calm state within us throughout the day. Showing up in this way supports our students' ability to achieve these calm states as they mirror us.

However, it is hard to teach what you don't practice. Having your own mindfulness practice is essential to being able to authentically share the tools discussed in this book. Your ability to embody stability, safety, and compassion facilitates your students' capacity to experience these states as well. Like Sam's therapist, learning such techniques alongside your student helps you to subtly attune to your student's internal state while also strengthening your capacity to remain calm and centered. When you radiate positive, calm energy, your students have the opportunity to coregulate and match these states.

Keenan-Mount and colleagues (2016) investigated the efficacy of mindfulness-based interventions in reducing stress and increasing positive behaviors in young people with ASD and their caregivers, such as their parents and teachers. We have observed this as well. Therapists and teachers become less reactive to students' behavior when they use the activities themselves. Keenan-Mount's study highlights an interdependent relationship between caregivers' level of mindfulness and their child's prosocial behaviors (Keenan-Mount et al. 2016). Furthermore, during parental participation in the Soles of the Feet program,

Singh et al. (2006) found that the mothers who practiced mindful tools along-side their child experienced a decrease in their child's aggression, noncompliance, and self-injury behaviors and felt higher satisfaction in their parenting skills and overall daily interaction with their child. Thus, this cultivation of self-awareness allows us to acknowledge our ability to use our own state of being as a therapeutic tool.

Research on *therapeutic presence* further supports what we have observed over the years. Eklund (1996) suggested that therapists may achieve effective therapeutic relationships with their clients when they are acutely aware of their own thoughts and feelings, feel confident, and value the interpersonal aspects of therapy. Practicing mindfulness activities can be an effective tool in cultivating one's therapeutic presence. A therapist can become attuned and responsive to the patient's needs and experiences through being fully engaged in the moment-to-moment interaction with the patient.

Practicing mindfulness also offers a shift in perspective in how we can approach our treatment from a seat of compassion and acceptance for ourselves and our students. It fosters our ability as teachers, therapists, or caregivers to notice an individual's strengths rather than focusing on his or her weaknesses. When we intentionally shift where we place our focus, we begin to notice more things that are aligned with that attention. Whether a child is verbal or non-verbal, the language of compassion and acceptance is universal and can be understood without the need for words to express the intention.

Zensational Kids: A Mindfulness Therapeutic Approach

We have both spent much of our careers in traditional school settings where the therapeutic model for service delivery is one to two sessions per week for 30 minutes of direct treatment. As Allison was developing the skills necessary for later forming the mindfulness-based therapeutic approach of Zensational Kids—an educational company that provides programs in which mindful practices are integrated throughout the day in classrooms—the initial implementation within her weekly occupational therapy sessions was essential. Working in the school setting allowed her to fully observe student responses and develop adaptations to increase accessibility for varied physical, cognitive, and communicative abilities. Although delivering this work in weekly sessions was initially helpful in the learning stage of building a model for a mindfulness-based therapeutic approach, it is not a model conducive to supporting students' daily use of the tools they have learned. Repetition is essential for taking advantage of students' natural neuroplasticity. For the students to become more familiar with states of calm—as opposed to states of anxiety, frustration or aggression—they needed more opportunities to be guided in practice on a daily basis.

For example, while participating in the traditional model of 30-minute sessions, Sam became better able to attend more fully to his learning in class on the day of his therapy session, but during the week, he still experienced the need to deescalate emotional discourse or refocus his agitated mind on an ongoing basis. Sam needed more frequent, routine measures for self-regulating during times of distress that would help him expand the toolbox he developed in therapy to instinctual, inner practice.

Developing a method of implementation to meet this need inspired Allison to create the Educate 2B: Tools for Engaged Learning and Living program as an integral part of implementing the approach of Zensational Kids and other mindfulness-based therapeutic approaches to the everyday classroom setting. This program is composed of 30 specific breath, movement, and mindfulness activities that can be completed in short, 1- to 2-minute practices several times each day in the classroom environment. During a 1-day training session, educators, school counselors, therapists, and classroom aides learn how to teach the exercises, which are offered in short classroom breaks. Educators often report that taking 2 minutes to stop and drop into a practice actually saves them 30–40 minutes in teaching time. There are often fewer disruptions and much more focused learning. In the initial trial phase of implementing the program, teachers reported that taking 2 minutes out of the daily schedule seemed reasonable and did not cause them to feel worried about the time commitment (Horbacewicz et al. 2017). They began to notice that these short breaks helped calm all of the students, especially those who often experienced anxiety. Disruptive behaviors began to decrease, and reports of improved attention circulated in the staff lunch room.

There are several benefits to this model. When used within a school setting, activities can easily be infused throughout the typical school day. No planning or setup time is needed. This model can be integrated into classified classrooms where all students have an Individualized Education Program (IEP) as well as in inclusive classrooms where neurotypical and neurodiverse students are educated together. Classroom breaks consisting of mindful exercises also provide additional opportunities for social connection and peer modeling in an activity that is not focused on achieving a specific goal and is noncompetitive in nature.

Along with the need to have more effective tools for students with ASD, there is an overwhelming incidence of mental health disorders in youth in general. Sharing these practices in classrooms can be both therapeutic and preventative for everyone. According to the National Alliance on Mental Illness (2018), one in five youth between ages 5 and 17 years have or will have a mental health disorder as an adult. With the Educate 2B model, every student in the class receives tools to reset his or her nervous system as well as create connections to engage executive function skills, cultivate positive emotional experiences, and activate a relaxation response more frequently because "what fires together, wires together" (Hanson and Mendius 2009). The more students practice these tools, the more hardwired they become in the brain, thereby becoming more readily available to help students achieve a calm, relaxed state.

Educate 2B: An Evidence-Based Intervention

A small pilot study on the effectiveness of the Educate 2B program for self-regulation techniques in the classroom setting of elementary children with ASD was completed by physical therapy doctoral students of Touro College in New York City (Morgan 2016) and presented at a poster session at the Combined Sections Meeting of The American Physical Therapy Association in 2017 (Horbacewicz et al. 2017). Although this study has not been published in a journal, it offers additional insight on mindful practices for ASD therapy. Whereas the current research in this area focuses primarily on observational or self-report methods, this study used a rigid experimental design to measure and compare the effects of an 11-week integration of Educate 2B mindfulness-based tools in improving behavior and motor function of elementary students with ASD in their regular classroom environments. Twenty participants between second and sixth grade with various severity levels of ASD (6 with mild severity, 11 with moderate severity, and 3 with severe ASD) were recruited from four classrooms of students in a New Jersey elementary school that specializes in special education.

In order to assess the impact of Educate 2B, a quasi-experimental design was used (Horbacewicz et al. 2017). Classrooms were randomly assigned to the experimental or control group. The experimental group (9 participants) were students who were taught to incorporate 15 of the 30 Educate 2B breath, movement, and mindfulness tools within their daily classroom participation. These tools were taught by their teachers and used three times per day for a total of 6 minutes per school day. Meanwhile, the control group (11 participants) did not receive Educate 2B practices instruction. All participants were assessed at the beginning of the school year and then postinstruction 11 weeks later using the Devereux Student Strengths Assessment–Mini (DESSA-Mini) to assess socioemotional intelligence and the Movement Assessment Battery for Children–Second Edition (MABC-2) to assess fine and gross motor function of participants. Each measurement has high internal reliability and construct validity. The DESSA-Mini assessments (20 participants) were scored by teacher observations, and the MBAC-2 assessments (18 participants, due to the inability of two participants to complete the testing) were evaluated by a licensed physical therapist blind to the study.

Although there was no significant difference between the experimental and control groups prior to testing in either of the assessments, findings indicated a significant difference between the control and experimental groups postintervention in both the DESSA-Mini assessment ($P=0.034$) and the MABC-2 assessment ($P=0.035$) (Horbacewicz et al. 2017). Students with ASD who received the Educate 2B mindfulness-based practices instruction in their classroom demonstrated improvements in both DESSA-Mini and MABC-2 scores. Students from the experimental group demonstrated improvement ($P<0.05$) in behavior and socioemotional learning. Although the experimental group did not show statistically significant improvement in gross and fine motor skills, the control group demonstrated a decline in motor skills. Furthermore, pretest and posttest evaluations indicated that the introduction of breath, movement, and mindfulness activities within the Educate 2B program in the classroom protected students from declining in their skills.

This preliminary study provided some scientific evidence of the potential effectiveness of integrating Educate 2B or other mindfulness-based approaches to a child's daily routine not only through therapy sessions but also through classroom activities (Morgan 2016). Results indicate that mindfulness-based programs can be easily implemented into the school setting as a practical intervention that may optimize classroom learning for children with ASD through improved behavior and motor function. Although the sample size for the study is considered relatively small, it is currently the only study including a control group for examining mindfulness-based approaches in assisting children with ASD. It is also worth noting that cluster random sampling was used for this study for convenience and not for statistical probability within the diverse population. However, the findings of this study may help other researchers in future studies to embark with larger sample sizes and randomization in a controlled environment for more scientifically significant data regarding the impact of mindfulness practices on the child's ability to self-regulate, reflect, and refocus. Future studies could also evaluate the impact that these in-classroom practices have on social integration with peers, overall classroom environment, and harnessing and maintaining essential life skills.

Conclusion

Research on the application of mindfulness therapeutic practices for children with ASD is beginning to point to promising benefits; however, we have a long way to go. The small sample sizes and lack of control groups in the current research limit the generalization of the findings to broader groups of individuals with ASD. Some of the studies were completed in India, a country where people are much more accustomed to mind-body practices than practitioners in our Western culture. Acceptance of these methods may contribute to their effectiveness. Because of the range of deficits within the diagnosis itself, there has been no investigation to determine which practices are more suitable and therapeutic for different areas of the spectrum.

Individuals with ASD receive services in groups as well as one-to-one intervention. Therapy can be conducted in homes, hospitals, schools, or clinics. Further identification of practices most conducive to these varied settings would assist professionals charged with care on individuals in these settings. We believe there is great potential for further research, and there is a great need. The costs associated with treatment for ASD is in direct proportion to the growth rate of the diagnosis itself. The burgeoning potential of using mindfulness as a therapeutic modality in multiple settings with ASD is exciting. It brings great hope and possibilities for the overall function and well-being of this population, as well as for the people working with and caring for them.

KEY POINTS

- Your own personal practice is an extremely important component when sharing the mindfulness tools you teach to children with ASD.
- Begin mindful practices with children through movement in the body, then explore the breath in order to facilitate stillness of the body and mind.
- Frequency rather than duration helps these practices stick and become everyday tools that are used independently or with little prompting.

Discussion Questions

1. In this chapter we discuss the human capacity to coregulate with another individual. Have you ever noticed how your regulatory state can shift the state of your patients or students (for better or for worse)? Have you ever considered that your emotional state and internal thoughts can influence your patients' or students' internal state of regulation, calm, and feeling safe?

2. In the beginning of the chapter, the story of Sam described the initial signs of his feeling overwhelmed. Have you recognized subtle changes that occur with your students or patients as they are becoming overwhelmed and dysregulated? What are some behaviors that serve as a signal to you that they may need to take a moment to calm them before a full-blown panic attack, outburst, or meltdown ensues?

3. A high percentage of individuals with ASD also have a diagnosis of anxiety disorder. For individuals who fit into this category, what tools have you used to address their anxiety? Have your patients been able to transfer these tools into their daily lives? Do you think that some of the practices mentioned in this chapter may help these youth?

Suggested Readings

Prizant BM: Uniquely Human: A Different Way of Seeing Autism. Reprint. New York, Simon and Schuster, 2016

Kuypers L: Zones of Regulation: A Curriculum Designed to Foster Self-Regulation and Emotional Control. San Jose, CA, Think Social, 2011

Wong C, Odom SL, Hume K, et al: Evidence-Based Practices for Children, Youth, and Young Adults with Autism Spectrum Disorder. Chapel Hill, NC, University of North Carolina, 2014. Available at: http://autismp-dc.fpg.unc.edu/sites/autismpdc.fpg.unc.edu/files/imce/documents/2014-EBP-Report.pdf. Accessed August 10, 2017.

References

Belardinelli C, Raza M, Taneli T: Comorbid behavioral problems and psychiatric disorders in autism spectrum disorders. J Child Dev Disord 2(11):1–9, 2016

Benson H, Klipper MZ: The Relaxation Response. New York, Avon, 1975

Bronson MB: Self-Regulation in Early Childhood: Nature and Nurture. New York, Guilford, 2000

Christensen DL, Baio J, Braun KV, et al: Prevalence and characteristics of autism spectrum disorder among children aged 8 years—autism and developmental disabilities monitoring network, 11 sites, United States, 2012. MMWR Surveill Summ 65(3):1–23, 2016 27031587

Cook-Cottone CP: Mindfulness and Yoga in Schools: A Guide for Teachers and Practitioners. New York, Springer, 2017

de Bruin EI, Blom R, Smit FM, et al: MYmind: mindfulness training for youngsters with autism spectrum disorders and their parents. Autism 19(8):906–914, 2014 25348866

Eklund M: Working relationship, participation, and outcome in a psychiatric day care unit based on occupational therapy. Scand J Occup Ther 3:106–113, 1996

Hanson R, Mendius R: Buddah Brain: The Practical Neuroscience of Happiness, Love, and Wisdom. Oakland, CA, New Harbinger, 2009

Horbacewicz J, Bensinger-Brody Y, Barresi J, et al: The effects of a yoga and mindfulness program on children with autism spectrum disorder in the school setting. Poster presented at the Combined Sections Meeting of the American Physical Therapy Association, San Antonio, TX, February 2017

Keenan-Mount R, Albrecht NJ, Waters L: Mindfulness-based approaches for young people with autism spectrum disorder and their caregivers: do these approaches hold benefits for teachers? Australian Journal of Teacher Education 41(6):68–86, 2016

Koenig KP, Buckley-Reen A, Garg S: Efficacy of the Get Ready to Learn yoga program among children with autism spectrum disorders: a pretest-posttest control group design. Am J Occup Ther 66(5):538–546, 2012 22917120

Loizzo J, Neale M, Wolf EJ: Advances in Contemplative Psychotherapy: Accelerating Healing and Transformation. New York, Routledge, 2017

Morgan A: Yoga and mindfulness for students: no mats required (blog post). Montvale, NJ, Zensational Kids, June 13, 2016. Available at: http://zensationalkids.com/2016/06/educate-2b-research-study-yoga-for-autism. Accessed May 16, 2018.

National Alliance on Mental Illness: Mental health facts: children and teens. 2018. Available at: www.nami.org/getattachment/Learn-More/Mental-Health-by-the-Numbers/childrenmhfacts.pdf. Accessed May 16, 2018.

Radhakrishna S, Nagarathna R, Nagendra HR: Integrated approach to yoga therapy and autism spectrum disorders. J Ayurveda Integr Med 1(2):120–124, 2010 21836799

Rosenblatt LE, Gorantla S, Torres JA, et al: Relaxation response-based yoga improves functioning in young children with autism: a pilot study. J Altern Complement Med 17(11):1029–1035, 2011 21992466

Singh NN, Lancioni GE, Winton AS, et al: Mindful parenting decreases aggression, noncompliance, and self-injury in children with autism. J Emot Behav Disord, 14(3):169–177, 2006

Singh NN, Lancioni GE, Manikam R, et al: A mindfulness-based strategy for self-management of aggressive behavior in adolescents with autism. Res Autism Spectr Disord 5(3):1153–1158, 2011

Spek AA, van Ham NC, Nyklíček I: Mindfulness-based therapy in adults with an autism spectrum disorder: a randomized controlled trial. Res Dev Disabil 34(1):246–253, 2013 22964266

van Steensel FJA, Bögels SM, Perrin S: Anxiety disorders in children and adolescents with autistic spectrum disorders: a meta-analysis. Clin Child Fam Psychol Rev 14(3):302–317, 2011 21735077

Appendix

Educate 2B Exercises

Heart Shining Breath
A practice to cultivate presence before you begin working with children
Sit with your feet on the floor, spine long, shoulders relaxed.

Place one hand on your heart and the other on your stomach. Begin to deepen your breath, noticing the movement of your hands as your lungs begin to fill with air and expand. Notice how your body contracts as you exhale and release the air. Simply notice the movement for a few breaths.

Imagine that in the center of your heart is a shining light. With each inhale, the light brightens and expands. With each exhale, the light moves throughout your body. Fill this light with compassion, kindness, patience, happiness, or anything else you feel you may need for today. Imagine this energizing and healing light traveling from your heart to all parts of your body. It fills every muscle, bone, and organ and every cell within your body. Continue growing your inner light with your breath.

Once you have become full of light, imagine the child you are about to work with seated in front of you. Use your breath to send rays of this light, moving from the center of your heart, to the center of this child's heart. Whatever you filled your light with is now shared with this child. Take a few more breaths with this visualization. When you are ready, open your eyes.

Energy Ball
A practice to build inner focus
Sit with your feet on the floor, spine long, shoulders relaxed.
Rub your palms together and create some heat.
Bring the fingertips of one hand to touch the respective fingertips on the other hand, making the shape of a ball with your hands.
Gently close your eyes or softly lower your gaze.

Imagine there is a glowing ball of energy in the center of the ball you just formed with your hands.

Use your breath to grow that energy. Take a deep breath in, imagining the ball of energy getting bigger and bigger. As the ball grows, gradually separate your hands to create more room for the energy within this expanding ball.

As you exhale, imagine you are containing that energy. Bring your fingertips back to meet, compacting the ball.

Continue using your breath to first inhale and grow the energy and then exhale and contain the energy. Your breath and movement happen at the same time.

Notice if your energy ball is a certain color. How does it feel? After you have practiced growing your energy, create a bowl shape with your hands and hold the energy ball in the bowl.

Now, notice your body. Is there any part of your body that can use some attention? Any part that feels tight or maybe feels some discomfort? Take your energy ball and gently place your hands over that part of your body, allowing that good energy to flow into those tight parts of your body. Remember to continue to use your breath.

Pause for a few seconds.

Bring your hands to rest on your lap. Take a deep breath in, pause, and then take a deep breath out.

Notice how you feel.

When you are ready, open your eyes.

Following this exercise, you may use the Feelings Worksheet (Figure 9–1) to mark down how this breath, movement, and mindfulness tool made you feel during this practice session.

Part III

Mindfulness Application to Specific Clinical Populations

Chapter

10

Immigrant Youth

Kristina C. Mendez, M.S.
Celeste H. Poe, LMFT
Sita G. Patel, Ph.D.

THE PURPOSE of this chapter is to inform mental health practitioners about how to culturally adapt mindfulness and yoga interventions for immigrant youth. We consider the best ways to make these adaptations, considering that first- or second-generation immigrants make up one-fifth of the U.S. population, and 25% of minors in the United States have a parent who immigrated to the United States (American Psychological Association Presidential Task Force on Immigration 2012). It is highly likely that clinicians, particularly those working in communities with higher immigrant populations, will be serving immigrant youth. Immigrant youth face unique, acute, and chronic stressors that mindfulness-based interventions may be well suited to address. In service of our goal of presenting you with clear methods to adapt your delivery of mindfulness, we also offer you select and specific scripts to guide you in facilitating.

We must also acknowledge that there are important distinctions between generations and subpopulations of immigrant youth, as well as other psychological factors such as level of acculturation, potential trauma history, context of reception, and immediate risk factors that need careful consideration in tailoring mindfulness interventions. We encourage readers to expand their study of these areas; a discussion of them is beyond the scope of this chapter. *Psychotherapy for Immigrant Youth* (Patel and Reicherter 2016) is a helpful resource for the reader to understand more about these complexities. We also include in Table 10–1 a summary of helpful resources to guide you toward further information in this area.

Ecological Theory as Guiding Framework

Immigrant youth may present with certain diagnoses such as depression, anxiety, and trauma, and researchers suggest that a broader ecological framework must be employed to understand and fully treat the breadth of these youths' complex symptom presentations (Staudenmeyer et al. 2016). Ecological theory is a comprehensive, holistic, and multisystemic approach to understanding the interacting realms of daily life that an individual inhabits (Bronfenbrenner and Ceci 1994). It is a useful tool when considering the complex stressors and challenges faced by immigrant youth across systems. This framework can be employed by assessing each youth's macrosystem, mesosystem, and microsystem both separately and as they might interact.

This holistic approach can offer useful insight to clinicians when formulating approaches to service provision. A stressor in one system may hinder a patient's progress in treatment if it is not addressed. It is also possible that youth and/or their families may feel more comfortable or willing to participate in an intervention in one system over another, such as working with a local religious leader or place of prayer to integrate mindfulness into religious or contemplative practice.

Given the myriad stressors faced by immigrant youth, ecological theory captures the many layers of challenges and support influencing all levels of functioning. The American Psychological Association Presidential Task Force on Immigration (2012) uses ecological theory as a guiding principle for work with immigrant adults and youth. The intervention approaches in this chapter also follow this ecological approach, which has been hailed as a culturally appropriate theoretical foundation for working with newcomer youth in particular (Staudenmeyer et al. 2016).

Mindfulness With Immigrant Youth

Mindfulness-based programming has been conducted with diverse youth, but research is generally limited, especially for newcomers and first-generation im-

TABLE 10–1. Summary of helpful resources

Reference	Focus	Summary
American Psychological Association Presidential Task Force on Immigration 2012	U.S. immigrant population	The task force focuses on spreading awareness for citizens, clinicians, and researchers regarding current and relevant issues concerning the U.S. immigrant population. It specifically highlights psychological treatment, research, and policy efforts for immigrant children, adults, older adults, and families.
Betancourt et al. 2017	Refugee children	The authors compare the clinical and service profiles of refugee youth with those of nonrefugee immigrant and U.S.-born youth. They also compare and contrast trauma histories, clinical profiles, and patterns of service use.
Bronfenbrenner and Ceci 1994	Ecological theory	The authors provide a theoretical framework for conceptualizing the way that the interaction between the individual and the environment influences that individual's life and well-being.
Ferreira-Vorkapic et al. 2015	Yoga-based intervention in schools	The authors examine current literature on yoga interventions implemented exclusively in school settings and explores the impact of yoga-based interventions on academic, cognitive, and psychosocial outcomes.
Frank et al. 2014	Yoga-based intervention in schools	The authors examine the effectiveness of a school-based yoga program for a diverse group of adolescents.
Frisby and Jimerson 2016	Immigrant youth in schools	The authors discuss the school-related needs of immigrant children. They aim to spread knowledge about current resources and also call for additional services for immigrant youth.

TABLE 10–1. Summary of helpful resources (*continued*)

Reference	Focus	Summary
Griner and Smith 2006	Historically disadvantaged racial and ethnic groups	In this meta-analysis of 76 studies, the authors provide support for the need for more culturally adapted treatment methods for disadvantaged racial and ethnic groups. Interventions that were more culturally focused were found to be four times more effective.
Lui 2015	Latinx[a] and Asian immigrants in the United States	The author examines acculturation, intergenerational cultural conflict, and mental health and educational outcomes in immigrant Asian and Latinx groups. Findings supported the view that an acculturation gap causes distress in these populations. In turn, this distress leads to internalizing problems and adaptive functioning. Sixty-one research reports were reviewed, with 68 independent study samples (41 and 27 Asian and Latinx samples, respectively; $N=14{,}453$).
Stern et al. 2016	Mindfulness programming for youth	This Internet resource provides open educational resources and curricula and includes a variety of training options such as daily classroom integration and stand-alone health and wellness courses.
Rettger et al. 2016	Immigrant youth	In this book chapter, the authors review the various ways that trauma and acculturative stress exist for immigrant youth. They also provide recommendations and effective treatments for addressing these concerns.
Staudenmeyer et al. 2016	Immigrant youth	In this book chapter, the authors provide definitions, highlight unique stressors, and give an overview of relevant concerns pertaining to the immigrant youth population.

TABLE 10-1. Summary of helpful resources (*continued*)

Reference	Focus	Summary
Suárez-Orozco et al. 2009	Newcomer immigrant youth	The authors outline the prevalence of newcomer immigrant youth in schools and examine the relationship between school-based relationships, academic engagement, and academic performance. Results suggest that school-based relationships play a significant role in academic engagement and performance.
Substance Abuse and Mental Health Services Administration 2015	Trauma-informed approaches	This resource provides information regarding a trauma-informed approach for treatment of PTSD and includes trauma-specific interventions.
Thorardson et al. 2016	Immigrant youth	In this book chapter, the authors emphasize the benefits of cognitive-behavioral therapy in the immigrant youth population.

[a]The term *Latinx* is used in order to be inclusive of all gender identities, including gender fluid and gender-nonconforming individuals of Latin American heritage. Latinx is used here instead of Latino or Latina in recognition of the gendered structure of the Spanish language and to support and include all youth regardless of their identity. When working clinically, the therapist might still choose to use Latino or Latina if the patient identifies as male or female, respectively, and identifies as Latino or Latina rather than Latinx.

Abbreviation. PTSD=posttraumatic stress disorder.

migrant youth. However, a meta-analysis of yoga-based programming in schools did highlight a particular study with a diverse group of teens on the West Coast (Ferreira-Vorkapic et al. 2015). The study yielded positive results, with significant improvements in areas such as emotion regulation, rumination, and emotional arousal (Frank et al. 2014). With less than 3% of students identifying as white, this study in particular is a promising step toward immigrant youth–specific research. Readers who are interested in additional research can refer to Chapter 3, "State of the Research on Youth Mindfulness." The following framework and intervention example provide insight into developing appropriately adapted mindfulness-based interventions for immigrant youth across generations and statuses.

Applied Example: Yoga With Newcomer Adolescents in Schools

The following is an applied example of a culturally adapted implementation of a manualized yoga-based curriculum taught at a public high school. The Pure Power Curriculum, developed by Pure Edge, has been used in schools across the nation and boasts physical education and socioemotional learning standards that can be integrated into the school day. The core components of the Pure Power Curriculum involve breath, movement, and rest (Stern et al. 2016). The first author (K.C.M.) taught the program to four physical education classes of newcomer immigrant youth ages 14–18 in 6-, 7-, and 8-week modules. In teaching the curriculum, K.C.M. made the following cultural adaptations.

    Bilingual delivery: K.C.M. sought out appropriate translations of curriculum concepts and vocabulary to Spanish, collaborated with the youth participating in the program to identify culturally salient terminology (because different regions of Latin America have different terms and dialects), and facilitated delivery of the curriculum in both English and Spanish (bilingual) to the physical education classes.

    Rapport building: The group of newcomer teens required rapport building and trust. K.C.M. had volunteered her time at the school for the previous 2 years and had become a familiar face to many of the students. When teaching the curriculum, she also shared that she is a second-generation immigrant to the United States so that the youth can relate to her interest in serving them. The youth often are very interested in knowing more about her, which leads to the creation of authentic and personal connections with these youth.

    Creating a safe space: All yoga, mindfulness, and school classes should create a safe space for students, particularly immigrant youth. In addition to the stressors associated with migration (before, during, and after) that these youth face, they live in an unwelcoming historical context. As appropriate, K.C.M carefully selected cues during rest pose, such as "This is a safe space just for you, where you can be completely at ease." Given the increased cultural tension since the commencement of the yoga programming in 2016, facilitators could consider stating more explicitly, "You are safe. You belong here. You are supported."

Practices for peace: K.C.M consistently introduced interactive components of the curriculum as tools to help the students feel calmer, regulate their emotions, and support their peers.

Facilitating Culturally Adapted Intervention

Because of the variety of immigrants in the United States, it is essential for clinicians to incorporate cultural knowledge into the assessment and implementation of interventions for this group. Important concepts that can differ from culture to culture and that should be acknowledged in treatment include gender roles, preferred language, and conceptualization of mental health issues (Rettger et al. 2016). Above all, it is important to remember that these immigrant youth and their families have overcome a great deal to be where they are, which underscores the importance of using a resilience framework when working with this population (Frisby and Jimerson 2016).

Intervention Considerations

Chronic Ecological Stressors

Although adolescence is typically a time of complex developmental processes, immigrant youth are confronted with unique stressors that may lead to negative psychosocial outcomes, such as intergenerational conflict, neighborhood violence, poverty, family separation, parentification, discrimination, acculturation, language acquisition, and legal status concerns. These numerous and often interacting stressors pose risk to physical, cognitive, and psychosocial health over time (Staudenmeyer et al. 2016). Poverty is one issue that can add compounding stressors, such as fear of safety, needing to work while in school, and not having basic needs such as food and shelter met. In 2014, approximately one in four first-generation immigrant youth and one in four second-generation immigrant youth lived below the federal poverty line (Staudenmeyer et al. 2016).

This is just one example of the ways in which an ecological approach to conceptualization can be useful in understanding which chronically stressed systems might need to be stabilized in order to proceed effectively with intervention.

ACCULTURATIVE STRESS

Acculturative stress, one of many stressors faced by immigrant youth, can have profound consequences on immigrant adolescent development. Acculturative stress is the stress experienced by most immigrants associated with balancing the demands of a new culture and challenges of adapting to social norms while also remaining familiar with the culture of their country of origin. The greater the similarities between an immigrant's new culture and culture of origin, the less acculturative stress is experienced. Greater cultural differences may require changes in beliefs, values, and behaviors, which can lead to an increase in risk for psychopathological issues (Lui 2015). With many immigrants coming from collectivistic cultures, it is no surprise that it can be particularly difficult for these groups to adjust to the more individualistic North American culture (Lui 2015).

CITIZENSHIP STATUS

Citizenship status is an important stressor to assess for because it has been linked to various behavioral and conduct problems in immigrant youth (Staudenmeyer et al. 2016). This is typically a very sensitive and personal topic for immigrant families, especially if they are from cultures that are targeted in anti-immigration policy. For this reason, rapport is an essential gateway for understanding whether additional stress is being caused by legal status concerns. This consideration is particularly relevant in light of current immigration policies, which may be daily stressors for these individuals. Therefore, an accessible, culturally relevant intervention is needed to address the distress caused by these very real concerns.

TRAUMA

Of further concern, first-generation immigrant youth are often subjected to a number of traumatic events and experiences throughout migration (Suárez-Orozco et al. 2009). It is important to consider the potential for varying types and severities of these events (Betancourt et al. 2017). A high number of first-generation immigrant youth are exposed to traumatic events, including torture, death threats, severe harassment, armed conflict, and extreme hunger (Rettger et al. 2016). Chronic, daily hassles such as discrimination or poverty-related issues also pose risk for compounding mental health problems (Staudenmeyer et al. 2016).

When examining service utilization in refugee youth in particular, Betancourt and colleagues (2017) found that this group often sought help for issues other than trauma, such as cultural adjustment and bereavement. This suggests that the interaction between chronic stressors and trauma can often be complex, and it is important to carefully evaluate the nuances between the two across ecological systems and timelines when implementing interventions with immigrant youth (Lui 2015). Despite presenting to treatment with socially normative complaints, these individuals may in fact be harboring deeper-rooted distress that they may or may not be willing to share until stronger rapport is developed. Mindfulness-based practice is an excellent coping skill to introduce outright in intervention if past trauma or ongoing chronic stressors are suspected. The mental health professional does not need to know if a trauma has or has not occurred to apply mindfulness practices from a trauma-informed approach, and we encourage all practitioners to view patients through this precautionary lens.

K.C.M has had success teaching mindfulness practices to combat insomnia with immigrant adolescents because this more concrete, physiological issue appears to be less stigmatizing. She offers these practices in both clinical and nonclinical settings (i.e., therapy and psychoeducation groups) and has noticed that among these youth, difficulty sleeping in particular has often been associated with acute traumatic experiences or chronic acculturative stressors. This does not mean that the trauma must be addressed outright, but again, it highlights the importance of facilitating interventions from a trauma-informed approach with this population.

PSYCHOSOCIAL NEEDS

Before beginning any formal intervention, it is crucial to evaluate the client's immediate needs from an ecological perspective. Immigrant youth, especially newcomers, refugees, and unaccompanied minors (see Patel and Reicherter 2016) may have acute psychosocial needs that require attention prior to starting treatment for psychological symptoms (Staudenmeyer et al. 2016). Mental health workers should know whether these youth have stable housing, access to school, and enough to eat, and whether they are currently subjected to ongoing stressors that may impact their ability to engage in intervention. By understanding cultural practice considerations for immigrant youth, mental health professionals can begin to connect local networks of resources across ecological systems to support their patients, enabling them to benefit optimally from intervention.

There is an ever-increasing need to advocate for this vulnerable population. Mental health professionals have an opportunity to advocate for these youth and families in contexts where they might be underserved or underrepresented, such as in schools without adequate translation services and when reevaluating individualized education programs. Mental health professionals should be flexible with treatment and mindfulness approaches in order to connect with the patient's own culturally informed values.

Effective Interventions

LANGUAGE ADAPTATIONS

Language should be considered a factor in a provider's competency to provide services and is crucial to address prior to or at the outset of intervention. Psychological intervention delivered in a patient's native language is twice as effective as interventions delivered in a second language (Griner and Smith 2006). It is therefore critical to consider language when evaluating the merits of an intervention. If an intervention is not available in the patient's native language, you should do your best to adapt the intervention to account for the fact that it is being conducted in the patient's second language. For example, facilitators must be aware of the particular language structure and how it might affect the delivery of the intervention. Often, translating a practice to another language may include additional cultural adaptations to integrate more relatable verbiage or metaphors. For example, the Spanish language uses grammatical gender, so translation requires knowledge of the gender attributed to each word. In addition, descriptors can come after a word: whereas in English one might say "a yellow dress," in Spanish, one would place the color designator after the word *dress*. This would read in English as "a dress yellow."

Depending on the youth's level of education, which may not be comparable to that of the youth's age peers in the United States, it is best to use caution when assigning traditional "homework" in the form of worksheets or written tasks. Even if the worksheets are in the youth's native language, assessment of the youth's literacy level in that language prior to administering such tasks is crucial. Consider supplementing therapeutic interventions with visual and tactile components as well as in-person practice if working with youth in a language other than their native language.

FLEXIBLE APPROACHES

As indicated throughout this chapter, immigrant youth often face a complex history of trauma, with acute and chronic stressors. Modular cognitive-behavioral approaches to treatment can be invaluable in working with complex symptom presentation as well as varying psychological stressors (Thorardson et al. 2016). It is advisable to use caution and flexibility if following manualized treatments that have not been studied with immigrant populations, especially newcomer immigrants. Such treatments may seem impersonal and disengaging to immigrant youth for whom a more individualistic and Western approach to intervention may not resonate.

In Latinx culture (see footnote for Table 10–1), *personalismo*, or developing a personable connection with another individual, is often an important and regular part of each session. With this population, agendas can seem oppressive, rigid, and impersonal. Homework can also be a challenge depending on the patient's level of education and experience in the educational system. *Homework is a Western construct in treatment based on Western values of education*, and it is important for mental health professionals to recognized it as such in case the concept of homework does not resonate with the patient's own culture. Even if the homework is as simple as taking 10 deep breaths before bed, it can be useful to create a regular bridge for the practice during session and to frame the practice in a less structured way to increase chances of patients practicing outside the intervention setting.

TRAUMA-INFORMED PRACTICE

Whether in treatment, intervention, or in community outreach and education, research supports the use of trauma-informed approaches when serving immigrant youth. The Substance Abuse and Mental Health Services Administration (SAMSHA) identifies four qualities of trauma-informed systems (Substance Abuse and Mental Health Services Administration 2015). Such systems

1. Realize the widespread impact of trauma and understand potential paths for recovery
2. Recognize the signs and symptoms of trauma in patients, families, staff, and others involved with the system
3. Respond by fully integrating knowledge about trauma into policies, procedures, and practices
4. Seek to actively resist retraumatization

SAMSHA additionally offers six transsystemic principles for trauma-informed care (Substance Abuse and Mental Health Services Administration 2015):

1. Safety
2. Trustworthiness and transparency
3. Peer support
4. Collaboration and mutuality
5. Empowerment, voice, and choice
6. Cultural, historical, and gender issues

The following considerations specific to immigrant youth are important supplements to trauma-informed care: nondiscrimination in regard to symptom severity, current political climate regarding immigrant youth, and culture-specific idioms of distress. When evaluating symptom severity, it is important to consider that immigrant youth, especially today, may feel more pressured to blend in to their surroundings. This pressure may influence the presentation of idioms of distress and the youth's willingness to describe personal information, which can differ significantly from culture to culture.

When applying mindfulness practices with immigrant youth, it is critical to first assess for trauma history. This includes assessment of premigration trauma, trauma during migration, and trauma experienced once the youth is settled in the new country. For youth who have trauma histories, mental health professionals must pay particular attention and take care when doing work involving movement, and work involving closed eyes or enclosed environments. It is also important to be transparent with the intention of each practice and to explain, using accessible language, the purpose of the exercises.

Relaxation and physiological training can be particularly effective with traumatized immigrant youth (Rettger et al. 2016). Interventions that can be used with immigrant youth in general include guided imagery, progressive muscle relaxation, breathwork, and mindfulness techniques (Rettger et al. 2016). Some techniques especially effective with traumatized immigrant youth include narration, coloring, drawing, and poetry (Rettger et al. 2016). K.C.M has found mindful listening to music and mindful coloring of mandalas to be appreciated among newcomer and first-generation immigrant youth that she has worked with over the years. It is important to note that symptom expression can vary across different cultures within the immigrant youth population. As such, one critical skill for mental health providers is the ability to interpret differences in symptom expression on the basis of culture and adapt intervention accordingly (Rettger et al. 2016).

Integrating Mindfulness Into Treatment

Mindfulness can be taught to the patient before embarking on formal treatment and can also be integrated throughout treatment, regardless of whether or not you use an overarching mindfulness-based approach. Immigrant youth can face significant stressors above and beyond the normative developmental experience of youth, with newcomers, refugees, asylum seekers, and unaccompanied minors being at particularly heightened risk of these stressors. Mindfulness can be taught right away as a coping tool to reduce stress and to help patients assume some level of self-agency over emotional dysregulation. Although many mindfulness practices are appealing because they are not bound to money, time, gender, religion, age, or ability, practices can and should always be adapted to meet the needs and values of patients.

The type of mindfulness practice will vary depending on a youth's cultural identity. For example, some youth may be willing to engage in yoga-based movement to release muscle tension, but for others this might be against their religion or cultural beliefs. If asking youth to close their eyes for a mindfulness practice, be sure that you have developed strong rapport with them. Closing one's eyes requires trust, especially if the youth has a history of trauma and/or acute or chronic stress. Many manualized treatments include some variation of a mindfulness practice, which can be adapted appropriately if needed to suit immigrant youth. K.C.M. has often adapted the delivery of mindfulness into modular interventions with immigrant families from Latin America. The following case study provides a real-life example of how to integrate mindfulness interventions into a modular treatment approach with an immigrant family.

Mindfulness and Acculturation Gaps

Case Example

Inez is a 38-year-old monolingual mother from a war-torn country in Latin America. Her U.S.-born daughter, Ariana, is 11 years old. In working with Inez and Ariana, K.C.M. tailored the practice significantly to meet the developmental, emotional, and acculturative needs of the family. Ariana is a preteen with low socioemotional awareness who speaks mostly English, and her mother experiences chronic stress surrounding her busy work schedule. Inez had had previous referrals to child protective services for hitting her daughter as punishment for bad behavior, which was culturally normative in her country of origin. Ariana was already being seen at school by K.C.M., and Inez actively pursued joint therapy in order to more appropriately work with her stress and manage her daughter's behavior. Inez reported a fear that any more reports might increase her risk of deportation and being separated from her daughter.

Already, we see multiple cultural considerations that warrant evaluation. These considerations can be addressed by using a trauma-informed approach, considering the impact of language issues, examining cultural differences, addressing population-specific stressors, considering the patient's developmental ability, and making use of available resources.

Trauma-Informed Approach

Inez's country of origin has been historically riddled with gang violence. This sanctions consideration of her status as a refugee or asylum seeker and possible trauma history premigration, during migration, or postmigration. Just as it is important to create a safe and supportive space for Ariana in the delivery of mindfulness interventions, it is also essential for the therapist to create a safe and supportive space for Inez. Trauma-informed care is not limited to our child patients or the child members of family systems work. This trauma-informed lens can assist the therapist in conceptualizing parent-child dynamics from a more compassionate, ecological perspective.

Language Considerations

Inez is a monolingual Spanish speaker. Therefore, it is essential for the therapist to 1) evaluate whether he or she can competently treat the family in Spanish; 2) consider acculturative stressors that may accompany being monolingual in the United States; and 3) consider acculturative disparities between Ariana (who speaks mostly English) and her mother (who speaks only Spanish), which might include potential language barriers in treatment.

Cultural Differences

Immigrant parents with a history of child protective services referrals are often villainized. It is essential to view such a history in the context of the parents' culture and to understand that they may be unfamiliar with or unaccustomed to U.S. laws. Mental health professionals can serve as an important source of compassionate, but unwavering, psychoeducation on appropriate methods of managing a child's behavior (while of course following our mandates to report abuse).

Population-Specific Stressors

Inez indicated a fear of deportation, which was a very real consideration at the time of treatment. Fortunately, during the course of treatment, she was granted citizenship, and this fear, along with many accompanying stressors, subsided. Many families are not as fortunate. When working with families fearing deportation, remember that they may be facing a very real, ongoing, and unpredictable threat. In teaching mindfulness to this demographic, the aim should never be to dispel fear of the chronic stressor because our training indicates that trauma cannot be treated if the cause of the trauma persists. This being said, families fearing separation and deportation can certainly benefit from training in mindfulness and yoga to manage their stress and to stay focused and present in their role as a caregiver. It is essential for these caregivers to have tools for returning to the present moment, especially in the face of stress, in order to best care for themselves and their families.

Developmental Ability

Developmental level and ability are essential considerations when choosing mindfulness practices, and they are not necessarily synonymous with age. For example, Ariana's socioemotional development was well below her age level. Practices can and should almost always be tailored to meet the patient where he or she is. This can be done through the use of metaphor, storytelling, videos, images, or audio recordings, to name a few. Often, including cues that include familiar experiences or vocabulary (e.g., "make your belly fill up like a balloon when you breathe in, and let all the air out of the balloon as you breathe out") is useful when working with children across the developmental trajectory.

Available Resources

Immigrant families of lower socioeconomic status may be limited in terms of the time they can spare for treatment. If undocumented, parents may have difficulty finding jobs that pay minimum wage or higher, and they can often be exploited to work long and undesirable shifts for less than minimum wage. This can cause stressors with regard to affording child care and also in practicing self care.

Case Example *(Continued)*

Following the ecological framework, all of the above factors were taken into consideration when planning treatment with Inez and Ariana. At the time, K.C.M. was in her second year of specialty training in bilingual therapy, with biweekly supervision in Spanish. In the first session, she immediately clarified language preferences to maximize treatment benefits for both the patient and her mother. Ariana said she did not speak much Spanish and preferred to speak in English. Inez preferred Spanish but could understand some English. Considering these differences in acculturation and language ability, K.C.M. conducted therapy bilingually with this family to accommodate both Ariana and Inez.

Given Ariana's low socioemotional development, K.C.M. and Ariana practiced some very simple mindfulness techniques for Ariana to use at school, such as taking three deep breaths to calm down. Ariana grasped this practice fairly easily and enjoyed it enough to share it with her mother. Inez then reported taking ten deep breaths before walking into her home after work. She indicated that it helped her destress and transition more easefully from work to home, allowing her to care more compassionately for her daughter. K.C.M. recognized that not only did this practice work for Ariana, she was able to grasp the practice enough to demonstrate it to her mother as well. Inez had time for this practice, and it seemed to make a meaningful difference in her day. K.C.M. therefore incorporated this strength into treatment and made it a daily homework assignment for both Ariana and Inez. She led this breath practice for the family in each session to refresh the practice and leave space for questions. As Ariana and Inez practiced deep breaths more and more, K.C.M. assigned it as a practice for them to complete together, and Ariana and Inez successfully integrated this practice into their regular routine.

Progress in mindfulness practice can be valuable in promoting communication and acceptability of acculturation for both youth and parent. In the case of Ariana and Inez, mindfulness practice served as a bridge for positive communication between youth and parent. The breath is an anchor that can be activated anywhere, anytime, for any amount of time. It is a simple tool that is always activated in some capacity, and mindfulness as a practice allows the practitioner to choose the method of activation. K.C.M. has found this practice of taking a set number of breaths to be successful, even with the most time-limited and resistant patients. Mindfulness does not have to be complex, and there is always room to build on the practice as the patient advances if he or she is willing.

Guided Meditations: Breathing and Grounding

In this section, we provide two sample meditations that can be taught to youth across the developmental trajectory. The overarching themes to be communicated when guiding immigrant youth through meditations and mindfulness practices are *breathing* and *grounding*. As we know, immigrant youth (or their parents) have been uprooted in some sense or another from their countries of origin, and often they have experienced some sense of uncertainty regarding where they stand in society. First- and second-generation immigrant youth and immigrant youth with bicultural identities may feel even less grounded because they often must choose which elements of identity from their culture are salient in any given situation. For these youth, the following practices are meant to establish a sense of grounding, security, and release. The initial focus on breath allows youth to purposefully access the parasympathetic nervous system and develop a self-regulating, self-soothing practice that lays a foundation for deeper work.

Ocean Breath

PREPARATION

Please begin by either closing your eyes or looking gently down. You can practice ocean breath lying down or sitting.

MEDITATION INSTRUCTIONS

Refer to Audio 3 (available online at www.appi.org/Carrion).

 Audio 3: Ocean Breath (6:41)

You have the power to nurture yourself with a practice that is so simple but we forget to do a lot of the time: by changing the way you are breathing. Notice your breath. No need to change it quite yet; just notice it. Imagine your breath like ocean waves. Is the breath like short, choppy waves crashing onto shore or smooth waves tiding in and out? When the breath is short, the body and the mind are tense. When the breath is big and slow, the body and mind can rest.

This is how you nurture yourself. We will spend 3 whole minutes noticing the breath and making it slow and big so that we can help calm the body and the mind [*note: the first minute is you reading the description that follows*]. Imagine your breath again as waves in the ocean. What kind of wave does your breath look like? If it is choppy or short, begin to slow it down. Begin to breathe deeper. Imagine your waves moving more slowly, peacefully, to shore, as you breathe in, and slowly, peacefully, back to the beautiful, calm ocean as you breathe out. Keep your focus on the breath, on each wave as it moves in and out. If your mind wanders to anything else, invite it back to the ocean waves. Keep practicing for 2 more minutes [*use bells or relaxing timer at the end of 2 minutes*]. Begin to notice your body in this room. Begin to notice the sounds around you. Take a big breath into your nose. Let that breath out through your mouth. Open your eyes when you are ready.

SUGGESTED DEVELOPMENTAL ADAPTATIONS

The Hoberman ball is widely used in the Pure Edge Pure Power Curriculum (Stern et al. 2016) as a visual, tactile breathing tool to assist in mindful breathing practices. The Hoberman ball is a colorful, spherical tool that manually expands and contracts. It is relatively inexpensive and can be found in different sizes online and in many toy stores. It is often used in the context of mindfulness practices as a metaphor for the diaphragm or, more simply, the body as it fills up with and releases the breath. This tool is especially helpful for nonverbal learners because it provides a visual and potentially tactile practice experience. As we know, the process of acculturation for newcomer and first-generation youth often involves English language learning. Therefore, nonverbal cues and teaching styles can be an engaging, culturally adapted approach to teaching mindfulness to these populations. The youth will breathe in as the ball expands and breathe out as it contracts. The facilitator can control the speed of expansion and contraction, similarly controlling the length of the breath. To make it a tactile learning experience, the facilitator can give the Hoberman ball to the participant or pass it among many participants to self-guide their practice. For a purely visual, more cost-effective variation, the facilitator can find computer-based models similar to a Hoberman ball (e.g., "Triangle breathing, 1 minute," available on YouTube at www.youtube.com/watch?v=u9Q8D6n-3qw). These free and accessible videos can serve as an excellent supplement to in-person practice for immigrant youth.

Earth Body Scan

MATERIALS NEEDED

For the earth body scan, you will need a relatively comfortable place to lie flat on the ground (i.e., yoga mat or carpet) or bed. If you are using the optional

activity after the meditation, a piece of paper and coloring supplies are also
needed.

MEDITATION INSTRUCTIONS

Refer to Audio 4 (available online at www.appi.org/Carrion).

 Audio 4: Earth Body Scan (9:29)

To begin, lie flat on the ground. Close your eyes, if comfortable, and practice ocean breath, the new tool learned earlier [*allow 1 minute for ocean breath*].
Now bring your focus to your feet. Let your feet become heavy and relaxed, supported by the earth beneath you. Breathe into your feet and imagine them relaxing more and more. Breathe into your legs. Imagine your legs becoming
heavy, relaxed. Release any tension from your feet and legs into the earth.
Breathe into your belly. Imagine your belly becoming soft, relaxed, and warm.
You are safe. You are supported. Notice your belly rise from the earth as you
breathe in, and release back down as you breathe out. Breathe into your chest
and into your heart. Imagine your chest is becoming relaxed, softening. Imagine
your heart growing roots into the earth. Let go of anything weighing down on
your heart as you breathe out. With each breath in, remember: you are safe; you
are supported. Breathe into your arms. Imagine your arms becoming heavy, relaxed. Breathe into your hands. Imagine your hands becoming heavy, relaxed.
Maybe you make a fist with your hands and then let them go. Imagine the most
loving and special person in your life is here with you, holding your hands. Relax
your hands, knowing that you are safe. You are supported. Let any tension left
in your arms and hands release down into the earth. Breathe into your neck.
Maybe rock your head slowly from side to side for a few breaths, gently stretching the muscles of your neck. Imagine the muscles in your neck becoming relaxed, at ease. Breathe into the muscles of your face. Soften your entire face. Let
your forehead and eyebrows become soft. Let your ears relax. Let your mouth,
your jaw, relax. Glide your tongue over the fronts of your teeth to relax the jaw.
Let your whole head become heavy, relaxed, supported by the earth. With each
breath out, let go of a thought that does not support you, even if it comes back
with the next breath in. With each breath out, let go of a thought that does not
support you. Let your worries release into the earth beneath you. You are safe;
you are supported. Gently come back to your ocean breath [*allow 1 minute*].

When you're ready, take a big stretch and roll off to one side. Pause with
one hand resting on the ground. Notice anything left over from the practice that
is not supporting you. Take a deep breath in. As you breathe out, release anything that is not supporting you into the earth. You are safe. You are supported.
Slowly rise up to sit

OPTIONAL ACTIVITY

Draw any reflection that came up in the practice. This can be words, a poem, a drawing, a feeling—anything that stuck with you from the practice.

Conclusion and Future Directions

Immigrant youth comprise a significant portion of the U.S. population, warranting special attention from mental health professionals nationwide. More bilingual work is especially needed in both treatment and intervention, and research on these themes would advance the field. In closing, we offer you a three-part call to action:

1. Culturally informed mental health professionals are needed trans-systemically in the field to implement mindfulness-based practices and interventions in response to the stressors faced by immigrant youth.
2. More research is needed that focuses on mindfulness-based interventions as both prevention and treatment with this specific demographic, including studies of the efficacy of bilingual delivery.
3. As the research becomes further established, mental health professionals must be on the forefront of advocacy. Through mindful presence and practice, we can help each youth we serve create an inner sanctuary.
   May we strive to bring peace to those who suffer.
   May we remember the urgency of now.

KEY POINTS

- An ecological approach to conceptualization supports a comprehensive understanding of intersecting influences of a child's supports and stressors.
- It is essential to assess for acute needs prior to starting treatment to ensure that basic needs are not a barrier to patient presence and healing.
- Trauma-informed practices is essential with this population, especially in creating and holding a safe space.
- A stance of cultural awareness and humility is encouraged. Mental health professionals should make an effort to be aware of best practices when working with immigrant youth and should understand that patients are an expert in their experience of their own culture.

- It is essential to recognize when you are practicing outside your scope. Seek consultation and training and refer out thoughtfully as needed.

Discussion Questions

1. How can we support immigrant youth with applied mindfulness practices through a trauma-informed approach?
2. How can we practice cultural humility in understanding what values are salient to each youth and his or her family?
3. How can we apply practices and interventions in a way that is culturally meaningful to the youth and his or her family?

Suggested Readings and Websites

For more information on culturally sensitive care of immigrant youth, trauma-informed psychotherapy, and developmentally tailored mindfulness scripts, please consult the following resources. Please note that this list is a selected sample and is nonexhaustive.

Hendricks A, Cohen J, Mannarino A, Deblinger E: Your Very Own TF-CBT Workbook, 1st edition [ebook]. New York, Guilford, 2006. Available at: https://tfcbt.org/wp-content/uploads/2014/07/Your-Very-Own-TF-CBT-Workbook-Final.pdf. Accessed May 15, 2018.
Mindful.stanford.edu: mindfulness blog with developmentally tailored meditation scripts, including audio and video recordings of select practices and recordings of select practices in Spanish.
Patel SG, Reicherter D (eds): Psychotherapy for Immigrant Youth. New York, Springer, 2016. Extensive review of important considerations for therapeutic work with the immigrant youth population.

References

American Psychological Association Presidential Task Force on Immigration: Crossroads: The Psychology of Immigration in the New Century. Washington, DC, American Psychological Association, 2012
Betancourt TS, Newnham EA, Birman D, et al: Comparing trauma exposure, mental health needs, and service utilization across clinical samples of refugee, immigrant, and U.S.-origin children. J Trauma Stress 30(3):209–218, 2017 28585740

Bronfenbrenner U, Ceci SJ: Nature-nurture reconceptualized in developmental perspective: a bioecological model. Psychol Rev 101(4):568–586, 1994 7984707

Ferreira-Vorkapic C, Feitoza JM, Marchioro M, et al: Are there benefits from teaching yoga at schools? A systematic review of randomized control trials of yoga-based programs. Evid Based Complement Alternat Med 2015:345835, 2015 26491461

Frank JL, Bose B, Schrobenhauser-Clonan A: Effectiveness of a school-based yoga program on adolescent mental health, stress coping strategies, and attitudes toward violence: findings from a high-risk sample. Journal of Applied School Psychology 30(1):29–49, 2014

Frisby CL, Jimerson SR: Understanding immigrants, schooling, and school psychology: contemporary science and practice. Sch Psychol Q 31(2):141–148, 2016 27243240

Griner D, Smith TB: Culturally adapted mental health intervention: a meta- analytic review. Psychotherapy (Chic) 43(4):531–548, 2006 22122142

Lui PP: Intergenerational cultural conflict, mental health, and educational outcomes among Asian and Latino Americans: qualitative and meta-analytic review. Psychol Bull 141(2):404–446, 2015 25528344

Patel SG, Reicherter D (eds): Psychotherapy for Immigrant Youth. New York, Springer, 2016

Rettger JP, Kletter H, Carrion V: Trauma and acculturative stress, in Psychotherapy for Immigrant Youth. Edited by Patel SG, Reicherter D. New York, Springer, 2016, pp 87–105

Staudenmeyer A, Macciomei E, Del Cid M, et al: Immigrant youth life stressors, in Psychotherapy for Immigrant Youth. Edited by Patel SG, Reicherter D. New York, Springer, 2016, pp 3–24

Stern E, McDowell C, Parker MJ, et al: 6–12 Power Curriculum. Palm Beach, FL, Pure Edge, 2016. Available at: http://pureedgeinc.org/wp-content/uploads/2016/10/Final-PureEdge_6-12.pdf. Accessed May 15, 2018.

Suárez-Orozco C, Pimentel A, Martin M: The significance of relationships: academic engagement and achievement among newcomer immigrant youth. Teach Coll Rec 111(3):712–749, 2009

Substance Abuse and Mental Health Services Administration: Trauma-informed approach and trauma-specific interventions. Rockville, MD, Substance Abuse and Mental Health Services Administration, 2015. Available at: www.samhsa.gov/nctic/trauma-interventions. Accessed May 15, 2018.

Thorardson MA, Keller M, Sullivan P, et al: Cognitive- behavioral therapy for immigrant youth: the essentials, in Psychotherapy for Immigrant Youth. Edited by Patel SG, Reicherter D. New York, Springer, 2016, pp 27–47

Chapter

11

Incarcerated Youth

Sharon Simpson, Ph.D.
Stewart Mercer, Ph.D.
Sally Wyke, Ph.D.
Michael Bready, M.A.P.P.

CRIMINAL offenses among young people are a concern worldwide. Young people who come in contact with the criminal justice system have usually experienced early childhood adversity and socioeconomic deprivation, have underachieved educationally, and have a high incidence of mental health problems. Impaired cognitive and emotional development; poor problem-solving skills; and challenging behavior, including impulsivity, are also common (Dodge and Pettit 2003).

Despite the challenges inherent in treating incarcerated youth and youth involved with the juvenile justice system, interventions that focus on rehabilitation have shown promise and have been associated with reduced offending. Specific training targeting emotion and behavior regulation and stress could conceivably augment existing rehabilitative strategies. In this chapter, we describe the development of a mindfulness-based intervention (MBI) designed specifically for use with incarcerated young men.

MBIs have been extensively applied in clinical and nonclinical settings, as described by our colleagues elsewhere in this book, and have generally been shown effective in improving psychological and emotional distress. As previously described in Chapters 1–4, mindfulness is a complex multicomponent intervention, thought to work by improving attention, enhancing emotional awareness and regulation, and facilitating a shift in perspective of the self. It might work for incarcerated young people by helping them deal with psychological and emotional difficulties via improving attention, emotional awareness, and regulation. The potential use of mindfulness approaches among incarcerated young people has not been widely studied, and their utility in this population remains largely unknown.

The Polmont Project: Background

In 2012 the Scottish Justice Department identified mindfulness as a potential treatment strategy to improve outcomes related to impulsivity, mental health, and resilience for incarcerated young people (see https://beta.gov.scot/about/how-government-is-run/directorates/justice). In response to this initiative, we developed a bespoke mindfulness course, delivered to seven consecutive groups of young men ($N=48$), ages 18–21 years, over a period of 19 months (Byrne 2017). The courses were iteratively tailored on the basis of stakeholder feedback to meet the complex needs of the youth. These courses were delivered at Her Majesty's Young Offenders Institute (HMYOI) in Polmont, Scotland, the national holding facility.

Methods Used to Develop and Optimize the Program

To develop and optimize the course, the mindfulness teacher tested out different teaching styles and techniques over the seven iterations, and the research team provided feedback using rapid appraisal methods. Rapid appraisal allowed preliminary understanding of data to be generated quickly yet systematically. Interviews with the young men were carried out 1 week after they had completed the course, and the findings then were used to modify subsequent courses.

The qualitative data were analyzed deductively to investigate positive and negative experiences of the course, as reported by the young men and the mindfulness teacher, to identify barriers to and facilitators for initial and sustained engagement. These findings were then fed back to the mindfulness teacher, who iteratively made the refinements and modifications to the course.

In the next section, we describe these refinements and modifications, justify these changes, and present the final optimized version of the course.

Core Therapy Interventions and Techniques

We established in a scoping review (Simpson et al. 2018) that no optimal MBI existed for incarcerated young men. We therefore started with the standard mindfulness-based stress reduction (MBSR) program (Kabat-Zinn 1990), with a view to modification and optimization as we accrued experience. Early discussions with the forensic psychology team in HMYOI Polmont had identified several potential difficulties in engaging young men in programs in this setting. These included the young men's difficulties with concentration, high distractibility, low levels of reading comprehension, and a tendency for manipulative behavior toward external teachers. Gang affiliations were also highlighted as a likely problem, potentially producing divisions, tensions, or even violence within groups.

On the basis of this information, some minor alterations to the MBSR program were made prior to starting the first course; these included a shorter session length (i.e., 90-minute sessions compared with the standard 150-minute sessions), omitting a full-day retreat at week six, and simplification in language and content of the educational components. Otherwise, the initial course that was delivered closely mirrored MBSR (Kabat-Zinn 1990) (see Table 11–1).

Modifications Made to the Course and Justification for Changes

Initially, many of the young men struggled to engage, and the mindfulness teacher was repeatedly confronted with disruptive behavior. This was consistent throughout the duration of all seven courses. However, the young men made many suggestions at the end of each course regarding how best to improve it and render subsequent courses more relevant. Along with the mindfulness teacher, they identified the following barriers (Byrne 2017).

1. They found the practices boring. One young man suggested that the program should be more engaging:

   The first couple of weeks it's boring [being]...asked to hold your breath.... [The teacher should] make it more exciting so people want to come back.

TABLE 11–1. Overview of the initial mindfulness practices delivered

Educational components	Core mindful components (duration)	Activities and exercises
Conceptual learning: what is mindfulness?	Body scan (progressing from 15 to 30 minutes; delivered in all sessions)	Weekly reflections on concepts discussed in session
Improving attentional abilities: introducing the wandering mind, automatic pilot, and present-moment awareness	Sitting practice (ranging from 15 to 30 minutes; delivered in all sessions)	Raisin exercise
Desire and aversion: why do we like or dislike things?	Movement (10 minutes; delivered during sessions 3 and 4)	Personal mission statement
Acceptance: developing a nonjudgmental attitude		Future aspirations and achievable goals
Dealing with stressful situations: adverse effects of stress		Reading selected poems
Compassion: exploring the idea of self-compassion		

Note. This overview is an example of session 1 of the mindfulness course.

2. They were restless and found it difficult to relax. One young man suggested the addition of breaks because mindfulness was not something they were used to:

> Short sessions—not shorter sessions; probably the same length but just a break in between, just a chance to go out the room and sort of go back to normal sort of thing, know what I mean? Because you're in here and you're pure relaxed, and likes of me it's something I'm not used to.

3. They had difficulty sustaining attention. The teacher commented that he was finding it difficult to cater to the wide range of attentional ability among the young men:

> The YO [young offender] with the attentional difficulties again found it difficult to tune into the story. It lasts about 6–7 minutes. This is a difficult challenge—differentiating between those YOs that can engage for longer periods and those that struggle to focus on any given task for more than 10 minutes.

4. They did not really see the value in doing the practices. One young man who did not complete the course commented that he thought there was a resistance to meditation:

> I think a lot of people would just say "it's a lot of shite"…it's just an attitude in here, you know what I mean, in other places you might be all right, It's just because this is a prison, you know what I mean, it's just it's a difficult place…people are very cold-minded.

On the basis of the feedback from the young men and observations from the mindfulness teacher and prison staff, the following changes were made.

1. A "taster" session was introduced to improve understanding and engagement with the course. This session was designed to help the young men learn what to expect from the course and to be sure they understood the level of commitment involved. Sessions were usually 1 hour in duration. However, the mindfulness teacher was responsive to the group's needs and temperament (i.e., if attention levels or levels of engagement were deemed to be low, then session duration would be shortened).
2. Course duration was lengthened from 8 weeks to 10 weeks to allow sufficient time for participants to settle into the practices. The mindfulness teacher felt that the young men needed more exposure to the mindfulness environment, language, and practices.
3. Mindfulness practices were shortened to match the level of engagement from the young men and applied flexibly, aiming for 90 minutes per session where possible. Shorter mini-meditations (2–10 minutes) were introduced, and the young men received these better.

4. Educational content was adapted to allow for low levels of reading comprehension, diverse learning styles, and low attention. More fun and games were introduced, including more simple exercises to illustrate psychological concepts and improve participants' understanding of mindfulness.

5. Sessions were tightly structured to manage problematic behavior and calm the young men. Strategies included trying to make the young men feel safe in the group environment (e.g., by avoiding a circular setup of chairs, which had been identified as intimidating), and an attempt was made to help the young men feel free to experience the practices without placing any unrealistic or stringent expectations on them. This was balanced with clear group boundaries so that participants knew they would be asked to leave if they displayed problematic or disruptive behavior.

6. Concepts from neuroscience were introduced to foster interest in the idea of neuroplasticity (i.e., being able to influence the way in which one's brain works) and how it can impact mental function and behavior.

7. Course content was tailored to the perceived needs of the young men. Focus was switched from *stress reduction* (which was not identified by the young men as important) to developing *character strengths* such as courage and resilience (which they identified as important).

8. Home practices and form filling were removed. None of the young men kept a record of home practices, so this aspect of the course was removed, allowing the young men to use the materials more flexibly, focusing simply on practicing techniques from the session they had attended and/or listening to the CDs provided as desired.

9. The course was pitched in a way that the young men could more easily relate to it. The course title was changed from Mindfulness for Wellbeing to Inner Strength Training, and concepts and predicted benefits from the course were likened to those derived from exercise or sports.

10. As an incentive to taking part, juice and chocolate were provided to help the young men relax and to encourage attendance. Certification was offered on course completion to acknowledge the time, commitment, and effort that participants had invested.

11. More fun was introduced; "icebreaker" activities were used to help the group relax and bond.

12. Regular breaks were incorporated into each session. The young men reported finding the practice quite intense. Thus, regular breaks allowed them time to digest their experiences and adjust to the novel way of learning.

13. A 100-minute challenge of continuous practice in silence gave the young men an opportunity to "test" themselves and develop a sense of self-mastery.

Additional Considerations for Mindfulness Teachers Working Within This Setting

It was also clear that working as a mindfulness teacher within HMYOI Polmont was very challenging, which is an important consideration when seeking to develop a bespoke course in this type of context. The teacher identified that it was particularly important to cultivate *intrinsic motivation and interest*, establish *group agreements*, and adopt a flexible approach while maintaining structure and boundaries. He also recognized the importance of a second facilitator to help with group management.

On reflection, having delivered three programs, the mindfulness teacher felt that the educational component was too analytical and believed that building rapport with the group was more important to gain trust, sustain attention, and cultivate participants' intrinsic motivation:

> One thing that I think makes a big difference is that I don't think the guys really respond to logic. I don't think they really respond to stories or analogies. They respond a little bit to activities, to games, but really, the thing that seems to make the bigger difference in terms of their engagement is the relationship, pure and simple.

Establishing rapport was not easy and required patience, tolerance, and concerted effort:

> So, it kind of suggested to me that the barriers and the threat systems in these young guys are really, really high. It takes a long time to build these relationships.

Problems with disruptive behavior and aggression were prevalent in the study, affecting group cohesion (Byrne 2017). The mindfulness teacher made reference to the volatile nature of one participant:

> He had divulged earlier that he feels ready to "burst and smash anybody at any time." He said that if somebody "threw a cup" at him right in this moment he would "batter them."

Later in the session, the mindfulness teacher said, the young man (here called James) had a dispute with an HMYOI officer:

> This kick-started a verbal shouting match between the officer and James.... This continued to escalate until the officer told James he wasn't going to his work party [a group where the young men learn vocational skills] but instead

was going to his cell. James said he wasn't going anywhere and challenged the officer to try and move him. Three more officers entered the room and a manager. Eventually, James got up and left the room—I thought he was going to punch the officer.

An undertone of vigilance, in particular, a sense of wariness or guardedness, was also apparent in the group settings. Safety concerns were raised frequently. For example, during one course, prison staff interrupted a session to search the young men. This revealed that one of the participants was carrying a knife.

Distrust, suspicion and angry outbursts were a frequent occurrence, with young men acting out frustrations on each other, refusing to participate with the mindfulness practices, or shouting at peers who were passing by outside the room. The young men spoke about this in the interviews:

> Aye, it was just hostile, man, for the first couple of weeks because all of us were just like that, not sure about each other with our eyes closed and all that.

The mindfulness teacher also perceived this in the way the young men initially related to him:

> To begin with, they were quite defensive is maybe too strong but maybe kind of just watch, just kind of like checking me out like, do I trust this guy?

Each of the groups was initially composed of 10 participants, but as the course progressed, numbers dwindled to 2–5 participants. Reasons for poor attendance and high dropout in this study were related to on-site organizational or logistic issues (such as booking errors or staff oversights) or young men being asked to leave because of their disruptive behavior or leaving to join a work party or attend an appointment (e.g., family visit, health checks). For a more comprehensive overview of the findings, see Byrne 2017.

In these smaller groups, the importance of group cohesion and connectedness became clear. A sense of belonging and connection at this point was described during the interviews, with the group format now providing the young men with an opportunity to meet new people, discuss aspects of life important to them, and share and make sense of their experiences. It was clear from participants' accounts that trust and safety acted as factors that enhanced a sense of cohesiveness and connection:

> It's going to sound kind of cheesy, but it felt like I was safe when I was coming to these mindfulness classes because I was safe from all the thoughts when I come here.

> I can let my guard down now in the group a bit more and be more feeling and that.

This cohesiveness was captured on the last day of delivery of the first course, when the mindfulness teacher and the participants shared a group hug, which was initiated by the members of the group. The mindfulness teacher described this in his notes:

> At the end of the session, as I shook the hand and half-hugged one of the young men, the other two came towards me to shake my hand. As I turned to shake the hand of another of the young men, the first opened his arms out and pulled everybody into a group hug. One of the YOs said, "Are we doing a group hug now?" and everybody laughed. There was humor and playfulness and a little bit of awkwardness in it, but I think it also reflected that genuine warmth and friendship that had developed over the 8 weeks of simply being together.

However, every group was different, and on occasion, certain group members needed to be excluded before a sense of cohesiveness could be established. Working guidelines and group agreements were introduced to help address problematic behavior. Establishing group agreements sought to provide a common standard for the young men (i.e., make explicit the behavior required, encourage personal responsibility for being in the group, and help them get the most from taking part). The mindfulness teacher felt that this also gave him authority, which was necessary at times when group members were disruptive:

> Taking time to establish commonly agreed upon guidelines would give me the legitimacy to intervene during times of conflict/aggression amongst the participants.

The mindfulness teacher strove to create an empathic, nonjudgmental, and therapeutic environment, where experiences were explored and the young men could feel supported as they engaged with these novel practices, observing themselves and reflecting on sometimes unpleasant experiences. As outlined earlier, this was at times quite challenging for the young men. The mindfulness teacher needed to be flexible in his approach and able to work within a structured institutional context, often in noisy surroundings and with limited teaching aids. He had to respond skillfully and sensitively to a challenging group of vulnerable and at times volatile young men.

In the study by Byrne (2017), a second facilitator to help with group management was suggested by the mindfulness teacher, but this proved difficult to arrange. Given the high prevalence of mental health concerns, some form of clinical training for teachers may also be necessary in this context. For example, one participant had mental health issues that were of concern to the mindfulness teacher:

> He seemed to describe symptoms of schizophrenia (though of course, I am not qualified to diagnose). He said he sometimes heard his mum talking to him like

she was in the room and he had had enough of it. He couldn't handle it anymore. He also said he couldn't control his anger. He was ready to explode at any moment.

In this instance, and throughout the duration of delivery of all seven courses, the mindfulness teacher worked under the supervision of the chief forensic psychologist and two clinical advisors with extensive experience in mindfulness, one of whom was a consultant psychiatrist.

It is important to consider the potential iatrogenic effects of mindfulness practice for incarcerated young men, many of whom have adverse childhood experiences and severe trauma histories. Potential harm and adverse effects of generic meditation practices have been discussed in the literature (Tangney et al. 2017; Van Dam et al. 2018). The biggest potential harms identified were unjustified claims of benefits, adverse effects, and the possibility of misleading patients who have serious medical conditions. The main adverse events recorded were meditation-related or "meditation-induced" psychosis, depersonalization, anxiety, panic, mania, reexperiencing of traumatic memories, and other forms of clinical deterioration.

In the study by Byrne (2017), the aim was to teach transferable skills (i.e., skills that could become embodied and accessible for the incarcerated young men in other settings) in a manner that was acceptable to the young men. It was also important to be inclusive of the social and cultural factors germane to this group (e.g., appreciating the adaptive and protective role of being vigilant within an environment that can be dangerous, hostile, and hypermasculine, in which any indication of weakness or vulnerability might be life-threatening). For this group, fighting and aggression can represent respect, honor, or status. Sam Himelstein, coauthor of Chapter 8, "Substance Abuse," has addressed this issue in his book *A Mindfulness-Based Approach to Working With High-Risk Adolescents* (Himelstein 2013). He advocates the importance of setting up group agreements and explicitly addresses the issue of safety. Here is an example of how he starts a new group:

> It is important that, if you feel angry, if you feel like you need to fight, that you tell me immediately and one of us will take you outside for a breather. Also, if we can't feel safe in here we will never learn anything. So, I'm really asking that everyone agree that, for this hour and a half each week, we do not get into a fight in this room. Okay?" (Himelstein 2013)

The courses in this study, therefore, were designed to be flexible enough to help participants manage their own, personally specific, problems and issues through the application of mindfulness skills. We explored whether the young men could transfer the mindful skills from the class environment to other settings such as their cells and other prison settings. We also asked, during the semistructured interviews, whether participants intended to use these skills once they were released back into the community. The young men gave concrete and practical examples of how they had independently adapted the practices, making them more relevant to the issues arising within the prison context. Examples of situations in which the young men recounted using the breathing practices to regulate distressing emotions included the following (Byrne 2017):

- Receiving news that a relative or friend had died (usually drug or gang related)
- Dealing with the stress and isolation of being incarcerated
- Dealing with posttraumatic flashbacks
- Dealing with the daily exposure to hostile and potentially threatening situations within the prison itself
- Dealing with potential peer conflict or disagreements with HMYOI Polmont staff

On basis of the needs and circumstances of the young men, course components were molded to render them more acceptable and accessible.

What Remained From Standard MBSR Following Optimization?

Many optimization changes were made, but each course retained the three core MBSR practices (breath awareness, body scan, and mindful movement). Table 11–2 presents the optimized mindfulness course, consisting of a set of 10 scripted sessions.

Comparison With the Existing Literature

In the Byrne (2017) study, sustaining attention and interest from the young men was challenging, with participants frequently describing the mindfulness practices as lengthy, boring, and irrelevant. Barnert et al. (2014) also found mindful meditation practices to be poorly received by incarcerated adolescents, who found them challenging and unhelpful. Mindfulness practices have often been met with initial difficulties in both clinical and nonclinical populations, especially where mindfulness is unfamiliar or practices are perceived as too long or difficult. Williams and Swales (2004) encourage anticipating "adverse reactions" when working with vulnerable groups because they may be overwhelmed by negative experiences or past traumas.

TABLE 11–2.   Optimized version of the mindfulness course

Session	Topic	Description	Activities
Introduction	Introductory taster session	Introduction to the core mindfulness practices; exploring the value of mindfulness	Drumming activity Lecture on neuroplasticity
1	We can train the mind	Introduction to the idea of self-directed neuroplasticity and how people can use mindfulness to change how their brain works	Core mindfulness practices Three questions icebreaker Video of football skills and neuroplasticity Establishing group agreements
2	Discovering attention	Exploration of the wild and unruly mind, which, like a puppy, needs to be trained	Core mindfulness practices Wheel of awareness Lecture on the monkey mind Thought experiment: "Don't think of a white bear" Video: Introduction to the wandering mind
3	Allowing	Learning how to recognize what's happening without resisting or reacting	Core mindfulness practices Cultivating an intention: What do you want? Pushing hands *Kung Fu Panda* movie: Master Oogway illustrates the mindful attitude—in particular, the quality of allowing. It also illustrates that when we allow experience to be as it is, the mind has a tendency to settle. Holding hands aloft exercise

TABLE 11–2. Optimized version of the mindfulness course *(continued)*

Session	Topic	Description	Activities
4	Beginner's mind	Being curious and open to what is happening, without old interpretations	Core mindfulness practices Box of mystery activity Mindful eating (2–3 minutes) Lecture on the beginner's mind Video of Jonathan (baby who hears for the first time) Listening for "the first time" exercise (5–10 minutes)
5	Willpower	Strengthening determination to practice without giving in to reactivity or distraction	Core mindfulness practices Activities: "Holding ice on the hand" and "Chill to be still"
6	Awareness of thoughts	Exploration of how thoughts lead to emotions and influence our behaviors and choices	Core mindfulness practices Story of John: illustrates how our mind creates thoughts and stories even though we may have very little information ABC model of emotion: shows how the thoughts and perceptions we have about an event influence the way we feel Awareness of breathing, sounds, and thoughts (15–20 minutes)
7	Awareness of emotions	Exploration of the nature of emotions and the impact they can have on our lives	Core mindfulness practices Discussion on emotions: what effects do they have in the body, mind, and actions? Who controls you? Lecture on how emotions are generated Exercise: allowing others to push our buttons

TABLE 11–2. Optimized version of the mindfulness course *(continued)*

Session	Topic	Description	Activities
8	Aspirations	Looking to the future	Core mindfulness practices Story of the two wolves: the story is a way of explaining that we can choose the habits we grow in the mind Subway story: shows the power of nonviolence and kindness to deescalate potentially violent situations Reflection: Who do you admire? Discussion of next week's 100-minute challenge
9	100-minute challenge	Practicing mindfulness for a sustained period of time	Core mindfulness practices 10 minutes sitting, 5 minutes movement, 30-minute body scan, 10 minutes walking, 10-minute break, 5 minutes sitting, 15 minutes walking/movement, and 15 minutes sitting
10	The power to create	Celebration of completion of the course, reflection on what has been learned, and inspiring participants to use what they have learned in the future	Core mindfulness practices Consolidating learning Mindfulness of breathing (including reflection on a positive future; 15 minutes) Discussion on a positive future Writing down three life goals Presentation of certificates Short body scan (10 minutes)

Note.   For a more depth explanation of these activities, see Byrne 2017.

In contrast to the Byrne (2017) study, Himelstein et al. (2012) reported that incarcerated adolescents were excited and curious about attending classes. It could be that Himelstein, having been incarcerated during his adolescent years, better matched course content to participants' needs or that the participants differed in some way from those in the Byrne (2017) study. Other differences in Himelstein et al.'s study were that participants were selected for the course by court order and/or probation staff and that Himelstein delivered the course and conducted the interviews himself, an important potential source of bias.

Problems with disruptive behavior and aggression were prevalent in the Byrne (2017) study, affecting group cohesion. Problems with disruptive behavior were also reported by Jee et al. (2015), who used MBSR to treat traumatized young people in foster care. They reported disruptive, aggressive, and volatile tendencies on several occasions, and participants brought weapons into the groups as a form of "protection." This led to young men being removed from courses. Jee and colleagues indicated that prevalent childhood adversity was a barrier to peer interaction and trust and suggested that background clinical information should be made available to teachers delivering the course.

The importance of mindfulness teachers being appropriately trained and qualified when working with specialized populations has been emphasized in the literature (Crane et al. 2010, 2012; Shafran et al. 2009). Although there are no statutory regulations, a UK voluntary code of conduct exists in this regard (https://mindfulnessteachersuk.org.uk/pdf/teacher-guidelines.pdf).

In the Byrne (2017) study, mindfulness sessions were reduced to 90 minutes; meditation practices were shortened; and simpler, more fun, and more interactive ways of learning and sustaining attention were introduced. Himelstein (2013) recommended integrating new and varied modes of learning in at-risk populations, keeping sessions "lively," "topical," and "interactive." He noted that variety is especially relevant in maintaining attention and interest because boredom is the "arch nemesis for many adolescents" (p. 126).

In the Byrne (2017) study, the program was lengthened from 8 to 10 weeks to allow more time for learning during shorter sessions. Similar developmental adaptations noted in the literature concerning young people include shorter session lengths; shorter and more frequent skills training techniques; defining "mindful" concepts more simply, preferably in a visual manner; and repetition to help facilitate lasting change, with emphasis on sensory observation (i.e., bodily sensations) over abstract experiences (i.e., thoughts), which is believed to be more grounding and tangible (Semple et al. 2010; Thompson and Gauntlett-Gilbert 2008).

It seems clear that learning styles and preferences have to be taken into account in delivering mindfulness training in this context. In 2013, the Young Offenders Survey (*N*=267) at HMYOI Polmont (McCoard et al. 2013) found that preferred ways of learning in the institute were through sports (58%) and practical workshops (57%) and that creating a relaxed learning environment was important. In the Byrne (2017) study, the young men struggled with psycho-educational components they often felt were less relevant to them. On the other hand, the young men reported more engagement and benefits with the body-based practices, such as the body scan or the breathing practices.

In the Byrne (2017) study, the young men reported very limited home practice. However, recent evidence has confirmed the importance of home practice as consistently contributing to better outcomes (Parsons et al. 2017), a finding echoed in incarcerated young people by Leonard et al. (2013). Therefore, future studies should attempt to better understand and improve acceptability and accessibility of home practice materials for this population.

For a summary of the literature, see Table 11–3.

Trauma-Informed Approach to Mindfulness Within Youth Offending Populations

A recent scoping review, evaluating existing evidence for MBIs among youth offending populations, reported it was not possible to determine the optimal approach in this context (Simpson et al. 2018). This was due to heterogeneity among interventions in terms of content, dose, and intensity. However, the authors noted beneficial effects across a range of outcomes, including mental health, self-regulation, problematic behavior, substance use, quality of life, and criminal propensity. No studies have reported on trauma-specific outcomes, highlighting an important gap in the knowledge base in this area.

In adult offending populations, the potential effectiveness of MBIs for trauma has been explored. In a pilot study, Simpson et al. (2007) evaluated whether participation in a 10-day Vipassana course had an impact on symptom severity in posttraumatic stress disorder (PTSD). Comparable improvements in substance use were demonstrated for individuals both with and without PTSD symptoms. How the Vipassana training may have influenced outcomes remains unclear. The study authors speculated that Vipassana may act by targeting and reducing "experiential avoidance." If this is indeed the mechanism of action, such an approach may potentially provide new skills for dealing with painful traumatic experiences, which is particularly relevant in PTSD. More research is clearly needed to better understand the potential role, effectiveness, and mechanisms of action of MBIs among people with PTSD.

Conclusion and Future Directions

Standard MBSR required substantial adaptation and flexibility in delivery to meet the needs of the young men who took part in the study by Byrne (2017). Necessary changes included introducing taster sessions, lengthening the course

TABLE 11–3. Summary of research literature

Study	Population	Intervention	Outcome
Randomized controlled trials			
Evans-Chase 2013	Male adolescents (*N*=59: 29 IBM, 30 control group) housed in a juvenile justice facility	IBM	The oldest age group (19–23) in the treatment group scored significantly higher in self-regulation ability (*P*<0.05) postintervention than their similarly matched control counterparts.
Himelstein et al. 2015	Male adolescents (*N*=27, assigned to either 1:1 mindfulness or TAU), housed at a juvenile detention camp	1:1	Treatment group showed significantly greater increases in quality of life (ES 0.60; *P*<0.05) and staff rating of good behavior (*P*<0.05). No difference was seen in self-regulation (ES 0.25; *P*>0.05), substance use (ES 0.32; *P*>0.05), and mindfulness (ES 0.09; *P*>0.05). Both groups showed significant improvements in decision making (ES 0.46; *P*<0.01).
Leonard et al. 2013	Male adolescents (*N*=264: 147 MBCT, 117 active control); treatment delivered at an urban correctional complex	MM-CBT	Overall task performance on the attention network test degraded in all participants. However, the magnitude of degradation was significantly less for the treatment group (ES 0.30; *P*<0.01).
Nonrandomized controlled trial			
Flinton 1997	Male adolescents (*N*=42: 23 SMP, 19 control), residing in a camp for juvenile offenders	SMP	Compared with controls, SMP group showed significant improvements in mental health (anxiety: ES 1.14; *P*<0.05) and in internal locus of control (ES 1.47; *P*<0.05).

TABLE 11–3. Summary of research literature (*continued*)

Study	Population	Intervention	Outcome
Pre/post studies			
Himelstein et al. 2012	Male adolescents (*N*=32), housed at a juvenile correctional facility in California	MBA	Participants showed significant improvements in mental health (stress: ES 0.42; $P<0.05$) and self-regulation (ES 0.60; $P<0.001$). No significant difference was found on self-reported mindfulness, although it did show a trend toward improvement (ES 0.22; $P>0.05$).
Khurana and Dhar 2000	Male adolescents (*n*=232) and female adults (*n*=30) incarcerated at Tihar Jail, India	VM	Significant improvement in subjective well-being ($P<0.01$) and decrease in level of criminal propensity ($P<0.01$) were seen for those who attended VM.
Le and Proulx 2015	Male and female adolescents (*N*=33), housed at a youth correctional facility	MBA	MBA participants showed significant improvements in mental well-being (stress: ES 1.00; $P<0.05$). Although not significant, a positive trend toward improvement was observed for impulsivity (ES 0.32; $P>0.05$), self-regulation (ES 0.29; $P>0.05$), and mindfulness (ES 0.40; $P>0.05$).

TABLE 11–3. Summary of research literature *(continued)*

Study	Population	Intervention	Outcome
Mixed methods			
Barnert et al. 2014	Male adolescents (*N*=29); treatment delivered at a juvenile correctional facility	MBA	Participants showed a significant increase in self-regulation (ES 0.44; *P*<0.05). Stress (ES 0.32; *P*=0.29), mindfulness (ES 0.20; *P*=0.31), and impulsivity (ES 0.20; *P*=0.30) showed a trend toward improvement but did not reach statistical significance. The young men spoke about feeling better, feeling more in control, having improved self-awareness, and having increased social cohesiveness. They also spoke about a resistance to the meditation practice and future use of the techniques.
Evans-Chase 2015	Male adolescents (*N*=61), housed in a juvenile justice facility	IBM	No significant difference found on self-reported mindfulness (ES 0.12; *P*>0.05). Participants described using class skills to regulate emotions and behavior and deal with conflict in the facility.
Himelstein 2011a	Male adolescents (*N*=48), housed at a juvenile correctional facility	MBSU	Results showed a significant decrease in impulsivity (ES 0.43; *P*<0.01) and a significant increase in perceived risk of drug use (ES 0.75; *P*<0.05) from pretest to posttest. No significant difference was found on self-regulation, although a trend toward improvement was shown (ES 0.25; *P*>0.05). From the focus group discussions, three major themes were identified: receptivity to the program in general, appreciation of the facilitator's teaching style, and learning about drugs.

TABLE 11–3. Summary of research literature *(continued)*

Study	Population	Intervention	Outcome
Observational studies and semistructured interviews			
Derezotes 2000	Male adolescent sex offenders; number of participants unclear	SMP	Participants reported feeling more relaxed, having improved concentration and improved impulse control, and being less disturbed by thoughts. Being treated with respect, care, and humanness was also identified as important. Parents and facilitators were supportive of the course.
Himelstein 2011b	Male adolescents (*N*=32), housed at a juvenile correctional facility in California	MBA	Main themes identified were increased well-being, improved self-regulation, increased awareness, and an accepting attitude toward the intervention.
Himelstein et al. 2015	Male adolescents (*N*=10), housed in a Californian detention center	1:1	Main themes identified were enhanced psychological mindfulness and well-being, development of worldview, novel experiences, challenging experiences, and future use.

Note.   1:1=one to one; ES=effect size; IBM=Internet-based mindfulness; MBA=mind-body awareness; MBSU=mindfulness-based substance use; MM-CBT=mindfulness meditation–cognitive-behavioral therapy; SMP=structured mindfulness program; TAU=treatment as usual; VM=Vipassana meditation.
Source.   Byrne et al. 2017.

from 8 to 10 weeks, shortening the meditation practices, adapting the educational materials, structuring the sessions to make them simpler and more accessible for diverse learning styles and levels of attention, and minimization of form filling.

Each delivery of the course retained the three core components of standard MBSR (awareness of the breath, body scan, and mindful movement), delivered in a format appropriate for the population in this setting. This required flexibility and responsiveness to the young men by the mindfulness teacher.

Development and optimization of the mindfulness course duration and content were a continuous and iterative process throughout the delivery of all seven courses. Future courses with this population should use the latest version of the tailored program. Future studies could specifically monitor adherence in relation to form (structure of how the course is delivered) and function (content of delivery and how it is received).

The results of the study by Byrne (2017) should be regarded as only the first step in formulating the evidence base for mindfulness with incarcerated young people. The optimal approach in this context remains unknown. It would be useful to explore the feasibility of delivering this type of intervention in a broader range of forensic settings, ranging from high-security, high-risk individuals to lower-risk community outpatient samples that can also involve families in a collaborative care approach.

Goals of future studies may be to create standardized mindfulness protocols and to use standardized outcome measures to facilitate comparison. Future large studies are required that include a control group for comparison of effects. Ideally, mindfulness should be delivered as a randomized control trial or, if randomization is not possible, then with a matched control group. Little remains known about how these interventions compare with other commonly used psychological interventions or how cost-effective they might be.

Further high-quality studies are needed to establish feasibility, effectiveness, and implementability of mindfulness programs with incarcerated youth. However, the challenges of conducting rigorous research within a prison setting must also be acknowledged and accommodated in future research in this area.

KEY POINTS

- At the initiation of the mindfulness course with incarcerated youth, the relevance and potential of the program to bring positive changes in young people's lives need to be made clear to participants in a way that promotes engagement.

- Facilitators can adapt the structure and length of sessions and tailor the specific mindfulness interventions in order to maximize participant attentiveness and engagement.

- Incarcerated young people have complex and diverse learning needs. Teaching materials will need to be adapted to match the developmental and educational level of the participants and to minimize form filling.

- When working with incarcerated young people, it is advisable to have at least two highly trained facilitators, one knowledgeable about mindfulness and the other knowledgeable about mental health, to navigate challenging and volatile behaviors and to promote a safe and positive learning environment.

- Further implementation research needs to be performed before this program is applied to other incarcerated populations (e.g., women, adult prisoners, sex offenders).

Discussion Questions

1. How could mindfulness be integrated with current rehabilitations strategies in young offenders?
2. How could support for mindfulness be continued after the young offenders are released from incarceration?
3. How could a definitive randomized control trial be designed for young offenders, and what would be the best primary outcomes to measure?

Suggested Readings

Himelstein S: A Mindfulness-Based Approach to Working With High-Risk Adolescents, Vol 35. London, Routledge, 2013

Shonin E, Van Gordon W, Slade K, et al: Mindfulness and other Buddhist-derived interventions in correctional settings: a systematic review. Aggress Violent Behav 18(3):365–372, 2013

References

Barnert ES, Himelstein S, Herbert S, et al: Exploring an intensive meditation intervention for incarcerated youth. Child Adolesc Ment Health 19(1):69–73, 2014

Byrne S: The development and evaluation of a mindfulness-based intervention for incarcerated young men. PhD thesis. Glasgow, Scotland, UK, Institute of Health and Wellbeing, University of Glasgow, 2017. Available at: http://encore.lib.gla.ac.uk/iii/encore/record/C__Rb3269060. Accessed May 14, 2018.

Crane RS, Kuyken W, Hastings RP, et al: Training teachers to deliver mindfulness-based interventions: learning from the UK experience. Mindfulness (NY) 1(2):74–86, 2010 23293682

Crane RS, Kuyken W, Williams JM, et al: Competence in teaching mindfulness-based courses: concepts, development and assessment. Mindfulness (NY) 3(1):76–84, 2012 23293683

Derezotes D: Evaluation of yoga and meditation trainings with adolescent sex offenders. Child Adolesc Social Work J 17(2):97–113, 2000

Dodge KA, Pettit GS: A biopsychosocial model of the development of chronic conduct problems in adolescence. Dev Psychol 39(2):349–371, 2003 12661890

Evans-Chase M: Internet-based mindfulness meditation and self-regulation: a randomized trial with juvenile justice involved youth. Journal of Juvenile Justice 3:63–79, 2013

Evans-Chase M: Mindfulness meditation with incarcerated youth: a randomized controlled trial informed by neuropsychosocial theories of adolescence. Int J Dev Neurosci 47(Pt A):3, 2015 29887072

Flinton CA: The effects of meditation techniques on anxiety and locus of control in juvenile delinquents. Doctoral dissertation, California Institute of Integral Studies, San Francisco, CA, 1997

Himelstein S: Meditation research: the state of the art in correctional settings. Int J Offender Ther Comp Criminol 55(4):646–661, 2011a 20332328

Himelstein S: Mindfulness-based substance abuse treatment for incarcerated youth: A mixed method pilot study. International Journal of Transpersonal Studies 30(1–2)1–10, 2011b

Himelstein S: A Mindfulness-Based Approach to Working With High-Risk Adolescents. London, Routledge, 2013

Himelstein S, Hastings A, Shapiro S, et al: A qualitative investigation of the experience of a mindfulness-based intervention with incarcerated adolescents. Child Adolesc Ment Health 17(4):231–237, 2012

Himelstein S, Saul S, Garcia-Romeu A: Does mindfulness meditation increase effectiveness of substance abuse treatment with incarcerated youth? A pilot randomized controlled trial. Mindfulness 6(6):1472–1480, 2015

Jee SH, Couderc J-P, Swanson D, et al: A pilot randomized trial teaching mindfulness-based stress reduction to traumatized youth in foster care. Complement Ther Clin Pract 21(3):201–209, 2015 26256140

Kabat-Zinn J: Full Catastrophe Living: How to Cope With Stress, Pain, and Illness Using Mindfulness Meditation. New York, Dell, 1990

Khurana A, Dhar PL: Effect of Vipassana Meditation on Quality of Life, Subjective Well-being, and Criminal Propensity Among Inmates of Tihar Jail, Delhi. Maharashtra, India, Vipassana Research Institute, 2000. Available at: www.vridhamma.org/node/2835. Accessed October 31, 2018.

Le TN, Proulx J: Feasibility of mindfulness-based intervention for incarcerated mixed-ethnic native Hawaiian/Pacific Islander youth. Asian Am J Psychol 6(2):181–189, 2015

Leonard NR, Jha AP, Casarjian B, et al: Mindfulness training improves attentional task performance in incarcerated youth: a group randomized controlled intervention trial. Front Psychol 4:792, 2013 24265621

McCoard S, Broderick R, Carnie J: Male Young Offenders 2013. 14th Survey Bulletin. Edinburgh, UK, Scottish Prison Service, 2013

Parsons CE, Crane C, Parsons LJ, et al: Home practice in mindfulness-based cognitive therapy and mindfulness-based stress reduction: a systematic review and meta-analysis of participants' mindfulness practice and its association with outcomes. Behav Res Ther 95:29–41, 2017 28527330

Semple RJ, Lee J, Rosa D, et al: A randomized trial of mindfulness-based cognitive therapy for children: promoting mindful attention to enhance social-emotional resiliency in children. J Child Fam Stud 19(2):218–229, 2010

Shafran R, Clark DM, Fairburn CG, et al: Mind the gap: improving the dissemination of CBT. Behav Res Ther 47(11):902–909, 2009 19664756

Simpson TL, Kaysen D, Bowen S, et al: PTSD symptoms, substance use, and Vipassana meditation among incarcerated individuals. J Trauma Stress 20(3):239–249, 2007 17597132

Simpson S, Mercer SW, Simpson R, et al: Mindfulness-based interventions for incarcerated populations: a scoping review. Mindfulness (NY) 9(5):1330–1343, 2018 30294385

Tangney JP, Dobbins AE, Stuewig JB, et al: Is there a dark side to mindfulness? Relation of mindfulness to criminogenic cognitions. Pers Soc Psychol Bull 43(10):1415–1426, 2017 28918714

Thompson M, Gauntlett-Gilbert J: Mindfulness with children and adolescents: effective clinical application. Clin Child Psychol Psychiatry 13(3):395–407, 2008 18783122

Van Dam NT, van Vugt MK, Vago DR, et al: Mind the hype: a critical evaluation and prescriptive agenda for research on mindfulness and meditation. Perspect Psychol Sci 13(1):36–61, 2018 29016274

Williams JM, Swales M: The use of mindfulness-based approaches for suicidal patients. Arch Suicide Res 8(4):315–329, 2004 16081399

Chapter

12

Trauma-Informed Yoga With Vulnerable Youth

Pamela Lozoff, M.S.W., RYT

Neurosequential Model of Therapeutics

A decade ago, I began working with The Art of Yoga Project (AYP), serving young women who are incarcerated and/or otherwise court involved through trauma-informed yoga and creative arts programs. The AYP had adopted a trauma-informed model for teaching yoga, which was largely influenced by the work of Dr. Bruce Perry, who pioneered the neurosequential model of therapeutics (NMT), a neurodevelopmental model for addressing complex trauma in children and youth (Perry 2006). In this model, Dr. Perry proposed therapeutic intervention and suggested that we have to regulate before we can relate or reason. This regulation occurs nonverbally and generally involuntarily within our physiology, except when we take conscious breaths to calm the nervous system. In this chapter, I outline various trauma-informed practices that have applications across many vulnerable populations of youth and for service providers as well.

Within the context of a yoga class with young people with complex trauma, this concept translates to first doing a warm-up exercise in which we regulate the nervous system through *tapping* at certain pressure points, *shaking* out each of the hands and then each foot while counting down from 10 or 5, or *twisting* side to side (to engage the brain contralaterally). Once the nervous system can begin to regulate, it then can signal to the brain that the body is safe from immediate external threats or harm. The brain can shift out of survival mode, and one can be ready to engage with others and learn new information.

Following the warm-up, we pose a check-in question to the group, asking them to share (with the option of passing) their name, how they are feeling, and a response to the question as it relates to the theme for the day. For example, this may include sharing a strength they have, some advice they've received for moving through a challenging time, or a person in their life who inspires them or "rocks their world." Once we have engaged in a relational activity, then we can move into the yoga practice, emphasizing movement with breath for self-regulation rather than the correct alignment or precision of the poses.

A recently released report out of the Georgetown Center on Poverty and Inequality stated that trauma-informed, gender-responsive, and culturally competent somatic interventions can lead to improvements in the following outcomes: self-regulation and other emotional development, neurological and physical health, and healthier relationships and parenting practices (Epstein and Gonzáles 2017). In this chapter, I describe yoga and other somatic-based interventions as promising interventions that can promote positive outcomes and are therefore an important area for further health research, especially concentrating on reversing the harmful effects of adverse childhood experiences and healing complex trauma.

For vulnerable youth, the practice of yoga is choice based, inviting the youth participants to tune into their own personal experience of the poses and make a choice about which poses to do, whether to use a modification, or whether to choose another pose. This approach to the practice allows participants to reclaim a sense of personal agency, which is at the core of addressing the impact of trauma, which often renders the survivor powerless and without a sense of personal agency (Emerson and Hopper 2011). Sometimes, youth will avoid more vulnerable poses in which the legs are spread wide apart or the hips are open. Sometimes, they will replay sexual trauma when coming into a pose, such as the goddess pose (also known as horse pose, which is a standing hip opener), standing with legs spread wide, bending through the knees. I have observed teen girls begin to thrust their pelvis while in this pose, either to get the attention of the other girls in the group or to get the attention of the guards or teachers.

In a context where, according to a report by the Office of Juvenile Justice and Delinquency Prevention, 75% of youth in the juvenile detention system have experienced traumatic victimization, to be trauma informed means to recognize that often, the behaviors we observe are a result of the trauma these young people have experienced (Finkelhor et al. 2011). As Sam Himelstein (see Chapter 8, "Substance Abuse") describes in his work, these behaviors are *traumatic adaptations* that have risen out of a response to trauma and as survival skills. What may look like acting out, defiance, or overt sexual behavior is often an adaptation to the type of trauma a young person has repeatedly been subjected to. Although this does not excuse the behavior, it can help us as practitioners to understand the behavior and where it is stemming from and then to address the young person from a place of compassion.

Rather than trying to correct the behavior by taking away a young person's coping mechanism or traumatic adaptation, we can offer new ways of coping through somatic-based tools. For example, after having a piece of notebook paper hurled at me by a young person who was having a particularly rough day, rather than telling her to never do that again, I named my feeling, telling her that I felt disrespected, and said, "I'm going to give you a new piece of paper, and I want you to see if you can trace the short side of the paper and inhale, and then trace the long side of the paper and exhale. If you don't want to join us for journaling, see if you can try this so that you are still participating in the group and I don't have to ask you to leave." She tried the breathing exercise one time, making sure to emphasize heavy and labored breathing for all of us to hear, and then she picked up a pen and started doodling.

Teaching Example: Coregulation and Self-Regulation

In one of the classes I was teaching, I encountered Joey, a transgender young person. Joey would often opt out of poses such as downward dog or lunges and would instead lie down on his belly with his arms bent, resting one cheek to the side and placing it on his stacked hands. I checked in with Joey consistently, and he always said he didn't like yoga, and he especially didn't like downward dog. I was not surprised, given his history of sexual abuse; doing a pose that requires you to fold forward and tilt your pelvis so your tailbone is the highest point in the pose can be triggering and make you feel unsafe in your body. Joey also would opt out of adjustments during our resting pose and in other poses, in which we would offer some suggestions and hands-on touch to find a version of the pose that works within one's own body.

After I had been teaching at the facility weekly for about 6 months, Joey called me over during resting pose and asked if I would adjust him on that particular day. I made my way over to him and began by holding his feet and swaying his legs side to side to lengthen through the hip flexor muscles. Then I moved to his head and placed my hands under his occipital lobe, cupping my hands behind his head, at which point there ensued a visceral response of tension releasing out through his jaw in waves of trembling.

I literally felt Joey's pain in this moment. I felt the pain as heat in my hands. I watched his breath move in staccato cadence, his chest heaving, while I placed my attention on my own breath and endeavored to keep it regulated and steady. As my breath deepened, Joey's breath began to deepen as well. As Perry (2006) described, we were coregulating, wherein my self-regulation through steady and even breaths signaled safety to this young person so that he could find a steadier breath for himself. Once a sense of safety had been reestablished within his nervous system, I could remove my hands, and he could begin to self-regulate.

Ultimately, as practitioners or service providers, we want to provide our patients with the tools to self-regulate and self-soothe. We want them to be able to steady their breathing, deepening their exhales to activate the parasympathetic nervous system through vagal toning and to deactivate the sympathetic nervous system. We want them to regulate their survival brain to be able to relate from their limbic/emotional brain and then be able to reason and learn from their cognitive brain. In fact, it is a hindrance to the therapeutic process if the youth are not regulated because it will impede the relational dimension of the therapy as well as their ability to engage in any form of cognitive processing or restructuring.

Joey's case provides a living example of the underlying trauma-informed teaching strategies that I present in this chapter. When giving instructions, make them *predictable*, *concrete*, and *invitational*.

1. **Predictable:** Let the students know how long they will be in the pose rather than being vague or uncertain. Give students a cue such as holding the pose for five breaths or repeating three times and invite students to count the breaths with you or for you.

2. **Concrete:** Keep the focus on physical sensations rather than abstract concepts. Bring students' attention to the muscle of the thighs working in the pose, the hands placed on the hips, or the core muscles engaging. Using concepts such as following a white light through the spine or feeling the energy at the crown of the head can be too esoteric and can lead students to dissociate because their attention doesn't have something to grab onto.

3. **Invitational language:** People with trauma have experienced a profound sense of powerlessness; therefore, the yoga space should be one where there is a sense of choice, not a power dynamic in which youth are being commanded to do something. Give options with structure. For example:

As you are ready, go ahead and step the foot forward to come into crescent lunge. Close your eyes in this pose or direct the gaze down and focused inward. Take a downward dog, or if that pose isn't for you, go ahead and take a child's pose.

Yoga Adaptations

Consideration of the youth's physical abilities is advised. For example, the youth may have physical injuries or other movement limitations that can present unique challenges for the yoga experience. Furthermore, with rises in obesity rates among youth, body image sensitivity, language, and cultural consideration, religion, and related physical challenges and resistances to practicing may arise.

Recommendations for Group Practice

Pay attention to how youth are placed relative to one another, facility staff, and their environment. The following are a few ways to create a trauma-informed group environment.

- Practice in a circle, horseshoe, or two rows facing each other. As much as possible within the space, configure the group so that students are practicing next to each other and not behind or in front of each other. This will prevent students folding forward toward someone else's pelvis or genital region and also sends a message of an inclusive and equitable space with everyone being seen and a part of the group.
- Notice where the entryways are into the room. Track where facility staff and other students enter and leave the room. Do your best not to have participants with their backs to a doorway so that they won't be startled if someone comes into the room. For your own safety as well, be sure that participants do not block the doorway.
- Position yourself so that students can see you. Practice in the circle or formation with the youth if possible. If you do need to move around the room, just ensure that you are not startling participants by coming up behind them unexpectedly. Let them know that you will be moving to a different part of the room.

Trauma-Sensitive Adaptation in Yoga Poses

It is suggested that instructors teach with sensitivity with respect to the physical shapes of yoga poses and how those shapes may be triggering for some students. These can include bound poses, such as those in which the physical body may feel trapped or restricted, or poses requiring the hands to be interlaced and placed behind the back, which may be bothersome because of a resemblance to handcuffing. Downward-facing dog pose can be a risky pose to teach to youth, particularly middle schoolers and older, because of the possibility that they may sexualize the pose. The same is true of seated or standing wide-angle poses, forward-folding standing poses, reclined butterfly, happy baby pose, and related variations.

In consideration of the important role of avoidance in feeding posttraumatic reactions, it is not recommended to forever banish these poses from your toolbox. However, it is advisable to introduce them slowly after the necessary time has been invested in establishing a strong treatment alliance and safety with the individual or group and unhelpful vulnerability is minimized (Emerson et al. 2009).

Working With Resistance

It is likely that in working with young people, you will encounter resistance. Across young populations, there may be considerable reports of somatic symptoms that may be psychological in nature, and these symptoms could serve as a resistance to practicing yoga. Here are a few helpful tips on how to work through resistance.

- Use rhythm and music and, when appropriate, incorporate suggestions from youth participants.
- Connect yoga to what inspires the youth—consider examples from professional sports or celebrities.
- Use challenge poses such as arm balances and inversions, practiced safely.
- Provide leadership opportunities and use more challenging youth as leaders.
- Use sensory objects such as a Hoberman sphere, fidgets, or tactile props to ground students.
- Provide experiences of success and mastery.
- Create structured choices. Provide several options for activities that are still within a relevant scope for participants to learn the skills, such as Zen tangles, coloring books, or clay, where clinically indicated.
- Give participants choices about postures. The poses should be invitational only, with other options provided for poses that may be triggering for some participants.
- In female-identifying adolescents, be aware that there may be menstrual cramping or discomfort. If this is the case, restorative poses such as reclined butterfly or gentle twists and use of bolsters or rolled-up yoga mats can be useful accommodations.

Therapeutic Setting and Duration

Depending on the setting, the length of the yoga program as an intervention may vary. Often, in my experience in treatment programs, the youth are there for 6 months and will receive yoga for the duration of their time. Some of the yoga service programs aim to offer yoga at least 2 times per week to emphasize learning through repetition and to create consistency and cohesion within the group. The sessions are between 45 minutes and 1 hour, and the group format creates a structure and container for youth to be able to know what to expect and begin to form a rhythm with the yoga practice as a group. Each group generally consists of an opening practice with movement and/or breathing exercises, a check-in, an asana or yoga practice, and then a checkout. Sometimes, journaling or other expressive arts activities will be folded into the session, depending on how engaged the youth are in the yoga.

Teaching Example: Holding Our Pain

Each of the young people in the girls' juvenile hall facility chose their final resting pose for our yoga class (either on their side, on their back, or on their belly), often crossing their arms or placing their hands in their facility-assigned sweatshirts so as not to lose their vigilance and awareness of their surroundings (or their street cred), often with their lower legs and feet remaining restless. After the participants indicated whether or not they wanted hands-on adjustments, I moved over to Joey, a transgender male-identifying young person, and kneeled by his head, placing my hands behind his neck to lengthen through his cervical spine. I cupped my hands at the base of his skull, following the protocol for using consensual and directed touch within the context of our classes in the juvenile hall settings. Joey's jaw began to tremble into my hands, sending currents of pain, transmitting information (which I had also acquired from our case conference meetings) about the abuse by his father and the sexual abuse by her uncle before she transitioned to identifying as male. I let him release these currents into my hands, and I held still.

"Are you doing OK?" I asked. Joey nodded silently. I watched the breath begin to slow and move into his belly while he lay there on his mat in resting pose. I slowly pulled away and moved to adjust the next young person, offering the same cranio hold, allowing the parasympathetic nervous system to release into its relaxation response.

My hands could hold the pain of this young person as it was being released out through his trembling jaw only because I have felt into the depths of my own pain—different pain, but pain nonetheless. I hold in my body the pain of a decade of restricting my food intake, of overexercising, of competitive gymnastics, of a mother struggling with depression, and of a nagging and persistent voice that has always told me I will never be good enough no matter how much I accomplish. First, I had to learn to have someone else hold my pain (physically and emotionally), and over the past decade of my own healing, I have had to learn how to hold and be with my own pain. In the next sections, I will share my learning and how I have applied it toward my work with youth in a range of community-based and therapeutic settings as a case manager, a social worker, and a yoga teacher.

Trauma-Informed Practice With Groups

For 2 years, I facilitated yoga groups two times per week at a therapeutic day school for high school–age youth, with 8–12 youth per group each day. Each of the group participants had a mental health diagnosis, and most had a history of trauma. Their presence at this school meant that mainstream school did not work for these young people, and they either were referred there after having been expelled from school for behavioral incidents or were referred by their previous school therapist to this more specialized setting.

Each group session began with one of the students volunteering to ring the chimes and all of the students taking 1 minute of silence together. Then, we moved to a check-in question and discussion, followed by the practice. The group format was always the same so that there was consistency and predictability—two key components of trauma-informed work, according to the model presented by Perry (2006). What students often remarked was most useful about this group was the opportunity to shift out of process-oriented therapy and, as one student put it, to "just have one place to be peaceful outside of the chaos and noise of all the rest of my life."

In group facilitation, there is quite a bit of rhetoric about creating a *safe space*, which often relates to participants feeling safe to express themselves and their opinions without judgment from the other group members. Safety cannot exist at the cognitive level without first being established by signaling to the body and survival brain through regulating the breath. In these yoga groups, participants experience what safety feels like within their own body. They choose what poses they want to do and the modifications they wish to take within the poses, and they have the right to pass when it comes to sharing in the check-in or checkout circle.

The group dynamic within the yoga group also presents opportunities for youth to lead one another through poses. Because of the repetition of the poses, a sense of mastery can be acquired through a consistent and regular practice. Within this group, after about 3–4 weeks, I first invited youth to go through a sun salutation, with each person in the group leading one part of the sequence. Next, I asked if anyone in the group wanted to lead their peers through a sun salutation. What I noticed was that the young people who were often the least participatory in the discussion or in the classroom (on the basis of their teachers' assessments) were the ones who volunteered to lead the sun salutations. These students learned kinesthetically, and after a few weeks of reinforcing the learning of the sequences, they felt competent and confident to lead a sequence. We always gave "snaps" as a form of applause after a young person led a sun salutation, and group members had the opportunity to recognize their peers for taking initiative and completing a task.

Exercises and Postures

In this section, we explore a few yoga postures with specific therapeutic functions and an NMT-based regulating practice. These practices are designed to regulate the nervous system, either down from hyperarousal or up from hypoarousal. When guiding the seated, standing, or reclined yoga postures described in the following subsections, always remind participants that they know their own bodies the best and instruct them to find the version of the posture that feels safest and most comfortable in their own bodies.

Note: When instructing postures, keep the attention on physical sensations that allow young persons to stay in their body and be aware of their breath in certain parts of the body or the weight shifting into certain places. Avoid esoteric instructions (e.g., "Imagine light filling up the rib cage as you breathe in") because they can take youth out of their direct experience of the posture and into memories or flashbacks.

Warm-Up and Regulating Exercises

FIVE-COUNT SHAKE-OUT

For this exercise, it is recommended that participants stand. Instruct youth to count down from 5 as they shake one hand overhead, then the other hand, and shake first one foot, then the other foot. Then count down from 4, then 3, then 2, and 1, after which instruct youth to shake everything out and then come to standing still, noticing the effects of the shake-out exercise.

BODY TAPPING

This exercise can be done seated or standing. Using the fingertips, begin at the scalp and gently tap the scalp, noticing the sensation, then moving to the face, the back of the neck, shoulders, and each arm, at which point the tapping can become firmer, reminding youth that they can choose how much pressure to apply. Then move the fingertips to the chest and belly, the low back, the hips, the thighs and back of the legs, and move down to the feet. Have youth then come to stillness and notice the effects of the body-tapping exercise.

Breathing Practices

1:2 BREATHING

In this exercise, make the exhale about twice as long as the inhale and count each part of the breath to focus the mind. For example, if inhaling for a count of 3, exhale for a count of 6; if inhaling for a count of 4, exhale for a count of 8. Instruct the youth to just do what count feels most comfortable according to their own breath and lung capacity. Most important is that the exhale is longer than the inhale; this slows down the heart rate and turns on the parasympathetic nervous system response.

RECTANGLE BREATH

Using a yoga block or a piece of paper as a visual for lengthening the exhales, inhale and trace the finger along the short side of the object, then exhale while tracing the finger along the long side of the object. Continue tracing the finger along the block or the paper for a few rounds of breath.

THREE-PART BREATH

This is a more advanced breathing technique to try after some time gaining an understanding of deep belly breathing and 1:2 ratio breathing. As you inhale, feel the breath moving into the chest and isolate the breath there. Next, feel the breath moving into the lungs and rib cage, isolating the breath there. Then feel the breath fill up the belly and isolate the breath at that location. On the exhale, reverse the route of the breath, following it from the belly to the ribcage to the chest, releasing all of the air.

Calming Poses for Anxiety

CHILD'S POSE

Begin on hands and knees with feet hips-width distance apart and palms underneath the shoulders. Begin to move the big toes toward each other, keeping knees wide, and shift the weight of the hips back toward the heels. Hips might not reach the heels, but the main objective is to turn the focus inward and use the weight of the body on the legs to begin to calm the nervous system. Arms can be outstretched or elbows bent, palms stacked or in fists, placing the forehead onto the palms or fists. The eyes can remain open or come to close. Invite youth to breathe in and out, noticing the breath as it expands and contracts through the rib cage.

FORWARD FOLD

Moving slowly, begin by standing and slowly tuck the chin toward the chest and then roll down and forward, folding slowly and bending the knees as needed to protect the low back and allowing the hands to come to the shins, to blocks, to the ankles, or to the floor. Let the head and neck be loose and the arms to drape down. You can bring in a sway of the arms back and forth, clasp opposite elbows, or clasp the hands at the back of the neck to traction the cervical spine. Remain in a forward fold for a few rounds of breath, taking any variation, and being mindful to roll back up slowly because the blood rushes to the head, and people sometimes can become light-headed following this pose.

Energizing Poses for Depression

RECLINED BUTTERFLY

When energy is lower, it is recommended to do poses that open through the chest and heart space, in contrast to a closed chest pose such as child's pose, for calming effects. For refined butterfly pose, if a bolster or rolled blanket is available, it can be helpful to place it lengthwise along the spine to aid in the chest opening. Place the bolster at the sacrum (low back area), with knees bent and feet on the floor, and begin to lean back over the bolster. Then begin to open knees wide and place the soles of the feet together, using blocks or blankets as support underneath the thighs. If no props are available, begin by lying on the mat with knees bent and soles of the feet to the floor. Then begin to open knees and press soles of the feet together. Arms can drape down by the side or hands can be placed on the belly to bring attention toward the breath.

FIERCE POSE OR CHAIR POSE

Activating the muscles in the legs can serve to bring energy up through the body. In this pose, stand with feet either hips-width distance apart or big toes touching. Raise the arms up over the head and begin to bend the knees as if sitting back into a chair. Keep the inner thighs hugging in toward each other and shift the body weight back toward the heels. Try lifting the toes up off the floor or mat, pressing into the balls of the feet and activating the muscles of the inner legs even more. From here, you can try inhaling while reaching the arms up at a diagonal, then exhaling to fold forward over the legs while reaching the arms back behind you and leaning tilted forward as if skiing. Repeat this dynamic movement three to four times, moving with the breath and bringing energy up through the body from the ground.

Other Poses

SEATED TWIST

This posture can be done in a classroom, courtroom, or other public setting. Shift forward in your chair so that the feet can be placed flat on the floor and you can find a tall spine. Inhale to lengthen through the spine, then exhale and bring one hand toward the opposite thigh, moving from the navel center to come into a gentle twist, revolving the shoulders around the spine, and opening through the chest and spine. Twists bring fresh oxygen and blood into the internal organs, thus detoxifying and promoting healthy digestion and blood flow.

LEGS UP THE WALL

This is a reclined, restorative posture to do before bedtime. Begin seated with one side facing the wall and knees hugging in toward the chest. Gently lower yourself down to the forearms and then begin to rotate the body to be square toward the wall, with the hips against the wall and the legs extending up the wall, forming an L shape. Arms can rest by the side or with elbows bent and hands at the belly, bringing attention to the breath. It is recommended to hold this pose for at least 2 minutes or roughly 20 rounds of breaths. Let youth know how long they will be in the pose so they can take charge of counting their own breaths.

Conclusion

In conclusion, I want to make clear that these postures are not just for the most marginalized youth experiencing the most complex forms of trauma; they are also for us as practitioners. Whether we are practicing with the youth or between patients or at the end of the day in the car before our commute home, we can use these tools for our own self-regulation practices as much as we are sharing them as tools with our patients. We are on the front line: we sometimes have the honor of bearing witness to people's stories as they are healing their wounds, and sometimes we have the hardship of having bits and pieces of their stories hurled at us between waves of rage, sorrow, and despair. We take in others' pain as it gets churned around with our own pain and with that of the broken systems with which we and the patients we serve interact.

On some days when I am teaching yoga, it seems that I, the teacher or facilitator, may need the practice as much as the group of young people do. We, as healers, need it because years of trauma work can take its toll. Secondary trauma can catch up with us, and therefore we must continue the practice ourselves. Ultimately, we must not forget that we offer these practices as tools for finding refuge within our own bodies, hearts, and minds in a world where sometimes the only place to turn is inward.

KEY POINTS

- Create choice within structure so patients can begin to regain a sense of personal agency through making choices.

- Understand that certain behaviors are traumatic adaptations or coping mechanisms, which we aren't trying to take away immediately. Rather, through the practice of yoga, we are introducing new coping mechanisms to promote behavior change.

- When a patient becomes dysregulated, practice steady and even breathing together to coregulate the nervous system, using your own self-regulated breathing to guide the patient toward his or her own sense of self-regulation.

Suggested Readings

Emerson D, Hopper E: Overcoming Trauma Through Yoga: Reclaiming Your Body. Berkley, CA, North Atlantic Books, 2011
Himelstein S: A Mindfulness-Based Approach to Working With High-Risk Adolescents. London, Routledge, 2013

References

Emerson D, Hopper E: Overcoming Trauma Through Yoga: Reclaiming Your Body. Berkley, CA, North Atlantic Books, 2011
Emerson D, Sharma R, Chaudhry S, et al: Trauma-sensitive yoga: principles, practice, and research. Int J Yoga Therap 19(1):123–128, 2009
Epstein R, Gonzáles T: Gender and Trauma: Somatic Interventions for Girls in Juvenile Justice—Implications for Policy and Practice. Washington, DC, Georgetown Law Center on Poverty and Inequality, 2017
Finkelhor D, Turner H, Hamby S, et al: Polyvictimization: Children's Exposure to Multiple Types of Violence, Crime, and Abuse. Juvenile Justice Bulletin. Rockville, MD, National Criminal Justice Reference Service, October 2011. Available at: www.ncjrs.gov/pdffiles1/ojjdp/232273.pdf. Accessed May 4, 2018.
Himelstein S: A Mindfulness-Based Approach to Working With High-Risk Adolescents. London, Routledge, 2013

Perry B: Applying principles of neurodevelopment to clinical work with maltreated and traumatized children: the neurosequential model of therapeutics, in Social Work Practice With Children and Families: Working With Traumatized Youth in Child Welfare. Edited by Webb NB. New York, Guilford, 2006, pp 27–52

Part IV

Mindfulness Settings

Chapter
13

Mindfulness at Home

Amy Saltzman, M.D.
Celeste H. Poe, LMFT

Theoretical Foundations

Let's begin with a definition of mindfulness. *Mindfulness* is paying attention here and now, with kindness and curiosity, so that we can choose our behavior. Paying attention here and now means doing our best to not dwell on the past, or worry or fantasize about the future, and simply paying attention to what's actually happening in *this* moment. And we pay attention with kindness and curiosity. Otherwise, we can often be incredibly hard on ourselves. As kids, teens, or parents (and health care providers), we tend to see only where we've "made a mistake" or "screwed up." Rather than judging and critiquing ourselves, with mindfulness we can practice bringing an attitude of kindness and curiosity to ourselves and our experience. Finally, when we bring our kind and curious attention to our thoughts and feelings, to the sensations in our bodies, and to

---

The majority of this chapter has been excerpted and adapted from my book, *A Still Quiet Place: A Mindfulness Program for Teaching Children and Adolescents to Ease Stress and Difficult Emotions* (Saltzman 2014).

the people and circumstances in our lives, then we have all the information we need to choose our behavior—that is, *respond* in the moment.

Before we begin to explore the moment-to-moment value of mindfulness in parenting and family interactions, it is important to note two things. First, as mentioned in Chapter 1, "Developing a Personal Mindfulness Practice," it cannot be emphasized enough that if you are going to share the skills of mindfulness with the youth and families that you serve, it is absolutely essential that you have your own mindfulness practice and an ongoing experience with using mindfulness in your day-to-day interactions. Second, this chapter provides a solid introduction and working foundation, but we must recognize that it is not possible to include all of the essential practices and comprehensive framework for sharing mindfulness with parents and families here.

Mindfulness Sessions

When I work with children and adolescents and their parents, a typical family or group series consists of eight sessions. When working with an individual child or adolescent, I allow the patient to choose if he or she would like his or her parent(s) to participate in the sessions. For the most part, young children choose to have their parents participate, and tweens and teens choose to have me summarize and offer any reflections to their parents at the end of our session. With younger children, having the parents participate has two advantages: 1) the parents learn the practices and can apply them in their parenting, and 2) the parents can reinforce the concepts and practices with their children. With teens, it is essential to honor their confidentiality, and it can be quite powerful for a teen to have an advocate suggest to the parents that they look at their own piece in the family dynamics.

Although I may modify the order of the elements on the basis of the issues with which the child, adolescent, or family present, a typical 8-week family or group model involves the practices listed in Table 13–1, several of which are described in further detail in this chapter.

Core Mindfulness Interventions and Techniques

WE ARE ALL IN THIS TOGETHER

In child-parent courses, both children and parents receive the same workbook and CD for home practice. The participants know that if a child picks up the parent's workbook or a parent picks up the child's workbook, they are exactly the same. This emphasizes that we are all in this together. At Stanford, I like to joke with the kids, telling them that Still Quiet Place is their first college course.

TABLE 13–1. Basic elements of family mindfulness practice

Practice	Application(s) and benefits	Audience/ practitioner	Materials needed	Notes
Resting in stillness and quietness	Parents, children, and adolescents	For all of the practices below, there are no materials, other than your own personal practice, that are absolutely needed. However, there are some items (e.g., river stones) that can be useful	It is not necessary for participants to be either still or quiet. A general rule of thumb is that they can rock, sway, wiggle, tap, or hum, as long as this behavior is not distracting others. If the behavior is distracting, the instructor can just sit beside them, or allow them to walk mindfully in the back of the room.	
Watching thoughts	The capacity to observe thoughts (especially those about family members) without believing them or taking them personally	Parents, children, and adolescents	Soap bubbles	The essence of this practice is to support participants in discovering that they can observe their thoughts without believing them or acting on them.

TABLE 13–1. Basic elements of family mindfulness practice *(continued)*

Practice	Application(s) and benefits	Audience/ practitioner	Materials needed	Notes
Befriending feelings	The capacity to have their feelings without their feelings having them	Parents, children, and adolescents	Crayons and paper	With this practice, it is helpful to mention that as with yoga, they can stretch into uncomfortable feelings, and it is important to know when to back off.
Understanding emotion theory	Understanding how the emotional waves of individual family members can create an emotional tsunami	Parents, children, and adolescents	Poster board with wave illustrations	It can be very helpful to introduce the idea of family tsunamis (upsets).
Being in the body	Recognizing the physical manifestations of emotions in the body	Parents, children, and adolescents		Again, it is not necessary for participants to be completely still or quiet during this practice. The practice will seep in even if they are wiggling or staring at the ceiling.
Responding vs. reacting		Parents, children, and adolescents		This is a key practice, especially for parents who have brought their children to learn mindfulness to address some issue. It is important that the parents practice responding rather than reacting when the issue arises.

TABLE 13–1.	Basic elements of family mindfulness practice *(continued)*			
Practice	**Application(s) and benefits**	**Audience/ practitioner**	**Materials needed**	**Notes**
Mindful communication	Especially helpful in moments of conflict	Parents, children, and adolescents	Worksheet	The essential element of this practice is for participants to let go of their agendas and listen for understanding.
Practicing lovingkindness		Parents, children, and adolescents		If relationships are extremely strained, it may be important to build this practice gradually. Family members should begin with someone inside or outside the family from and toward whom it is easy for them to feel caring and love.

I usually offer child-parent courses only to children 13 years and younger. If the group is large, with 20 or more participants, you should encourage the children to be the primary speakers and have the parents take a secondary role so that the discussions don't exceed the children's capacity for sitting and listening. If the kids are wiggly and need to do some movement, take them outside for a movement practice and leave the parents with a discussion question such as "What subtle feelings did you notice over the week?" "What are your common holes (problematic situations and reactions) with your children?" "What different streets are you discovering?"

For teens and parents, much of their stress comes from interacting with each other, and it is often difficult for them to speak honestly about the stress caused by family dynamics if they are all in the same room. If you are inclined to share mindfulness with teens and parents, I recommend that you partner with another teacher and that one of you teaches the teens while the other teaches the parents. Then, once both groups have some fluency in mindfulness, you can bring them together to explore common family holes and difficult communications.

LETTING GO

In social settings, many parents feel obligated to manage their children's behavior. (If you are a parent, you may recognize this behavior in yourself.) Because mindfulness is about being with what is rather than managing, I encourage parents to allow me to be responsible for and responsive to the children and their behavior during the session. I say something like "As parents, we often feel that we have to modify, correct, manage, and generally control our children's behavior, especially in new group settings. To the best of your ability, see if for this hour and a half you can let that go and allow me to guide, redirect, set limits, create consequences. If I need your help, I'll let you know." Many parents find this both a challenge and a relief. The habits of intervening are ingrained, and the opportunity to simply be present with one's children in a group setting without feeling responsible for their behavior is rare.

During the last 15 minutes of class, give the parents time to ask questions and have an adult discussion about applying mindfulness to the joys and challenges of parenting. Remember, this is a time to offer compassion for those moments when we are not the parents we intend to be and simultaneously to encourage the parents to pay attention, here and now, with kindness and curiosity, and then choose their behavior, especially in challenging moments with their children.

Parents really appreciate this time and often want to stay well past the end of class—and beyond their children's willingness to stay. During this time, the children can draw pictures of their experience of the still quiet place, write haikus or poems, or play inside or outside. Inside games that engage mindfulness include pick-up sticks and Jenga. In Jenga, blocks are placed in a stack, and then each player in turn pulls a block from the middle of the stack and places it on the top of the stack, with the object being to not topple the stack.

PARENTAL AGENDAS

Most children and teens do not spontaneously and enthusiastically choose to learn mindfulness. Youth usually come to our offices and groups because their parents want them to learn mindfulness to improve their ability to focus, to alleviate their stress, to build their resilience, or to manage their anger. Parents enroll their children because either the child or the parent is suffering from the effects of the child's attention-deficit/hyperactivity disorder, anxiety, depression, physical illness, or stress-induced physical symptoms, (e.g., tension headaches, migraines, stomachaches). Parents of some tweens and teens may also be desperately seeking a remedy for ongoing self-destructive behavior, including eating disorders, cutting, substance abuse, acting out, and suicidal behavior. These parents love and care for their children; they are often deeply concerned or truly afraid regarding their children's mental health, general well-being, behaviors, and choices. Simply put, parents usually bring their children to us with understandable agendas. Parents bring their children to us for the specific benefits being documented in the research. However, parents can get quite attached to the outcome.

To further complicate things, the parents may or may not have clear insights into their own habits, issues, and contribution to the family dynamics. Let me share an example. In the third session of the first course in a child-parent research study at Stanford, one parent asked, "What if my children don't want to come?" On the basis of how the question was asked and other interactions I had had with the mother, implicit in the question was the hope that I would "make" the children attend. This particular course was in the context of a research study, and research doesn't like dropouts. However, my response was, "Mindfulness is about accepting what is, and not about forcing anything. Therefore, it's contrary to the practice to force anyone to participate."

The question prompted me to solicit suggestions from both the children and the parents about the class format to help ensure that classes were appealing and inviting for the children. The children suggested more movement and less talk. As a group, we agreed that the suggestions would be incorporated into the upcoming classes; that the children who didn't want to continue would attend two more sessions; and if at that point they still didn't wish to participate, they would stop coming to class.

After the large group discussion, in the closing discussion with just the parents I shared the following thoughts in response to the mother's question. First, as parents, our practice is to notice when we want our children to be other than they are and when we have an agenda. There is a distinction between supporting children in developing useful skills and trying to change or "fix" them. Once we realize our true intentions, we can make a wise choice about how to proceed. Perhaps living mindfully and being present with and responsive to our children moment by moment is more important than *getting* them to practice mindfulness.

Second, the first two sessions had provided children with an experience of mindfulness and the still quiet place and vocabulary for sharing their experience. Before starting the course, the children had no experience with mindfulness and didn't know that they had a still quiet place. By the time the children would be allowed to drop out, they also would have developed some capacity for observing their thoughts and feelings. Perhaps the benefits of experiencing the still quiet place, learning to observe their thoughts and feelings, and developing a common family language were enough for now.

Third, introducing mindfulness to children and parents is like planting seeds, and seeds grow and eventually blossom in their own time. A child who is uninterested in mindfulness now may choose to apply this learning 6 months from now, before taking the SATs, or during a particularly difficult time in college. (As an aside, many college health services are now offering instruction in mindfulness to their students.)

In closing, I reminded the parents that although they might have enrolled in the mindfulness class "for Susie or Patrick," their children would benefit if the parents developed their own mindfulness practice. In fact, research indicates that parental stress contributes significantly to child stress and related issues (Crum and Moreland 2017). Thus, if parents use mindfulness to reduce their stress, they will simultaneously reduce their children's stress and provide a living demonstration of the value of mindfulness in daily life. I encouraged the parents to practice mindfulness "out loud" in front of their children in the course of daily life. For example, a parent might demonstrate mindfulness of feelings and reactivity and pause to consider a more mindful response in this way: "Wow! That e-mail from your coach really upset me. I'm going to take some time to notice my thoughts and feelings and then choose what I want to say before I write back." These comments helped the parents remember that in the first class, many of them had acknowledged that they were taking the mindfulness course not only for their child but also to cultivate patience, kindness, clarity, gentleness, and wisdom within themselves.

Before moving on to some practice examples and scripts, let's review the current science regarding the benefits of offering mindfulness to parents and families.

Evaluation of the Approach

PARENTAL STRESS AND CHILDREN

The intergenerational consequences of parental stress have been well established in the literature. Children of parents with increased levels of stress frequently demonstrate psychological outcomes that often last into adulthood

(Snyder et al. 2012). In addition to the increased risk for psychological problems in children, additional potential consequences of parental stress include harsh parenting, physical abuse, and emotional hostility (Crum and Moreland 2017). Although parenting styles can vary across many contexts, the presence of parental stress tends to result in harsher, more authoritarian parenting styles regardless of other factors. Additionally, Nair and colleagues (2003) found that increased stress in parents is linked to increased child abuse potential. A possible consequence of child maltreatment and/or emotional hostility is emotional or behavioral issues in the child. In turn, this can often add to the stress of the parent, thereby creating a cycle and increasing the likelihood of abuse.

Parental stress is a cause for concern because it impacts not only the psychological well-being of the parent but that of the children and the family system as a whole. Research on parental stress and child outcomes demonstrates that children of parents with high levels of stress tend to experience emotional and behavioral problems such as depression, aggression, anxiety, difficulty coping, disruptive behavior, and impaired social cognition (Crum and Moreland 2017). The mechanism by which parental stress is linked to these outcomes in children may lie in maladaptive parent-child interactions. High levels of stress can compromise parents' ability to show empathy to their child, impair their ability to recognize and meet the emotional and physical needs of their child, and influence them to use emotionally hostile means of communication.

Biologically, stress is regulated in the human body through the hypothalamic-pituitary-adrenal (HPA) axis. However, as a result of chronic stress or abuse, when hyperactivated, the HPA axis develops a greater sensitivity to stress. The implications for children and teens who are chronically subjected to stressful environments and parental interactions are great, and hypersensitivity of the HPA axis has been linked to various negative outcomes, including depression and anxiety (Brand et al. 2010).

PARENTAL MINDFULNESS

Protective factors. Researchers have demonstrated that external forces are not the only factors at play when mitigating the often stressful experiences of having children (Smith et al. 2017). In recent studies on parental well-being, the focus has shifted to more internal factors, which may act as buffers to emotional distress and enhance parent-child interactions (Snyder et al. 2012). Mindfulness is one approach that has shown positive results. Research on the effectiveness of meditation and mindfulness programs has demonstrated significant results across various populations in the reduction of psychological distress, disturbances in affect, and depression and anxiety and an increase in emotion regulation (Snyder et al. 2012).

Mindfulness investigators have demonstrated numerous mechanisms by which mindful parenting creates positive mental health outcomes for both parents and children. Mindfulness skills help to minimize reactivity to stress by modulating the interaction between the sympathetic and parasympathetic nervous systems (Amihai and Kozhevnikov 2015). Although the sympathetic nervous system (SNS) protects us by activating our fight-flight-freeze response to threatening stimuli, this process becomes maladaptive when it is triggered in response to emotionally threatening situations, such as parental stress. In opposition, the parasympathetic nervous system (PNS) works to bring a calming effect to the body by reducing heart and breathing rates and by bringing us a sense of safety. Parental mindfulness provides parents with a buffer to the fight-or-flight response in one of two ways: 1) through reducing SNS activation or 2) by improving PNS response (Amihai and Kozhevnikov 2015).

Additional mechanisms for positive outcomes include attunement, intentionality, attention to variability, and reperceiving (Townshend 2016). Incorporating intentionality and emotional awareness, *attunement* allows parents to be able to focus their attention on the experience of their child. Mindfulness reinforces these skills by cultivating embodied, kind, and curious attention and heartfelt presence. *Attention to variability* refers to the ability to actively make distinctions between stimuli in one's awareness. This focused attention allows parents to be more perceptive and mentally flexible when interacting with their child. The focusing of attention also allows parents to focus on their emotional experiences in real time. This skill is vital in the ability to regulate one's emotions, an important piece of effective parenting. *Reperceiving* is the ability to have an outside perspective on one's thoughts, without placing judgment or reacting to them (Townshend 2016). The incorporation of mindfulness into parenting has demonstrated positive results across various contexts, including parents of children with disabilities, parents of preschool children, and parents of older children with conduct issues (Townshend 2016).

Parental mindfulness and children.

The link between parental mental health and the mental health and well-being of their children has long been established. As mentioned in the previous subsection, mindfulness facilitates the ability to regulate psychological arousal, which creates positive benefits for the parents. Coregulation can be defined as the dynamic process between two people in which the emotional expression of one affects and is affected by the other. Because of the process of coregulation, children depend on the emotional regulation capabilities of their parents. Exposure to effective emotion regulation strategies, especially while young, lays a foundation for long-term positive psychological outcomes in children.

However, parents who fail to fulfill the role of an attuned, responsive caregiver can often demonstrate abuse, hostility, and disengagement. Although this is true for both mothers and fathers, research has demonstrated that in particular, mothers who cannot fulfill this role have been found to have deficiencies in proper attunement and restricted affect and overall have more negative interactions with their children (Snyder et al. 2012). The literature has also demonstrated that often, this takes place in mothers who suffer from depression and/or have trauma histories. Children who do not receive appropriate emotion regulation modeling, attunement, and responsiveness often display socioemotional deficits themselves, including behavioral problems (Snyder et al. 2012). These maladaptive ways of relating can lead to negative psychological outcomes in children, such as depression, anxiety, attachment disorders, and conduct disorders (Townshend 2016). A study conducted by Corthorn and Milicic (2016) found that parental distress had a significant negative relationship to mindful parenting. This was particularly true for the role of being a mother, parents' interactions with their children, and their perceptions of their child.

The parental ability to demonstrate appropriate regulation, attunement, and responsiveness to a child can have critical consequences for a child's socioemotional development. Research has also demonstrated that increased parental mindfulness has positive effects on parent-child relationships and results in a decrease in behavior problems in the child (Siu et al. 2016). Siu et al. (2016) noted that mindful parents are considered to be parents who focus on the present and have the ability to express compassion and kindness while parenting their children. Additional positive child outcomes include empathy, prosocial behavior, and the ability to self-soothe. Ultimately, parental mindfulness can have many positive consequences, including an increase in psychological well-being for the parent as well as the child, and in turn allows for more positive parent-child interactions.

An additional benefit to parental mindfulness is the modeling that takes place for children. Mindfulness for children is a growing field that has been producing more and more positive outcomes. A meta-analysis examining the integration of mindfulness into K–12 schools found academic improvements such as increases in working memory and attention, as well as socioemotional benefits such as emotion regulation, positive self-esteem, and mood improvement (Meiklejohn et al. 2012). Just as with parental mindfulness, the benefits of children practicing mindfulness are bidirectional. With positive outcomes for child mood and relational abilities, mindful children can experience more positive child-parent interactions, thereby providing a benefit to parents as well.

Adolescence can be a particularly stressful developmental period for children. The physiological, neurological, and psychological changes that take place during this time can have a significant impact on social roles and relationships. Research examining coping with stress in teenagers highlights both external and internal characteristics that can protect against the negative effects of stress as mentioned in the subsection "Parental Stress and Children." Further demonstrating the advantages of parental mindfulness, Skrove et al. (2013) found that teens with families from which they gained support and stability demonstrated greater resilience to stress. Alternatively, inner resources such as flexibility when approaching new challenges and self-compassion appear to act as buffers against the development of stress in teenagers (Bluth et al. 2016). Bluth and Eisenlohr-Moul (2017) found a mindfulness program with teens, Making Friends With Yourself, to be beneficial in reducing perceived stress and significantly increasing resilience, gratitude, and exploration.

FAMILY MINDFULNESS

Although the incorporation of mindfulness techniques into psychotherapy is most often described in the individual therapy literature, there is a growing body of work offering these techniques in group formats. As mentioned in the previous subsection, emotion regulation plays a critical role in the psychological well-being of all family members. Emotion regulation has a major relational component, is often bidirectional in nature, and can impact the entire family (Brody et al. 2017). Because of the natural proximity to and time spent with most family members, each member of the family is vulnerable to one another's regulation and expression of emotions. This suggests that family interactions can be especially important because of the transmittable nature of emotion. The focus on the here and now in mindfulness makes it a viable option for targeting deficits in effective emotion regulation that occur in families. Interpersonal mindfulness-based practices can be used to enhance family outcomes, including improvement in negative communication patterns, decreasing areas of high conflict, and increasing family cohesion (Brody et al. 2017).

Physiological arousal, a popular area of intervention in family therapy, is often demonstrated in families through such behaviors as physical and/or verbal aggression, blaming, and criticizing. Although some traditional forms of therapy focus on altering behavior patterns within the family, mindfulness aims to increase awareness of the process of that behavior (Brody et al. 2017). This increased awareness is among the strengths of this type of approach.

Additionally, this approach stresses the growth of skills in self-regulation that can be demonstrated intrapersonally and interpersonally. Teaching mindfulness skills to families provides members with the ability to navigate emotionally taxing situations with less distress. Interpersonal conflicts can be handled in more adaptive ways when there is nonjudgmental awareness and less impulsivity. In highlighting relational awareness, mindfulness allows families to develop greater awareness of dysfunctional patterns of interaction, the ability to slow down emotional responses, and alternative ways of functioning. Through increasing prosocial skills such as empathy, compassion, and connection to others, mindfulness-based skills can improve overall family functioning and family coregulation (Brody et al. 2017).

Despite the fact that the inherent structure of the family system leaves members vulnerable to the negative patterns of others, this very structure allows for positive ways of interacting to be experienced by all members. For this reason, parental mindfulness provides a practical and accessible intervention that can benefit all members of the family and family functioning as a whole.

Research Areas for Development

As an intervention for individual growth and increased awareness, mindfulness provides a useful tool for increasing internal resources, constructive communication, and responsiveness in challenging situations. As we learn more about the profound implications for attachment and the impact that childhood distress can have on the developing individual, we recognize a need for more interventions that target families through mindful parenting and provide a means for positive child and adolescent development. Future research can target families, paying particular attention to the ways in which mindfulness interventions can be accessed by parents and children early in order to help mitigate the impact of stress in childhood, adolescence, and adulthood. Future research can also take an ecological approach to understanding how internal resources such as mindfulness counteract the pressures and barriers among the various systems of which families and communities are a part. Ultimately, these systems contribute to either poor or beneficial mental health outcomes.

Practice Examples and Scripts

The following are practice examples that demonstrate the use of child, parent, and family mindfulness.

Rest Practice

As with many mindfulness programs, developing present-moment awareness begins with resting attention on the breath, like the following practice geared for tweens and teens. Parallel practices for younger children are available in the book from which this practice is excerpted (Saltzman 2014) and on a CD available from the first author (A.S.).

> Give it a rest. For the next few minutes, give it a rest, all of it—homework, parents, the hallway gossip, your inner gossip, the next new thing. Let everything be exactly the way it is. And rest.

Let your body rest. If you feel comfortable, allow your eyes to close. If not, focus on a neutral spot about a foot in front of you. Feel your body supported by the chair, the couch, or the floor. Allow the muscles in your body and your face to rest. Maybe even let out a long, slow sigh.

And let your attention rest on the breath—the rhythm of the breath in the belly. Feel the belly expand with each in breath and release with each out breath. Narrowing your attention to the rhythm of the breath, and allowing everything else to fade into the background. Breathing, resting. Nowhere to go, nothing to do, no one to be, nothing to prove.

Feeling the in breath, from the first sip all the way through to where the breath is still, and the out breath, from the first whisper all the way through to where the breath is still. Now see if you can let your attention rest in the still quite place between the in breath and the out breath. And rest again in the still space between the out breath and the in breath.

Breathing, resting, being. It is more than enough. Just hanging out with the breath and the stillness.

Feeling the stillness and quietness that is always inside of you.

And when your attention wanders, which it will, gently return it to the experience of breathing—feeling the rhythm of the breath in the belly.

Choosing to rest. Choosing to focus your attention on the breath. Allowing things to be just as they are. Allowing yourself to be exactly as you are. Nothing to change, or fix or improve.

Breathing and resting. Resting and breathing.

As this session comes to a close, you may want to remember that in our fast-paced, media-driven world, resting is a radical act. With practice, you can learn to breathe and rest anytime, anywhere: When you're putting on your shoes. When you're struggling in class. When you're hanging out with friends. Even when you're arguing with someone. This kind of resting and breathing is especially helpful when you're nervous, depressed, bored, or angry. So give yourself permission and rest.

Befriending Feelings Practice

After children, adolescents, and parents have practiced resting their attention on the breath, they can be supported in resting in stillness and quietness (also known as *pure awareness*) and observing their thoughts and feelings. It is especially helpful for all ages to recognize how feelings (emotions) manifest in the body. The following practice supports people in "having their feelings, without their feeling having them"—in other words, being aware of their feelings so that their feelings don't cause them to say or do things they regret.

Sit or lie in a comfortable position, find your breath in your belly, rest in the stillness and quietness, and then simply note the feeling or feelings that are present. Some feelings may have ordinary names such as angry, happy, sad, excited, and others may have more unusual names such as stormy, bubbly, fiery, or empty. Some feelings may be small (subtle) and kind of shy or big and powerful (intense). There may be layers of feelings.

Gently notice where the feelings "live" in your body: sitting in the chest, stirring in the belly, resting in the big toe. See if you can really feel how the feeling feels in the body. Is the feeling small, heavy, hard, warm, wiggly, jagged?

Do you best to simply bring your kind and curious attention to whatever you are feeling. If any instruction shifts you into thinking about rather than experiencing the feeling, simply breathe and return to being with the feeling.

Notice if or imagine that the feeling has a color, or colors, perhaps dark red, pale blue, or bright green. Listen to discover if the feeling has a sound, such as giggling, groaning, or whining.

It is enough to end the practice here:

As this practice comes to a close, take a few more minutes to simply breathe and rest in stillness and quietness.

If you wish, you may suggest that participants ask the feeling what it wants from them, noting that usually feelings want something simple such as attention, time, or space. Ask participants if they are willing and able to give the feeling what it asked for. There is a highly skilled way to address whether the feeling wants something that is unwise, unkind, or unhealthy, but that is beyond the scope of this chapter. To learn more about this skill, please refer to "Dialog with Emotions" in Saltzman (2014, p. 97).

Mindful Communication

After family members have learned to breathe, rest in stillness and quietness, watch their thoughts, recognize when and how feelings manifest in the body, and befriend their feelings, they have the basic skills they need to practice mindful communication.

Whether we are young children or "grown-ups," much of our stress, unhappiness, and difficulty arise because of our less than skillful communication with others. To complicate matters, our less than skillful communication with others often contributes to their stress, unhappiness, and difficulty. The skills presented in this section support people of all ages in listening deeply to themselves and others and then communicating more clearly and compassionately.

This exercise is designed to support family members during difficult communications by helping them learn to pause to consider what they feel and want, what another person feels and wants, and how they might work things out. In combination, these steps nurture empathy and compassion for oneself and others and lay a foundation for creative problem solving and true cooperation (literally, operating together).

You may introduce the exercise by saying something along these lines:

When we are upset, in the heat of the moment, and at the peak of an emotion, we often react and just blurt out thoughts and feelings as they appear. If the person we are (interacting) with does the same thing, soon, we find ourselves being tossed about on big waves of reactivity and drowning in a shared tsunami of thoughts and feelings.

So let's try something different. Close your eyes, take several slow deep breaths, settle into stillness and quietness, and remember a recent family disagreement or argument. Now let's work our way through the practice. The first step in the process of communicating skillfully is asking yourself, "What did I feel? What did I want?" When you have remembered what you wanted and how you felt, write it down. Just a few brief words are fine.

Sometimes the answers to these questions are quick and clear. At other times, it may be helpful to slow down and to really listen to what is true for you. This takes practice, and it is important to understand how you feel (your emotions) and what you want (your desires) before moving on to the next steps.

The second step in the process is considering what the other person feels and wants. Without this step it is very difficult to communicate and move toward a solution. So take some time, let go of what you felt and wanted, and *really* consider what the other person felt and wanted. When you feel you understand the other person, write down a few brief words or phrases.

Now that you have a better understanding of what you wanted and felt and what the other person wanted and felt, how might you resolve this issue? What are some creative solutions? If you have some ideas, write them down. If you feel stuck, we will explore possible solutions in a minute.

In moments of difficulty, the combination of paying attention to our own feelings and wants and then considering the feelings and wants of others helps us be kinder to ourselves and kinder to other people.

If you are working with one family, you can fairly easily facilitate a conversation. I almost always begin by having the parents listen, *really* listen, to their children. I encourage them to do their absolute best to let go of any anger from the past and fears about the future and simply hear their child freshly in this moment.

Mindful Communication for Child-Parent Groups

If you are working with a group, have each young person pair with a parent and each parent pair with a young person who is *not* in their family or a close friend of the family and then share their family difficulty. Let them know that if the original circumstances they reflected on feel too private (embarrassing, tender, intense), they may choose a slightly "easier" difficulty instead. Once everyone has a partner, designate who will be partner A and who will be partner B. There are many simple ways of designating partners: for example, the person with the shortest hair is partner A, or the person whose name comes first alphabetically is partner A.

Explain that partner A will begin by sharing his or her difficult communication while partner B practices mindful listening, listening with his or her heart and attention, as well as with the ears. To support the process, it is helpful if you read the following prompts, allowing partner A about a minute to respond to each question. All pairs will work simultaneously as you offer the prompts to the group.

- What was the difficulty? Describe it to your partner briefly.
- How did you feel during the difficulty?
- What did you want?
- How do you think the other person felt?
- What do you think the other person wanted?
- What ended up happening?
- Looking back on it now, what were possible solutions, ways of resolving the difficulty?

When partner A is done sharing, partner B may practice mindful speaking—speaking with kindness and curiosity, asking questions, or offering observations based on what he or she heard. Then the partners switch roles.

Once the participants have shared with their partners, you can facilitate a discussion with the entire group: "Raise your hand if you are willing to share your difficulty and what you wrote down with the group or if you struggled to find a creative solution and would like some help from the group."

Something close to miraculous happens in this process as an event is reported, in a supportive setting, from the perspective of *a* child, rather than *my* child, or *a* parent rather than *my* parent. Participants usually report that they are able to share their feelings, desires, and needs clearly and simply and to hear and really understand what the other person felt, wanted, and needed. Then they are able to respond with kindness and compassion rather than reacting out of habit, fear, defense, or the need to control. In general, these role-plays tend to be much more skillful than most families' usual fraught communications on touchy subjects; they tend to be characterized by mutual respect and trust—essential ingredients for mindful communication and positive outcomes. This kind of communication can help children convey what's important to them while also helping parents avoid long, drawn-out negotiations. This can help highlight the benefits of finding a neutral time to discuss problematic situations and make family agreements about how to handle them.

It is important to support participants in discovering and speaking their truths, even if they are not "politically correct." For your own practice, please pause and notice your thoughts, feelings, and physical reactions in response to the following sentence: "I was so angry I just wanted to hit him."

Did fear arise? Did you begin to judge? Did you find yourself wanting to correct or fix? If so, are you now judging your fear and judging and attempting to fix your desire to fix? Remember that, ideally, as facilitators and as human beings doing the best we can, our role is to first *make space for ourselves and others to be exactly as we are.* Are you willing to admit that at times you have been so angry you have thought about harming another person?

Inevitably, you'll encounter an individual who will honestly tell you "I wanted to hit him." When a person speaks so honestly, rather than making that person wrong, thank him or her. Meet the person where he or she is in the moment and say something along these lines:

> Thank you for being so honest. I understand. Like you, I have sometimes been so angry I wanted to harm someone. Being honest about these feelings and wants can help us choose our behavior. Sometimes when we pretend we aren't angry, then the anger sneaks out and we do something we wish we hadn't. So it is very brave and helpful to be honest with ourselves.

Paradoxically, this type of comment acknowledging the intensity of anger and the impulse to attack or defend when we feel threatened normalizes this very common human experience and demonstrates that it is possible to feel intensely angry, to want to cause harm, and then to *choose* otherwise.

That said, it is equally important not to leave participants stuck in their feelings and wants and to support them in moving through the subsequent steps of considering the other person's perspective and then choosing their own behavior. It is essential to remind family members that engaging in mindful communication doesn't mean that they will get what they want.

Sometimes, participants may move through the process and discover that they want something other than what they thought they wanted. This can be a good time to remind them that suffering = pain × resistance and that when they are busy wanting things to be different than they actually are, they are contributing to their own upset. Simultaneously, it is important not to imply that they shouldn't want what they want or shouldn't take steps to create the outcome they desire (as long as it will not cause harm to someone else). Ultimately, this process is about understanding how we really feel and what we really want and what others really feel and want so that we have the best chance at coming up with choices that allow us, and others, to be as happy as possible.

You can also introduce the idea of "one finger pointing out, three fingers pointing back." This short saying invites us to explore that often what we find most difficult in another person is a reflection of our own behavior. If a participant says, "He was so busy arguing, he didn't even listen to me," you may ask, "Can you see where you were so busy arguing, even if it was just in your head, rather than out loud, that you didn't listen to him?"

The benefits of repeatedly engaging in this process of working with difficult communications are increased self-awareness (participants may even be able to recognize patterns of behavior); increased perspective taking, empathy, compassion, and resilience; more effective communication; enhanced conflict resolution and cooperation; and, ultimately, greater energy for engaging in learning and living.

Conclusion

In summary, the self-awareness, empathy, compassion, and resilience that children and parents can find in mindfulness practice have many long-lasting positive outcomes. Although the essential practices and comprehensive framework for sharing mindfulness with parents and families are far too extensive to have been covered here, ideally, with this foundation one can provide space for introducing mindfulness to parents, children, and families. The provision of an appropriate space for mindfulness practice begins with promoting a *come as you are* attitude, allowing both parents and children to leave pressure and responsibility at the door.

Despite developmental differences between parents and children, it is possible to create this space for both, allowing children to be primary speakers at times and being flexible with expectations. Although it can be beneficial for a parent to be involved, it can be just as critical to allow children and adolescents to choose their own experience. By allowing this, we emphasize the power of choice, thereby highlighting the process by which mindfulness allows us greater opportunity to choose our behavior during challenging moments. Remember, introducing mindfulness to children and parents can sometimes be like planting seeds: when allowed the appropriate space and nurturing, they can develop and evolve in their own time.

KEY POINTS

- As facilitators, and as human beings, it is essential we first *make space for ourselves and others to be exactly as we are.* This requires that we cultivate our own mindfulness practice and ongoing experience with using mindfulness in day-to-day life.
- Mindfulness is about being aware of both inner and outer experience and skillfully choosing our behavior.
- Pushing anyone to participate is counterintuitive. As facilitators, or parents, our practice is to notice when we want our group members, or children, to be other than they are.

- We are all in this together. Parental mindfulness fosters mindfulness in children and vice versa, creating more positive outcomes for the entire family.

Discussion Questions

1. What is the most essential element for skillfully offering mindfulness to families, parents, children, and adolescents?

2. When offering mindfulness to families and/or child-parent combinations, what potentially counterproductive parental behaviors should the facilitator be aware of?

3. When offering mindfulness to families and/or child-parent combinations, what practices and ways of being does the facilitator encourage?

4. What are the benefits of offering mindfulness to parents, children, adolescents, child-parent combinations, and entire families?

Suggested Readings

Greenland SK: The Mindful Child: How to Help Your Kid Manage Stress and Become Happier, Kinder, and More Compassionate. New York, Free Press, 2010

Saltzman A: A Still Quiet Place: A Mindfulness Program for Teaching Children and Adolescents to Ease Stress and Difficult Emotions. Oakland, CA, New Harbinger Publications, 2014

Saltzman A: Still Quiet Place: let's talk about your practice: qualities and qualifications for sharing mindfulness with youth, December 15, 2016. Available at: www.stillquietplace.com/lets-talk-practice-qualities-qualifications-sharing-mindfulness. Accessed September 8, 2017.

Willard C, Saltzman A, Greenland SK: Teaching Mindfulness Skills to Kids and Teens. New York, Guilford, 2015

References

Amihai I, Kozhevnikov M: The influence of Buddhist meditation traditions on the autonomic system and attention. BioMed Res Int 2015:731579, 2015 26146629

Bluth K, Roberson PN, Gaylord SA, et al: Does self-compassion protect adolescents from stress? J Child Fam Stud 25(4):1098–1109, 2016 26997856

Bluth K, Eisenlohr-Moul TA: Response to a mindful self-compassion intervention in teens: a within-person association of mindfulness, self-compassion, and emotional well-being outcomes. J Adolesc 57:108–118, 2017 28414965

Brand SR, Brennan PA, Newport DJ, et al: The impact of maternal childhood abuse on maternal and infant HPA axis function in the postpartum period. Psychoneuroendocrinology 35(5):686–693, 2010 19931984

Brody JL, Scherer DG, Turner CW, et al: A conceptual model and clinical framework for integrating mindfulness into family therapy with adolescents. Fam Process June 7, 2017 [Epub ahead of print] 28590541

Corthorn C, Milicic N: Mindfulness and parenting: a correlational study of non-meditating mothers of preschool children. J Child Fam Stud 25(5):1672–1683, 2016

Crum KI, Moreland AD: Parental stress and children's social and behavioral outcomes: the role of abuse potential over time. J Child Fam Stud 26(11):3067–3078, 2017

Meiklejohn J, Phillips C, Freedman ML, et al: Integrating mindfulness training into K-12 education: fostering the resilience of teachers and students. Mindfulness 3(4):291–307, 2012

Nair P, Schuler ME, Black MM, et al: Cumulative environmental risk in substance abusing women: early intervention, parenting stress, child abuse potential and child development. Child Abuse Negl 27(9):997–1017, 2003 14550328

Saltzman: A Still Quiet Place: A Mindfulness Program for Teaching Children and Adolescents to Ease Stress and Difficult Emotions. Oakland, CA, New Harbinger, 2014

Siu AY, Ma Y, Chui FY: Maternal mindfulness and child social behavior: the mediating role of the mother-child relationship. Mindfulness 7(3):577–583, 2016

Skrove M, Romundstad P, Indredavik MS: Resilience, lifestyle and symptoms of anxiety and depression in adolescence: the Young-HUNT study. Soc Psychiatry Psychiatr Epidemiol 48(3):407–416, 2013 22872359

Smith SL, DeGrace B, Ciro C: Exploring families' experiences of health: contributions to a model of family health. Psychol Health Med 22(10):1239–1247, 2017 28425318

Snyder R, Shapiro S, Treleaven D: Attachment theory and mindfulness. J Child Fam Stud 21(5):709–717, 2012

Townshend K: Conceptualizing the key processes of mindful parenting and its application to youth mental health. Australas Psychiatry 24(6):575–577, 2016 27354336

Chapter

14

Mindfulness in Schools

Lisa Flook, Ph.D.
Meena Srinivasan

THE FOCUS of this chapter is on mindfulness in education as a preventative or early intervention strategy to promote well-being. Schools are an opportune platform for offering mindfulness practices for staff and students given the amount of time that children and educators spend in the classroom and the potential for mindfulness to support learning goals, both academic and socioemotional in nature. The research on mindfulness in education is still nascent, but initial findings show promise across a variety of outcomes. For a review of mindfulness focusing on school psychology, we refer the reader to Felver et al. (2013).

Education Initiatives

Two recent education initiatives, the multitiered system of supports (MTSS) framework and the Every Student Succeeds Act (ESSA), may impact the use and dissemination of mindfulness in school settings.

Multitiered System of Supports

MTSS is a framework commonly adopted by schools for aligning and integrating initiatives that seek to promote equitable access and opportunity for students' academic, behavioral, and socioemotional success (see Figure 14–1). Supports are classified into three tiers representing the breadth of their intended reach. Tier 1 supports are universal and typically are adopted schoolwide to create positive conditions for learning for every child. Tier 2 interventions are those geared toward a smaller group of students who need additional support above and beyond those offered through standard instruction. Tier 3 interventions provide intensive support for students who have more need, often on an individual basis.

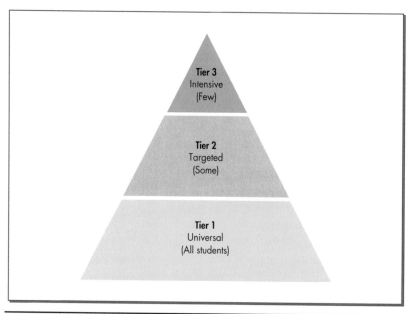

FIGURE 14–1.   Multitiered system of supports diagram.

The predominant approach to mindfulness as introduced in school settings is consistent with tier 1, as a practice that is introduced for its potential benefit to all students. Mindfulness as a strategy for tiers 2 and 3 has not received as much attention—only a handful of studies have worked with clinical populations or youth with specific needs, although not necessarily within a school setting (for a review, see Zoogman et al. 2015).

Every Student Succeeds Act

From an education policy lens, the ESSA calls for schools to use evidence-based interventions as the foundation for education programs and interventions (U.S. Department of Education 2015). The emerging body of research on mindfulness in school settings can help inform educators about the promise of these practices. There are four tiers of intervention defined according to the level of research rigor that supports them (California Department of Education 2018) School improvement plans are required to apply interventions meeting criteria from the top three levels of evidence.

- Tier 1: strong evidence—supported by at least one well-designed and well-implemented experimental study
- Tier 2: moderate evidence—supported by at least one well-designed and well-implemented quasi-experimental study
- Tier 3: promising evidence—supported by at least one well-designed and well-implemented correlational study with controls
- Tier 4: demonstrates a rationale—includes evidence building and ongoing efforts to examine effects

Extant research on school-based mindfulness falls into tier 3, showing promise, with a handful of randomized controlled trials that meet standards for high-quality research (Grant et al. 2017; What Works Clearing House 2018). It is important to acknowledge that the research base on youth is nascent, and even the strongest studies involve relatively small samples and bear replication. Notwithstanding the current limitations, the research to date does suggest promise for mindfulness with youth and needs larger samples of 350 or more participants from multiple sites in a rigorously designed experimental study showing positive effects to meet criteria for strong evidence (U.S. Department of Education 2016).

Education Initiatives and Mindfulness

Mindfulness is most compatible with an MTSS tier 1 approach that provides access to all students as a universal practice. ESSA provides opportunities to introduce mindfulness in schools through considering a broader definition of student success and as a potential research-informed method for addressing school improvement.

In this chapter we discuss ways that mindfulness complements and can be integrated with existing school practices as a universal practice for all students and highlight relevant research and implementation recommendations with attention to the importance of making mindfulness accessible to diverse communities. We also name two potential misconceptions that have been described in the recent press that can impact mindfulness in schools. Further, we provide examples of practices for teachers and students. Last, we address the limitations of current school research and explore directions for further research and practice.

School-Based Applications

Schools are a complex system comprising many interconnected parts. For example, students are embedded within a classroom where they interact with teachers and peers and are shaped by the broader school environment. In order to address the entire system, training that is inclusive of educators as well as students is necessary. School-based intervention research indicates that the greatest impact occurs when classroom teachers who themselves have adequate preparation are involved in delivering the intervention for students (Durlak et al. 2011). Extrapolating from this, and consistent with suggestions from other authors in this book (e.g., see Chapter 1, "Developing a Personal Mindfulness Practice," and Chapter 13, "Mindfulness at Home"), teachers who themselves have direct experience with mindfulness practice can gain familiarity with and reap the potential benefits of practice for themselves and, in turn, provide support for their students in learning and integrating mindfulness throughout the school day.

Although mindfulness can be presented as a set of lessons or a curriculum, it is not intended to be an intervention that is practiced only during discrete times of the day. Rather, the greater potential of mindfulness is as a foundation, a way of being that is infused throughout the school culture and embodied by the adults and leaders in the school setting through their interactions with one another and with students. In this way there is an implicit component to the transmission of mindfulness. This foundational view of mindfulness can be augmented through formal training and even woven into core academic content to support transferability of skills to life beyond and outside the classroom.

Other school personnel, including the school counselor, social worker, positive behavior intervention specialist, or other mental health provider, can support a school's mindfulness initiative. Individuals in these roles may bring special expertise that lends itself to supporting school-based mindfulness initiatives; however, the impact is constrained if classroom teachers are not involved. Finding ways for classroom teachers and other school personnel to coordinate can help to reinforce the practices and instantiate a mindful way of being into the school culture, resulting in greater impact throughout the school community than if only support personnel are involved. Schools where implementation has been most successful use teacher professional development time to train the entire staff, with periodic follow-up and check-ins. Although school counselors may find mindfulness to be a useful MTSS tier 2 or tier 3 intervention strategy, labeling mindfulness as primarily a mental health intervention is unnecessarily limiting.

Implementation Recommendations

Working With Teachers and Educators

Mindfulness initiatives are frequently brought into schools as either stand-alone programs or short, discrete practices (such as mindful breathing during transitions) that are introduced at various points throughout the school day. Before implementing mindfulness with students, schools are advised to take at least a year to develop teachers' personal mindfulness practice.

In fact, in the past 10 years it is estimated that more than 25,000 educators, administrators, mental health professionals, and school community members have been trained in mindfulness (see the Mindful Schools website, www.mindfulschools.org). Some research has specifically examined applications of mindfulness with teachers. Training geared toward educators can be adapted to take into consideration specific issues around the teaching profession, such as stress, burnout, and effectiveness in the classroom. For a recent example of research, readers can refer to Jennings et al.'s (2017) study of teachers' social and emotional competence and classroom interactions. Supporting teachers is critical because of their significant role in youths' overall educational experience.

A school-wide approach that starts with adults helps teachers and school leaders model what they want to see in their students. "Putting your own oxygen mask on first" is a popular way of describing the importance of having adults first gain an experiential understanding of mindfulness before they bring mindfulness into their classrooms. A strong model for programs focuses on supporting teachers in developing, growing, and deepening their own mindfulness practice so they can create the conditions for a supportive learning environment while also nurturing their own well-being. On the basis of our experience with programs, schools where mindfulness initiatives have had the most success have strong leadership support while simultaneously emphasizing the growth and development of the teacher's own mindfulness practice. Involving other stakeholders such as parents, school staff, and administrators to provide input on developing a program is critical to take into account the school's unique context, needs, and resources. Community-building efforts can be strengthened by inviting all of those involved to the mindfulness practice as well.

Extension to Children in Schools

Mindfulness training can be extended to youth in schools through numerous methods. Prioritizing training and ongoing practice for adults who support children is a good place to start. Much is communicated through everyday student-teacher interactions. Adults who are grounded in the practice themselves are more able to provide support and model this way of being for students.

There are different levels of involvement with mindfulness practice that can range from specific exercises practiced for discrete periods to fully integrating mindfulness into the academic and social activities and climate of the classroom. There has also been interest in apps as a means to disseminate training. Apps may complement in-person training, but more research is needed to determine their impact. Dedicating a class period or portion thereof to mindfulness training and activities is one format for training. This may occur, for example, as part of physical education time or special class electives. However, the more that practices can be incorporated throughout the day, the more opportunities there are to reinforce and generalize mindfulness as a habit. There may be ways to include school-wide practice time, for example, at the beginning and end of the day and as part of transitions between classes. Mindfulness may also complement other programs that are being implemented, such as those described in the next section.

A search of the PsycINFO database, one of the primary sources for cataloguing studies in the field of psychology, reveals that the number of published studies on mindfulness has grown exponentially over the past decade (see Figure 14–2). By comparison, as an indicator of how nascent research on mindfulness in education is, the first empirical study on mindfulness training with school children was published in 2005. Readers interested in more specifics on current research in youth and schools can refer to Chapter 3, "State of the Research on Youth Mindfulness."

As mindfulness continues to grow in schools, scholars and practitioners are calling attention to the need to examine issues of race through a mindfulness lens (e.g., Magee 2016). Therefore, the extension of mindfulness training to youth in schools must be culturally relevant, respectful, and tailored to the community. Evidence suggests that mindfulness may reduce implicit biases (Kang et al. 2014) and promote positive mental health and coping outcomes in at-risk settings (for recent examples, see Frank et al. 2017; Sibinga et al. 2016). This initial evidence provides promising data that mindfulness, if adapted appropriately for diverse school communities, can help with existing efforts to promote constructive change. Readers interested in cultural adaptations of mindfulness can refer to Chapter 10, "Immigrant Youth," for a more in-depth discussion.

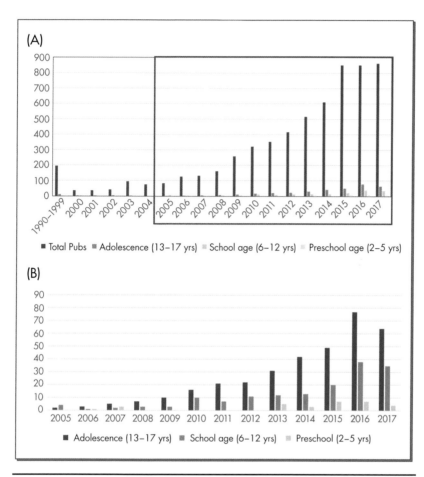

FIGURE 14-2. Figure 14-2. (A) Trends in mindfulness publications from 1990 to 2017 and (B) number of mindfulness publications by age group from 2005 to 2017.

Complementary Approaches to Mindfulness

Social and Emotional Learning

A commonly recognized social and emotional learning (SEL) framework from the Collaborative for Academic, Social, and Emotional Learning (CASEL) identifies five core competencies that are aimed at developing intrapersonal and interpersonal skills: self-awareness, self-management, responsible decision making, relationship skills, and social awareness (see https://casel.org/core-competencies). Arguably, self-awareness is the foremost skill on which the other skills rely. Although SEL as a framework recognizes the importance of self-awareness, the practices and tools available (e.g., emotion recognition and management) tend to emphasize the other competencies, with a bent toward positive psychology and valuing positive emotion. SEL is described as taking an outside-in approach, with a focus on teaching explicit skills, whereas mindfulness is said to work from the inside out (Lantieri and Zakrzewski 2015).

There is increasing interest in developing mindfulness and SEL in tandem and how both approaches can reinforce and enhance each other. Mindfulness has the capacity to help students manage stress, regulate their emotions, and focus their attention so they can be available for academic, social, and emotional learning. Several evidence-based SEL programs have already begun incorporating mindfulness into their programming. Although many of these programs lack a daily mindfulness practice, the fact that well-established evidence-based SEL programs are incorporating mindfulness signals the growing importance of these practices to the SEL field.

Restorative Practices

Restorative practice is an approach to discipline that focuses on repairing harm through a dialogue that includes all parties and is a growing practice in schools. When implemented well, restorative practices have the potential to shift discipline from punishment to learning and to strengthen the sense of community. By incorporating mindfulness, restorative practice educators are better equipped to hold a nonjudgmental, open-hearted stance through the process, which involves engaging in deep listening and cultivating compassion.

Social justice education complements mindfulness approaches. Skills and competencies central to social justice include interdependence, social responsibility, perspective taking, multicultural literacy, and community engagement (Hamedani et al. 2015). From a mindfulness lens, we also recognize our deep interconnectedness and nonseparateness from the rest of life (interdependence), and in recognizing our fundamental interdependence, we cultivate value and care for other beings (social responsibility). The lessening of self-reification through mindfulness practice can support perspective taking. Habits of mind cultivated through mindfulness can inform skillful action and engagement—compassion is a cherished virtue in the contemplative traditions and aligns with community engagement from a social justice perspective.

Misconceptions

Behavior Management

The skillful application of mindfulness is an important consideration that should be factored into implementation efforts. Caution is warranted around mindfulness being used as a behavior management tool in schools. This can be seen as problematic, especially in schools with predominantly children of color. As researchers and practitioners, we are called on to examine potential biases and color-blind presuppositions behind mindfulness initiatives.

Overemphasizing the "Self"

Mindfulness has been criticized in the popular press as an individually oriented practice, a form of "navel-gazing" that promotes self-absorption and indifference (Joiner 2017; Wright 2017). Much research attention has been focused on the effects of practice related to attention and cognition. However, the intrapersonal dimension represents only one side of the coin—the interpersonal dimension is equally profound, and school-based research that incorporates measures of relationship skills, compassion, and socially engaged mindfulness will enable the field to grow and uncover latent capacities.

Example Practices

Teacher Practice

Teaching is a high-stress profession, rated even more stressful than most other professions. To help cope with this stress, teachers can easily integrate the following two practices into their day:

1. One daily activity (e.g., the three Ts) done with mindfulness—The three Ts refer to tea time, transitional time, and toilet time. You can choose one of the Ts to engage in mindfully. With tea time, through simply engaging in mindful breathing and truly tasting your tea or coffee, you can practice mindfulness. Transitional time refers to all the time we spend waiting—in line at the grocery store, stuck in traffic, waiting for our Internet to load, and so on. If you live to be 70 years old, you will have spent 3 years of your life waiting. Imagine if that time were spent practicing mindfulness. Depending on how long your trips to the bathroom last, you might spend between 1.5 and 4 years on the toilet during your lifetime; for teachers, this is often the only time they get during the school day when they can be alone.

Everyone has to use the bathroom. Relieving ourselves instantly brings us back into our bodies, which presents a ripe opportunity to practice mindfulness.

2. Sending good wishes to oneself and students—This is a beautiful practice that can be done before you start your teaching for the day. For example, you can follow this script:

> Get into a comfortable seated position. Gently place your hands on your abdomen or chest. Close your eyes if it feels safe to do so and bring a half smile to your face. Breathing in, say silently to yourself, "I'm aware I'm breathing in." Breathing out, say silently to yourself, "I'm aware I'm breathing out." Silently say to yourself, "in" on the in breath and "out" on the out breath 5 times. Breathing in, say silently to yourself, "I calm my body." Breathing out, say silently to yourself, "I send peace through my body." Silent say to yourself, "calm" on the in breath and "peace" on the out breath 5 times. If it feels available to you, you can now send feelings of peace to your classroom. If you feel that you need more time to cultivate calm and peace in yourself, continue to do so for the next 10 breaths.

Teacher-Student Practice

Teachers can easily practice mindfulness with students to begin the day, during transitions, or before tests by inviting students to bring awareness to their breathing. The practice can be as simple as three to five breaths. Students can place a hand on their belly or chest, and the teacher can either ring a bell or simply cue students to relax their body and feel the natural flow of their breath. Students may need practice relaxing and feeling rather than thinking about breathing or thinking about whether or not they are doing it "right." A useful prompt is "Feeling breathing in, feeling breathing out." For older students, perhaps you can add, "So your bodies are here, notice where your mind is. Is your mind still at lunch or still in your last class? Bringing your mind to your body, feeling the breath in your belly."

Engaging in mindfulness of breathing can support students in connecting their minds and bodies in the present moment. Once students have engaged in some focused breathing, the teacher can offer the following simple prompts for students to share in groups of three or, depending on class size and available time, as a full class: "What did you notice? What did you feel? Is there anything that would help you be present to what's happening right now?"

Conclusion

Programs targeting youth vary in frequency of lessons, length of sessions, duration of overall program, and program activities. Empirical research using randomized controlled trials and other designs is beginning to emerge and suggests feasibility and potential benefits. One of the purposes that research can serve is to help guide curricular decisions and understand for whom, how much of, and when specific types of training may be most helpful. At the same time, at its core, mindfulness is a practice for liberation, and this should remain at the center of scientific inquiry and practice.

There are two parallel movements unfolding around bringing mindfulness into schools. On one side, there has been a vast proliferation of programs offering training for teachers and students. On the other, the research to understand the mechanics of mindfulness and best practices is much slower to catch up. Much of the current research available is on programs that are targeted directly at students. There are still many questions that remain to be investigated, including the following: 1) How much practice is needed and how often should it be done in order to show benefits? 2) Are there characteristics of individuals that predict which practices they will respond to best? 3) How can mindfulness be adapted and incorporated across development to support students? 4) What are the long-term effects of practice? The push to scale in both research and practice needs to be carefully balanced with maintaining the integrity of practice through skillful training and consistency. Going a step further, as a standalone, mindfulness training for students has benefits. However, this does not take into account the full complexity of the school system. A stronger model going forward would be building student training on top of a teacher training component so that mindfulness is ecologically embedded and supported.

There is also a tension between the value placed on randomized controlled trials to demonstrate the efficacy of mindfulness training and the value placed on systems-level change. By design, random assignment of individual students or classrooms is more tractable than random assignment of entire schools or districts for research. However, focusing solely on individuals or classrooms as the unit of change overlooks the importance of the school system as a whole. Shifting the entire culture of a school is likely needed to effect long-term, widespread changes in practice. Research designs that examine school-wide approaches would add to our understanding of transformation at a broader level. In addition, although this chapter focuses on schools, given the embedded nature of children's development and interactions across multiple contexts that support children's growth, involving families is another important facet to complement and potentially increase the impact of school-based approaches.

As the research we point to suggests (also see Chapter 1), mindfulness practice has the potential to further the aims of the education system in terms of boosting cognitive and self-regulatory skills that are conducive to learning and academic achievement. However, mindfulness is not limited to the potential cognitive and academic benefits. As an end in themselves, this would limit the potential scope and depth of what the practices might offer. In addition, mindfulness can be (mis)applied to further competition and individual gain (e.g., if used instrumentally for the primary purpose of increasing productivity) or as a practice to help youth see through the filters of conditioning and limiting impressions.

As described by one of the pioneers in bringing meditation practices into the mainstream culture, "The difference between misery and happiness depends on what we do with our attention" (Salzberg 1995, p. 12). Learning to use our attention and any benefits derived from practice to connect with compassion to the fundamental humanity of ourselves and others is a noble education.

KEY POINTS

- Mindfulness fits within a multitiered system of supports framework as a universal intervention for students.
- Existing research on mindfulness in education with youth shows promise, although research is still at an early stage and more rigorous research is needed.
- We recommend that anyone interested in bringing mindfulness into school settings begin with training for educators so that the adults gain firsthand experience and familiarity with practices.
- Mindfulness training for educators is associated with benefits for teachers both personally and professionally and provides a foundation for introducing practices to students.
- Teachers are encouraged to sustain practice for themselves and their students by finding ways to integrate practices throughout the school day and forming communities of practice with colleagues.

Discussion Questions

1. What are ways to build a professional learning community around mindfulness to support my own practice?
2. What are possible ways that I can incorporate mindfulness into my own school day?
3. What is my intention for practicing mindfulness?

Suggested Readings

Jennings P: Mindfulness for Teachers: Simple Skills for Peace and Productivity in the Classroom. New York, WW Norton, 2015

Rechtschaffen D: The Way of Mindful Education: Cultivating Well-Being in Teachers and Students. New York, WW Norton, 2014

Treleaven D: Trauma-Sensitive Mindfulness: Practices for Safe and Transformative Healing. New York, WW Norton, 2018

Willard C: Growing Up Mindful: Essential Practices to Help Children, Teens, and Families Find Balance, Calm, and Resilience. Boulder, CO, Sounds True, 2016

References

California Department of Education: Evidence-based interventions under the ESSA. Sacramento, CA, California Department of Education, 2018. Available at: www.cde.ca.gov/re/es/evidence.asp. Accessed May 17, 2018.

Durlak JA, Weissberg RP, Dymnicki AB, et al: The impact of enhancing students' social and emotional learning: a meta-analysis of school-based universal interventions. Child Dev 82(1):405–432, 2011 21291449

Felver JC, Doerner E, Jones S, et al: Mindfulness in school psychology: applications for intervention and professional practice. Psychology in the Schools 50(6):531–547, 2013

Frank JL, Kohler K, Peal A, et al: Effectiveness of a school-based yoga program on adolescent mental health and school performance: findings from a randomized controlled trial. Mindfulness 8(3):544–553, 2017

Grant S, Hamilton LS, Wrabel SL, et al: Social and Emotional Learning Interventions Under the Every Student Succeeds Act: Evidence Review. Santa Monica, CA, RAND Corporation, 2017

Hamedani MG, Zheng X, Darling-Hammond L, et al: Social Emotional Learning in High School: How Three Urban High Schools Engage, Educate, and Empower Youth—Cross-Case Analysis. Stanford, CA, Stanford Center for Opportunity Policy in Education, 2015

Jennings PA, Brown JL, Frank JL, et al: Impacts of the CARE for Teachers program on teachers' social and emotional competence and classroom interactions. J Educ Psychol 109(7):1010–1028, 2017

Joiner T: Mindfulness would be good for you. If it weren't so selfish. Washington Post, August 25, 2017. Available at: www.washingtonpost.com/outlook/mindfulness-would-be-good-for-you-if-it-werent-all-just-hype/2017/08/24/b97d0220-76e2-11e7-9eac-d56bd5568db8_story.html?utm_term=.28bf35a2b5d0. Accessed May 17, 2018.

Kang Y, Gray JR, Dovidio JF: The nondiscriminating heart: lovingkindness meditation training decreases implicit intergroup bias. J Exp Psychol Gen 143(3):1306–1313, 2014 23957283

Lantieri L, Zakrzewski V: How SEL and mindfulness can work together. Greater Good Magazine, April 7, 2015. Available at: https://greatergood.berkeley.edu/article/item/how_social_emotional_learning_and_mindfulness_can_work_together. Accessed November 1, 2018.

Magee RV: Community-engaged mindfulness and social justice: an inquiry and call to action, in Handbook of Mindfulness: Culture, Context, and Engagement. Edited by Purser RE, Forbes D, Burke A. New York, Springer, 2016, pp 425–439

Salzberg S: Lovingkindness: The Revolutionary Art of Happiness. Boston, MA, Shambhala, 1995

Sibinga EM, Webb L, Ghazarian SR, et al: School-based mindfulness instruction: an RCT. Pediatrics 137(1):e20152532, 2016 26684478

U.S. Department of Education: Every Student Succeeds Act. Washington, DC, U.S. Department of Education, 2015. Available at: www.ed.gov/essa?src=ft. Accessed May 17, 2018.

U.S. Department of Education: Non-regulatory guidance: using evidence to strengthen education investments. Washington, DC, U.S. Department of Education, September 1, 2016. Available at: www2.ed.gov/policy/elsec/leg/essa/guidanceusese investment.pdf. Accessed May 17, 2018.

What Works Clearing House: Standards Handbook, Version 4.0. Washington, DC, Institute of Education Sciences, 2018. Available at: https://ies.ed.gov/ncee/wwc/Docs/referenceresources/wwc_standards_handbook_v4.pdf. Accessed May 17, 2018.

Wright R: Is mindfulness meditation a capitalist tool or a path to enlightenment? Yes. Wired, August 12, 2017. Available at: www.wired.com/2017/08/the-science-and-philosophy-of-mindfulness-meditation. Accessed May 17, 2018.

Zoogman S, Goldberg SB, Hoyt WT, Miller L: Mindfulness interventions with youth: a meta-analysis. Mindfulness 6(2):290–302, 2015

Chapter

15

Mindful Nature Practices

Nicole Ward, M.S.

MINDFULNESS, in a variety of settings, can be an effective and meaningful intervention for youth. In fact, one of the things I appreciate most about mindfulness is that with practice, the benefits are readily available and can be accessed in any moment. Although any setting works, natural settings are particularly well suited to mindful practice because nature itself is restorative. Moreover, focusing on nature as a central component transforms the practice into something that warrants its own category of intervention: mindful nature practices.

In this chapter, I introduce three predominant theories and present a brief literature review, highlighting existing therapies that involve mindfulness in nature as well as adventure therapies, horticultural therapies, and mindful walking interventions. Next, I explore possible reasons young people are spending less time in nature. The therapeutic framework, goals, and assessment strategies of mindful nature practices are discussed. I then recommend some specific practices that are presented alongside their theoretical foundations and provide two scripts of mindful nature practices. Confidentiality and risk management concerns are outlined, and developmental and cultural differences are considered. A home practice worksheet, key concepts, discussion questions, and suggested readings are included at the end of the chapter.

Theoretical Foundations

A growing body of research indicates that nature-based interventions may be effective at reducing symptoms of mental illness (Maller et al. 2006). Health professionals are becoming more aware of the positive impact contact with nature can have, but the theory behind why time in nature is so beneficial is less well known. Attention restoration theory (ART) is the most prominent theory to date (Kaplan 1995). According to ART, people experience "directed attention fatigue" after spending a significant amount of time attending to voluntary, goal-directed stimulation, such as paying attention in class (Kaplan 1995). ART suggests that nature allows individuals to involuntarily notice beauty in the environment, which then rests directed attention and dissipates fatigue. For example, while writing this chapter, I suddenly noticed a hummingbird stop in front of me and pay a visit to a nearby flower. This moment of awe provided me with a short directed-attention break and allowed me to return to writing feeling more restored.

Another prominent theory is stress reduction theory (SRT), which claims that nature immediately and preconsciously elicits positive emotions and reduces physiological arousal (Ulrich et al. 1991). Proponents of SRT argue that this quick-onset, positively toned affective reaction is critical to restoring psychological and physiological states and that this emotional response precedes all cognitive processing (Ulrich et al. 1991). Yet another important theory is the biophilia hypothesis (Wilson 1984). The biophilia hypothesis asserts that humans have a genetic predisposition to affiliate with other forms of life such as plants and animals and that affiliating with other life forms results in psychological benefits (Wilson 1984). These three theories are not mutually exclusive and together inform this area of inquiry.

Literature Review

Ambrose-Oji (2013) examined 37 research studies that discussed the theoretical links between mindfulness and nature environments and found five different approaches for practicing mindfulness in forests: *shinrin-yoku* (the Japanese concept of "forest bathing"), forest walking, mindfulness and cognitive-behavioral therapy in a forest setting, forest therapy, and ecopsychology. The outcomes from these studies revealed a number of positive benefits such as depression remission, stress reduction, and feeling refreshed. Although these approaches provide possible frameworks for how to practice mindfulness in nature and outline some potential benefits, overall, the evidence base on these approaches is limited, particularly with children and adolescents.

Research on youth explicitly practicing mindfulness in nature is sparse. However, researchers have questioned if living near nature may be enough to positively impact children's well-being. Wells and Evans (2003) found that children who lived near nature had significantly lower levels of distress. They discovered that the proximity to nature had a buffering effect, reducing the psychological distress caused by stressors encountered by the children. Their findings suggest that nature moderates the relationship between stressors and buffers the impact that stress can have on a child's life. The stress moderation that can be found in nature may be particularly well suited for children who deal with many stressors in their lives. This is an idea that could have broad implications: integrating nature into the everyday life of a child, even in small ways, can be meaningful. Not every child and his or her family are able to have nature nearby, but there are many other ways to use nature's benefits for a path to well-being.

A significant portion of the research on nature-based interventions for youth examines adventure or wilderness therapies. The formats and overall goals of adventure therapies vary greatly. However, a commonality seen throughout these programs is the use of experiential learning in a natural environment to help youth manage their psychosocial problems (Bowen and Neill 2013). In a meta-analysis of 197 studies, the majority of which had participants in the 10- to 17-year age range, adventure therapies were compared with alternative treatment and no-treatment groups. The results indicated a moderate positive short-term effect on psychological, interpersonal, emotional, and behavioral domains for groups who engaged in adventure therapy. In addition, the authors found that these positive changes were maintained at follow-up (Bowen and Neill 2013). Specifically, adventure therapies might be most impactful for youth who want to build skills in overcoming challenges and gaining independence. Clinicians working with adolescents who might benefit from adventure therapies could consider referring patients and their family to already-existing reputable programs.

Horticultural therapy may be a more accessible nature intervention, particularly for mental health professionals working in schools or at a center with groups such as hospitals, juvenile detention centers, or community mental health centers. Children who participated in a year-long school garden program increased their self-understanding, ability to work in a team with their peers, and overall life skills (Robinson and Zajicek 2005). One horticultural probationary program in San Antonio, Texas, was as effective at reducing recidivism as traditional probationary programs and provided program participants with the additional benefits of gaining new job skills and giving back to their community (Cammack et al. 2002).

An even less resource-intensive practice is a mindful nature walk. Mindful walking, also known as walking meditation, is one of the practices taught in Jon Kabat-Zinn's highly successful mindfulness-based stress reduction program, which prompts participants to walk slowly, with awareness focusing on the sensations of walking (Kabat-Zinn and Hanh 2013). Mindful walking can be done in any setting; however, this style of walking may be particularly valuable in a natural setting. Shin and colleagues (2013) determined that meditative walking in a forest was the most effective at increasing happiness compared with meditative walking in a gym and athletic walking in a forest or a gym.

Furthermore, increasing cognitive engagement with the natural environment while walking may provide additional psychological benefits. In a study by Duvall (2011), participants were randomly assigned into either a standard care group or an engagement group. Both groups were asked to commit to and schedule three 30-minute walks each week for 2 weeks. In addition, the engagement group was asked to engage in self-selected awareness activities, such as focusing on their senses, while on the walk. The engagement group showed improved attentional functioning, increased feelings of contentment, and reduced feelings of frustration. The psychological benefits that can be experienced by meditative walking in nature and from walking while paying attention to your environment are promising; however, the participants in these studies were all older than 18 years, demonstrating the need to try mindful walking in nature with children and adolescents.

Although the research on youth intentionally practicing nature interventions with mindfulness is limited, the nature interventions outlined in these studies, such as adventure and horticultural therapies, are likely already eliciting participants to engage in mindfulness without explicitly mentioning mindfulness per se. Future research should examine psychological outcomes with youth practicing mindfulness in nature, particularly mindfulness practices where the focus of the practice is on the outdoor environment itself. With a better understanding of the intersection of mindfulness, nature, and mental health, clinicians can better incorporate these findings into their therapy services.

Relevance to Youth Today

Existing theories and research posit that natural environments are captivating, stress reducing, and innately pleasing to us, but nevertheless children are spending less and less time outside in nature (Juster et al. 2004). Richard Louv coined the term *nature deficit disorder* to describe the current generation's move away from nature (Louv 2008). There are many possible contributing factors, such as movement to urban areas, the rise in structured after-school activities, and increased concerns for safety. However, with the rapid advances and increased accessibility of technology today, it seems particularly important to look at the evolving relationship between youth and their technological devices. A new study from the Pew Research Center found that 92% of teenagers go online daily, with 56% going online several times a day and 24% reporting that they are online almost constantly (Lenhart et al. 2015). This indicates that a considerable percentage of youth seem to be more interested in spending time on their smartphones than spending time outside.

One way to understand this preference is by discerning the difference between "soft" and "hard" fascination. Natural settings are referred to as *soft fascination* environments, which essentially are any pleasing environments that gain attention effortlessly while not providing so much stimulation that it impacts the ability to reflect (Herzog et al. 1997). This differs from *hard fascination* environments, such as an engaging sports game, which replenish directed attention but do not invoke reflection (Herzog et al. 1997). For today's youth, attention gets pulled toward hard fascination entertainment activities such as watching TV or playing a computer game. These activities naturally capture attention and allow directed attention to rest, but they may be too stimulating to allow for reflection or to facilitate mindful awareness.

The tendency of technology to soak up the time of young people makes the practice of connecting to nature all the more important. Spending time in nature is not something that happens automatically in the present world. Many young people are being deprived of the benefits of spending time outdoors by the default way modern life is structured and the compelling nature of technology. Reversing this trend through mindful practices focused on nature is something that must be done intentionally to regain the benefits of being outside. That way, the stress-reducing and attention-restoring characteristics of nature can be harnessed and applied to create a more balanced life.

Therapeutic Framework, Expectations, and Goals

The therapeutic framework of mindful nature interventions is flexible and can vary greatly on the basis of therapist comfort, patient factors, and available resources. However, there are several overarching goals that mindful nature interventions have in common:

- When first introducing a practice, the therapist should be explicit about the intention of the practice, and this intention should align with the therapeutic goals that have already been created with the patient. Common therapeutic goals of mindful nature interventions include restoring attention, reducing stress, and broadening perspective.

• The therapist should engage in the practice with the patient and simultaneously act as a guide throughout the intervention.

• A natural element should play a role in the practice. Although being outdoors is ideal, an indoor space with a window or indoor plant is a great way to incorporate a natural element when access to the outdoors is limited.

• After the therapist finishes a mindful practice with the patient, there should be enough time for processing questions and reflection. Depending on the intervention format, this can be done through writing in a personal journal, sharing with a group, or talking with the therapist.

Assessments

The primary type of assessment used to measure psychological outcomes of nature interventions is a self-report measure given before and immediately after the intervention. Sometimes, the same measures are given again weeks or months later to determine if effects have been maintained. Self-report measures are cost-effective and easy to administer and replicate, but participants' biases and imperfect memories can have an impact on the results. Physiological measures of stress such as cortisol levels, heart rate variability, and blood pressure are other common assessment types used to measure nature exposure outcomes that are not impacted by bias and memory. Physiological measures may reliably measure stress, but they do not capture other potential benefits of engaging with nature.

One self-report measure, the Connectedness to Nature Scale, is a 14-item scale that was developed to determine how connected an individual feels to the natural environment (Mayer and Frantz 2004). Using this scale, two studies that controlled for social desirability bias found that nature connectedness was positively correlated with psychological and social well-being (Howell et al. 2011). Providing this scale alongside other measures of interest when assessing nature therapies may reveal additional information about the relationships between these measures.

To further understand the reasons that nature interventions are beneficial, it is helpful to be able to measure and classify different aspects of the natural environments themselves. Currently, there is no standard system for measuring the benefits of nature. This is not surprising because there are many different benefits and the research in this area is young. However, the theories indicate that measurements of stress, attention, and connectedness to nature may be particularly informative areas to assess.

In a meta-analysis that analyzed 10 U.K. studies, Barton and Pretty (2010) compared different environment types and determined that waterside habitats showed the greatest improvements in self-esteem and mood compared with urban space, countryside, and woodland habitats. Although this meta-analysis broadly categorized different environments, techniques can be applied to neighborhoods and homes to determine the exact level of naturalness that they possess. The Naturalness Scale is a four-item scale that assesses how natural a home environment is by recording different aspects of the home such as the view from living room and bedroom windows, how many living plants are in the room, and what material the yard is made of (Wells and Evans 2003). These types of assessments could be used to control for differences between natural environments, and by applying these two different ways of examining nature settings, we may be able to more easily identify the ideal setting for a given intervention.

Mindful Nature Practices Based on Existing Theories

Theories provide us with the framework and context needed to help us consider and select the most appropriate treatment options to match the patients we work with. Often, this process happens quite naturally. For example, a therapist might encourage a depressed patient to engage in meaningful and pleasurable activities because the therapist trusts the theory that the ways we think, feel, and act all interact with one another. It is similarly helpful for therapists who plan to provide mindful nature practices to keep in mind the theories behind what make these practices effective. Thus far, the theories on why spending time in nature is beneficial suggest that simply being in a natural environment can restore attention, reduce stress, and increase feelings of connectedness to the natural world. In this hands-on section, I recommend specific types of practices on the basis of the following three theories, which were outlined earlier in the section "Theoretical Foundations": ART, SRT, and the biophilia hypothesis. Table 15–1 provides a content guide to help you navigate the resources for each theory.

Sensory Nature Practices to Restore Attention

With so much to focus on, being out in nature lends itself to sensory mindfulness practices. With intention, it can be quite easy to feel the temperature of the air on your skin, smell nearby flowers, or hear the sounds of the wind. Nat-

TABLE 15–1. Recommended practice type and script based on theory

Theory	Practice type	Script
Attention restoration theory	Sensory nature practices	Sensory Nature Walk
Biophilia hypothesis	Engaging with nature	Planting the Seeds for Transformation
Stress reduction theory	Incorporating breath, movement, and freeform exploration	

ural interventions capture attention effortlessly through the senses, so it follows that cueing youth to use their senses can facilitate attention restoration. The script "Sensory Nature Walk" is for those who have access to a natural environment nearby and is inspired by Jon Kabat-Zinn's version of walking meditation and meditations that focus on the senses. This practice has a particular focus on using the senses to bring awareness to the natural environment.

SENSORY NATURE WALK

Intention: Restore attention through tuning into the senses while in nature
Time: 15–30 minutes
Script: On this mindful nature walk, we are going to use our eyes, ears, nose, mouth, and hands to help us pay attention. Before we start walking, we are going to do a few things that will help prepare us. Start by planting your feet firmly on the ground, standing up tall like the trees around us. Let's take three deep breaths. Now I am going to ask a few questions that I don't want you to answer right now. You can just think in your head about what I am asking, and we will have time at the very end to share our experiences. First, I want you to look around. What types of things are you seeing? Notice the different shapes and textures. Look at the colors around you, noticing the many different shades that exist even for just one color. Now let's shift our attention to what type of things we can hear. Can you hear any birds, or maybe you can hear the sounds of the wind? What types of things can you smell? What does the air here smell like? You may even be able to notice the "taste" of the air. Last, we tune into our sense of touch. How does it feel to have your feet on the ground? You may even wish to take your shoes off and feel the connection of your bare feet with the grass or ground beneath them. What types of things can you touch in this area? If there is something you can reach and touch or pick up right now, go ahead and do so. Does it feel rough or smooth, warm or cool? If you picked something up,

place it back right where you found it. Now that you get the idea of how we are going to use our senses of seeing, hearing, smelling, tasting, and touching, you are going to get a chance to do this on your own. Let's take 5 minutes to walk quietly and slowly, and we will meet back here to share our experiences at the end.

REFLECTION QUESTIONS

1. What caught your attention on this walk?
2. How are you feeling?
3. Did you walk slower or faster than you normally do? How did that change your experience?

TIPS

- Ask that all cameras, phones, and anything else that could distract from the present moment are left behind.
- Adjust the language on the basis of your nature location (e.g., "Can you hear the sounds of the ocean?").
- Keep the pace of the walk slow through modeling and redirecting if needed.
- You may need to provide additional instructions about the types of things you can and cannot touch in this exercise.
- Make clear what the boundaries are of the independent walk and provide developmentally appropriate supervision.

Although getting outside into a natural environment is ideal, even having a window with a natural view can have restorative effects (Ulrich et al. 1991). Some additional ways to bring sensory nature practices indoors are listening to audio recordings of nature sounds, smelling natural aromas, tasting natural foods, viewing nature photos or videos, and feeling the breeze from an open window. For a more complete list of indoor sensory nature practices, see Appendix A, "Bringing Nature Indoors," at the end of the chapter.

Engaging With Nature to Increase Connectedness

According to the biophilia hypothesis, humans have a natural inclination to connect with nature. This connection seems especially prevalent in mindful nature practices, in which people are in direct contact with natural elements. During my time assisting with elementary school garden classes, I observed a great sense of pride and accomplishment from the children, whether they were tasked with harvesting sunflower seeds, planting potatoes, creating fairy gardens, or picking the perfect flower to hand to their teacher. The outdoor environment and inter-active lesson plans not only served as an outlet for the high-energy children but also got classmates to work together as a team toward a common goal. The experience of touching the dirt and plants paired with the opportunity to nurture and foster growth make gardening practices particularly effective at increasing feelings of connectedness with nature. The following script, "Planting the Seeds for Transformation," is geared toward working with one child in a therapy office, but it can be adapted for groups in any setting.

PLANTING THE SEEDS FOR TRANSFORMATION

Intentions: Increase connectedness to nature through interacting with natural materials and increase patient's understanding of the therapeutic process through engaging in this hands-on metaphor

Materials: Planter box or pot, soil, seed or small plant, window with sunlight or outdoor area

Script: We are going to start today by doing some gardening. First, put some soil into the gardening pot. The soil in the bottom of this pot is going to be the foundation for the plant. We hope that it puts its roots into this soil to keep it stable and strong. Next, hold the seed in your hand, and let's set an intention for this seed to grow into a healthy plant. Setting an intention means that we are going to set a goal that we are going to take steps to accomplish. Now place the seed in the soil and cover the seed with more soil. Next, pour some water on top of the soil. We will need to water the seed each time we see each other if we want the seed to grow into a healthy plant. Now pick a place for the seed to live on my office window. Nice work; you have planted the seed! You may notice that right now all you can see is a pot of wet soil. That's because growth doesn't happen instantly. Gardening takes time, patience, our attention, and hard work. Each week when we water the seed, we will pay attention to how it grows. Since you have already put in the hard work of planting the seed, it is now up to the seed, soil, sun, and water to do the work of growing. The plant might grow fast or slow. The plant might look different than you expect it to. Weeds might sprout up. The plant may never take off, and we may need to try again and plant another seed. Setting an intention or goal helps to keep us focused so that even if we run into some challenges along the way, we can continue to notice the plant and check in each week about what we should do next.

REFLECTION QUESTIONS

1. Here we made the intention for this seed to grow into a healthy plant. What are some other intentions you would like to make in your life?
2. What other things in your life require attention, time, patience, or hard work?

3. How does it feel to not be able to control how the seed will grow?

4. Has anything in your life ever turned out different from how you expected it to? What did you do?

TIPS

- Do a little research about what type of plant to get depending on whether you are keeping the plants indoors or outdoors, the weather, and your desired level of maintenance.

- With parent permission, you could have the child take the plant home to keep in his or her room to take care of at home. This may increase feelings of connectedness and responsibility.

This script not only tries to elicit connectedness with nature but also serves as a metaphor for the therapeutic journey. Metaphors are frequently used throughout therapy to illustrate concepts and help shift perspectives by visualizing something in a new way, and nature-related metaphors are common. For example, as a way to explain cognitive defusion in acceptance and commitment therapy, patients are asked to imagine that they are placing their thoughts on leaves floating down a stream or on clouds floating across the sky. Mindful nature practices have the unique ability to merge a hands-on practice such as gardening with a helpful metaphor such as growth, which can be particularly engaging for children. When providing nature practices, don't be afraid to be creative and come up with your own metaphors that are relevant to the individuals you work with.

Incorporating Breath Movement, and Exploration to Reduce Stress

Considering the stress-reducing physiological effects of meditation, practicing mindful breathing in a natural environment may be particularly stress reducing. Similarly, engaging in movement while in nature may be especially helpful in releasing tension because of the ability of exercise to lower cortisol levels and decrease our stress. Even more, the pairing of breath and movement in a nature environment may also bring about a calm state. Guiding patients to synchronize their breathing patterns with their walking stride is an effective way to shift the focus from the patient's thoughts to the present experience of breath while walking in a natural environment. This breath and movement pairing can also be done with other nature activities, such as rowing a boat or swimming. *Qigong*, a traditional holistic Chinese practice often practiced in outdoor nature locations, demonstrates another way that the breath and coordinated body movements can be used together for relaxation.

Simpler still, eschewing all structure can provide a profoundly healing nature experience. When you are your own guide, you can do whatever feels comfortable (e.g., sitting, exploring, lying down). Being truly unbound by expectations or goals and allowing yourself to follow curiosity or desires as they come up can provide relief from the hyperstructured modern lifestyle. When you offer a practice that is free of structure, it can be helpful to include some practical guidelines, such as designating an area to stay within or identifying any hazards or fragile areas to avoid.

Confidentiality

Confidentiality and its limits are particularly important to discuss when moving the therapeutic setting outside. Before engaging in outdoor mindful nature practices, providers should talk with their patients about the potential reduced privacy that can arise. The possibility that other people will be in the same outdoor space and therefore may be able to observe or overhear the provider and patient should be made clear. Guidelines on how to proceed if another person attempts to interact, or even join the practice, should be decided ahead of time. This may be particularly relevant in settings where it is likely that the provider and patient will cross paths with someone they know. To mitigate issues with confidentiality, personal content should not be discussed when outside the therapy room. Instead, the focus should be on the mindful nature practice itself.

Risk Management

There are additional risks to consider when engaging in outdoor practices, and these risks vary greatly depending on setting and practice. For example, engaging in a gardening practice right outside your therapy office poses different risks than guiding a large group in a nature walking practice on uneven terrain in a location without cell phone service. When selecting a nature setting, choose a location that has cell phone service and make sure all important safety numbers (e.g., emergency contacts, nearest hospital, police) are easily accessible in case of an emergency. If you are going to a location without service, consider purchasing a satellite phone. Many outdoor nature interventions will require additional adult support to help supervise at an appropriate ratio to the group size (minimum of 1:10 for day practices and 1:6 for expeditions). If the outdoor practice is strenuous or takes place in a remote area, it may be advised to have a medical professional or wilderness guide. Always get permission from parents or guardians beforehand and always let another responsible adult know your destination, return time, and contact information.

Developmental Considerations

Mindful nature practices are accessible for all ages; however, specific adaptations may need to be made depending on the developmental stage of the child. It is important that the type of activity is engaging enough to hold a child's interest and that the language and style being used to guide the practice are age appropriate to ensure comprehension. For example, if the treatment goal is to teach a group of kindergarten to third-grade children how to understand different perspectives, you could engage them in an exercise in which they pretend to be a living thing they see in nature, such as a squirrel or a tree. This type of play is active, fun, and accessible for this age group. However, it may be more difficult to engage in this same activity with a group of junior high or high school students because they might feel the activity is too silly and potentially embarrassing to do in front of their peers. Instead, teenagers may be more willing to write a poem from the perspective of an animal that they observe in nature.

The time frame and format of a nature experience should be adjusted for the developmental stage of the child. Multiweek wilderness experiences are usually geared toward adolescents and transitional-age youth (ages 16–24), for whom an extended time in the wilderness setting can foster a sense of independence and help build self-confidence. However, this same format may not be appropriate for younger children because it could be very overwhelming. The same theory could also be applied to single-day experiences: an older participant may be willing to stick with a single activity for a long time, whereas it may be helpful to change activities frequently with young participants.

Adaptations and Cultural Considerations

Longer nature interventions, such as staying at overnight camping facilities, can still be highly valuable to a wide age range and for children with a variety of disabilities or health concerns. This was demonstrated in my experience working with children at Camp Okizu, a camp that provides support and recreational services to children ages 6–17 with childhood cancer, their siblings, and their families. Camp Okizu adapts its recreation activities to be inclusive of all kids, regardless of their abilities. Children in wheelchairs are able to spend time out on the lake in a large raft and can participate in the ropes course in a swing that can be operated by another person. Children with ports are able to go out in designated dry boats and can participate in camp games because these games are designed to be less physical. For 1 week, these accommodations allow children who have had to spend so much of their lives thinking about their poor health and limitations to experience a sense of normalcy and fun in the outdoors.

Access to nature varies with socioeconomic class, and it may be much more difficult for youth living in urban areas to safely be in outdoor spaces. For populations with limited access, using more indoor nature practices or orienting families to safe local green spaces may be indicated. At an elementary school that I worked with in East Palo Alto, California, many parents were unfamiliar with the local green spaces that were nearby. To familiarize them with these beautiful resources, the school partnered with a local environmental education and restoration agency and co-led mindful nature walking events for the families. The local environmental agency created nature scavenger hunts to assist the children and their families in noticing the wildlife native to their home. We found that providing this type of event not only served as an introductory exercise for families to feel comfortable bringing their children to these spaces but also provided the environmental agency with an opportunity to interact with families who do not often get out to the parks and to consider how to make these locations more accessible.

How to Get Started

The hope is that after reading this chapter, providers will feel comfortable incorporating mindful nature practices into the therapies they already provide. One simple way to get acquainted with these practices is to select a couple of ideas from Appendix A, "Bringing Nature Indoors"; simply adding a plant or nature photo to your office can be the first step toward incorporating nature into your practice. Another easy way to get started is to develop a list of local and reputable resources to refer your patients to, which could include adventure therapy programs, community gardens, environmental agencies, and outdoor education organizations.

Before guiding some of the more hands-on practices, look to the earlier sections "Therapeutic Framework, Expectations, and Goals" and "Assessment." It is important to review the patient's therapeutic goals and consider developmental and cultural factors before selecting the practice type and assessments measures. In addition, it is essential to assess risk and confidentiality concerns before leading a practice. If applicable, use the mindful nature practice scripts in this chapter and the worksheet in Appendix B, "Home Practice: Plant Mindfulness." Last, give yourself permission to be creative. No two mindful nature practices will look exactly the same. Similar to other interventions, adaptations will have to be made, so allow yourself enough agency so that you can provide the most appropriate and helpful practices for the youth you serve.

Conclusion

Applying mindfulness practices in natural settings is a simple, cost-effective way to improve well-being for children, adolescents, and their families. The research supporting this combination has just begun to emerge, but it already illuminates the potential applications and benefits for young people that can be achieved through cultivating mindfulness in nature. The practices discussed in this chapter provide clear examples of how to promote mindful awareness through fostering a connection to nature. However, these practices are far from comprehensive, and many more variations can be created to adapt to any young person's particular needs. Mindful nature practices are versatile and effective, and we hope clinicians will incorporate these practices into the therapies they provide for youth today.

KEY POINTS

- The focus on nature itself is the central component of mindful nature practices.
- Attention restoration theory, stress reduction theory, and the biophilia hypothesis are three of the predominant theories on the effects of spending time in nature.
- The existing research on youth explicitly practicing mindfulness in nature is sparse. However, there is growing research on the potential applications and benefits for young people that can be achieved through cultivating mindfulness in nature.
- Mindful nature practices for youth are versatile and effective, and you can incorporate these practices into the therapies you provide.

Discussion Questions

1. How can we integrate mindful nature practices into existing mental health services for youth?
2. What are the key patient characteristics and presentations that indicate that mindful nature practices might be beneficial?
3. How do we make mindful nature practices accessible to low-resource, at-risk urban communities?

Suggested Readings

Louv R: Last Child in the Woods: Saving Our Children From Nature-Deficit
  Disorder. Chapel Hill, NC, Algonquin Books, 2008
Khan IL: Mindfulness in Nature: Teaching Mindfulness Skills to Kids and
  Teens. New York, Guilford, 2015, pp 256–274

References

Ambrose-Oji B: Mindfulness Practice in Woods and Forests: An Evidence Review. Re-
  search Report for the Mersey Forest, Forest Research. Surrey, UK, Alice Holt
  Lodge Farnham, 2013
Barton J, Pretty J: What is the best dose of nature and green exercise for improving men-
  tal health? A multi-study analysis. Environ Sci Technol 44(10):3947–3955, 2010
  20337470
Bowen DJ, Neill JT: A meta-analysis of adventure therapy outcomes and moderators.
  Open Psychol J 6(1):28–53, 2013
Cammack C, Waliczek TM, Zajicek JM: The Green Brigade: The psychological effects
  of a community-based horticultural program on the self-development characteris-
  tics of juvenile offenders. Horttechnology 12(1):82–86, 2002
Duvall J: Enhancing the benefits of outdoor walking with cognitive engagement strat-
  egies. J Environ Psychol 31(1):27–35, 2011
Herzog TR, Black AM, Fountaine KA, et al: Reflection and attentional recovery as dis-
  tinctive benefits of restorative environments. J Environ Psychol 17(2):165–170, 1997
Howell AJ, Dopko RL, Passmore HA, et al: Nature connectedness: associations with
  well-being and mindfulness. Pers Individ Dif 51(2):166–171, 2011
Juster FT, Ono H, Stafford FP: Changing Times of American Youth: 1981–2003. Ann
  Arbor, MI, Institute for Social Research, University of Michigan, 2004, pp 1–15
Kabat-Zinn J: Full Catastrophe Living: Using the Wisdom of Your Body and Mind to
  Face Stress, Pain, and Illness. New York, Bantam, 2013
Kaplan S: The restorative benefits of nature: Toward an integrative framework. J Envi-
  ron Psychol 15(3):169–182, 1995
Lenhart A, Duggan M, Perrin A, et al: Teens, Social Media and Technology Overview
  2015. Smartphones Facilitate Shift in Communication Landscape for Teens. Wash-
  ington, DC, Pew Research Center's Internet and American Life Project, 2015
Louv R: Last Child in the Woods: Saving Our Children From Nature-Deficit Disorder.
  Chapel Hill, NC, Algonquin Books, 2008
Maller C, Townsend M, Pryor A, et al: Healthy nature healthy people: 'contact with nature' as an upstream health promotion intervention for populations. Health Pro-
  mot Int 21(1):45–54, 2006 16373379
Mayer FS, Frantz CM: The connectedness to nature scale: a measure of individuals'
  feeling in community with nature. J Environ Psychol 24(4):503–515, 2004
Robinson CW, Zajicek JM: Growing minds: the effects of a one-year school garden
  program on six constructs of life skills of elementary school children. Horttechnology 15(3):453–457, 2005

Shin YK, Kim DJ, Jung-Choi K, et al: Differences of psychological effects between meditative and athletic walking in a forest and gymnasium. Scand J For Res 28(1):64–72, 2013

Ulrich RS, Simons RF, Losito BD, et al: Stress recovery during exposure to natural and urban environments. J Environ Psychol 11(3):201–230, 1991

Wells NM, Evans GW: Nearby nature: a buffer of life stress among rural children. Environ Behav 35(3):311–330, 2003

Wilson EO: Biophilia. Cambridge, MA, Harvard University Press, 1984

Appendix A

Bringing Nature Indoors

Sight

🌿 Hang up nature photos or artwork.

TIP: *Display photos that you have personally taken or artwork you have created yourself.*

🌿 Place plants thoughtfully around the indoor space.

CONSIDER *planting them yourself in containers you like.*

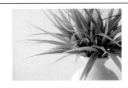

Sound

🌿 Listen to recordings of nature sounds.

CONSIDER *downloading an app that plays nature sounds on your phone.*

🌿 Listen to an indoor water fountain.

NOTICE *how you are feeling.*

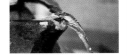

Smell

🌿 Fill the room with natural aromas through use of nature-scented essential oils or candles.

NOTICE *if these scents elicit any memories and then gently bring yourself back to the present moment.*

🌿 Keep flowers in the indoor space.

TIP: *Both freshly cut and dried flowers can offer lovely aromas.*

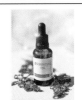

Taste

🌿 Engage in a mindful eating practice with a natural food.

CONSIDER *the journey this natural food item has taken to get from the ground to your taste buds.*

🌿 Sip a cup of herbal tea.

TIP: *Pick fresh herbs for your tea.*

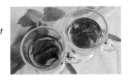

Touch

🌿 Plant an indoor container plant.

FEEL *the textures of the dirt, water, and plant.*

🌿 Open the window and feel the air and temperature on your skin.

FEEL *the sensations of a gust of wind or the heat of the sun.*

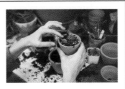

Appendix B

Home Practice: Plant Mindfulness

Before starting the activity, check in with yourself. How are you feeling?
Circle below and/or write in your own feeling words:

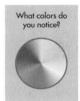

What colors do you notice?

Afraid	Angry	Bored	Confused	Confident	Curious	Disappointed
Disgusted	Excited	Embarrassed	Frustrated	Guilty	Happy	Hopeful
Hopeless	Jealous	Loved	Nervous	Proud	Refreshed	Silly
Shy	Thankful	Tired	Worried			

Directions: Choose a plant to use for this activity. It can be as small as a
blade of grass or as big as a tree. Use the mindfulness skills we have been
practicing to fill out this worksheet.

Draw the plant in the box below (be detailed!):

What about this plant caught your attention?

_____

_____

_____

_____

_____

_____

How do you feel after completing this worksheet?

What does the plant smell like?

Afraid	Angry	Bored	Confused	Confident	Curious	Disappointed
Disgusted	Excited	Embarrassed	Frustrated	Guilty	Happy	Hopeful
Hopeless	Jealous	Loved	Nervous	Proud	Refreshed	Silly
Shy	Thankful	Tired	Worried			

Chapter

16

Mindful Movement in Schools

Catherine Cook-Cottone, Ph.D.

THE term *yoga* is derived from the Sanskrit verb *yuj*, which means to join, connect, or unite. Yoga is both a philosophy and a set of practices. Philosophically, yoga is rooted in the belief that all human suffering is the result of our minds ruminating about the past; feeling distressed about the future; and not being *connected to*, or present and engaged in, the current moment (Bryant 2015; Cook-Cottone 2017). Practically, yoga is offered as an antidote to this suffering. That is, yoga practices serve to *connect* us to the present moment through physical postures, breathing exercises, relaxation, and meditation, simultaneously relieving us of rumination and distress (Cook-Cottone 2017). Moreover, the nature of the connection is critical in yoga practice. As stated in the yoga stutras (see Bryant 2015), physical and mental practices help us connect with the present moment by continuously cultivating lovingkindness, compassion, equanimity, and joy throughout the practice (Cook-Cottone 2017). It is both the nature of the practice and the practice itself that is believed to promote connection to the present moment and the positive embodiment of self within the present moment (Cook-Cottone 2017; Cook-Cottone et al. 2017c).

Researchers are working to understand the potential benefits of yoga and the aspects of the practice and specific mechanisms that promote change (Butzer et al. 2016). It is theorized that the practices of yoga (i.e., postures, breathing, meditation, relaxation) facilitate the development of mind-body awareness, self-regulation, and physical fitness, which in turn supports the development and expression of prosocial behaviors, an improved mental state, and increased performance for students from kindergarten through college (Figure 16–1) (see Butzer et al. 2016).

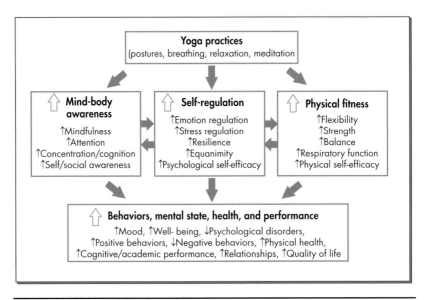

FIGURE 16–1. Model of yoga practice and outcomes.

Source.   Reprinted from Butzer B., Bury D., Telles S., et al.: "Implementing Yoga Within the School Curriculum: A Scientific Rationale for Improving Social-Emotional Learning and Positive Student Outcomes." *Journal of Children's Services* 11(1):3–24, 2016. Used with permission.

How does this happen? Yoga practice appears to help students positively and effectively negotiate both their inner (i.e., physical sensations, emotions, and thoughts) and outer (i.e., family and close friends, school and community, and culture) experiences of self (Cook-Cottone 2017). For school children and adolescents, the inner and outer domains of self can function as a support (e.g., predisposition to good health, a peaceful and loving home, a good school system) or a challenge (e.g., predisposition to anxiety symptoms, alcoholic parents, a violent neighborhood). Most students experience a mix of support and challenge that shifts from day to day and year to year. Further, during these developmental years, children are on a discontinuous and sometimes unpredictable path of growth and development both physically and mentally (Cook-Cottone 2017). They are negotiating an incredible number of daily challenges before they even walk into the classroom. Yoga offers a set of tools and practices that help children and adolescents increase awareness of their bodies, emotions, and cognitions and learn to internally self-regulate while effectively engaging with their ever-changing world (Cook-Cottone 2017). In particular, research indicates that yoga can help improve physical fitness, manage stress, improve focus, regulate emotions, increase positive behaviors, and enhance learning outcomes (e.g., Butzer et al. 2016). Accordingly, yoga is being offered in schools across the United States, and the number of schools offering yoga is increasing steadily (Butzer et al. 2015).

Provision of Yoga in Schools

Yoga, when taught in schools, helps students develop and practice a set of mind and body tools that support well-being (i.e., stress management, self-regulation, and enhanced health) so that they are ready to connect to the present moment and engage in learning in the classroom (Childress and Harper 2015; Cook-Cottone 2017; Serwacki and Cook-Cottone 2012). In schools, yoga aligns well with the three-tier model of prevention and intervention (Cook-Cottone 2017). (For a discussion of the multitiered system of supports, see Chapter 14, "Mindfulness in Schools.") Specifically, yoga practices can be provided as a tier 1, or universal, prevention program. This can be done through classroom-based and after-school yoga sessions along with implementation of mindful movement and breathing breaks in class. At tier 1 (focus on all students, often serving 80%–90% of the students), yoga is often implemented schoolwide as part of the school's socioemotional learning curriculum and physical education programs. At tier 2 (focus on students at risk, serving 10%–15% of the students), yoga is offered in smaller groups, aimed at specific skill development for vulnerable students in need of self-acceptance and whose self-regulation and attentional capacity are underdeveloped. At tier 3 (focus on students in need, serving about 1%–5% of students), specific yoga skills such as calming breaths and systemic relaxation can be taught one on one for students who do not respond to whole-school or small-group interventions.

Therapeutic Frame

Yoga is a mind and body practice affecting both the physical experience of self and the mental (emotional and cognitive) experience. Yoga asanas, breath work, relaxation techniques, and meditation may function somewhat like both aerobic and anaerobic forms of exercise, with benefits tied to continuous and steady practice over time. Research has yet to answer the questions "Do the benefits of yoga practices stop when the student is no longer practicing?" and "Do the skills that are internalized through practice shift the way a student experiences his or her world in a way that endures over time, even without practice?"

The answers to these questions may be difficult to sort out using current school-based yoga programs. Many school-based yoga programs integrate yoga and psychoeducational skills known to have enduring effects, such as stress management, emotional awareness, self-regulation, and healthy relationships (e.g., Cook-Cottone 2017; Frank et al. 2017). Accordingly, there is no set, universally accepted dosage for yoga (i.e., How much? How often? How long?); no particular identified type of yoga known to be most effective; no specific sequence of poses and practices known to work best for certain students or struggles; and no context for the provision of yoga (e.g., small group, classroom, whole school) that is best (Cook-Cottone 2013, 2017).

Dosage questions can be answered in two ways: by looking at typical practice or by noting trends in the research. In practice, many schoolwide yoga programs are delivered year round, offering yoga sessions one to three times per week along with classroom-based yoga breaks and yoga skill practice (e.g., deep breathing and mindfulness practice before a big test or energetic yoga poses to invigorate the room after a long study session). In this way, along with the standard yoga sessions, teachers use yoga practices to help students manage their energy levels and focus in the classroom. In typical research protocols, programs tend to run from 8 to 12 weeks in duration, with some research programs implementing yoga for the full school year (Butzer et al. 2016; Ferreira-Vorkapic et al. 2015; Khalsa and Butzer 2016; Serwacki and Cook-Cottone 2012). Studies with positive outcomes tend to offer programs 2–4 days a week, with sessions as long as 30–60 minutes (Cook-Cottone 2017).

Structured yoga sessions typically begin with a centering activity such a breathing or a short guided meditation. Next, students practice physical postures, with some programs integrating a theme such as gratitude, compassion, the effects of breath, or the power of body awareness. Although there is variety across programs, physical postures (described in more detail in the subsection "Physical Postures") are frequently delivered in an intentional sequence moving from warm-up to challenging poses to more calming poses. Last, the sessions typically end with a guided relaxation and mindful meditation practice. The sequence of the yoga session components also varies from program to program. For example, some programs offer psychoeducational content just prior to the yoga asana practice; some offer it after. For an in-depth review of yoga programs for schools, see Cook-Cottone (2017), and for a best practices guide for yoga in schools, see Childress and Harper (2015).

Training

Currently, there are no generally agreed-on training or professional standards for teaching yoga in schools. Yoga Alliance Foundation is a not-for-profit group that offers guidance for training by registering programs that meet their standards. Yoga Alliance offers a specific designation, or specialization, for the teaching of yoga to children (see www.yogaalliance.org). Although there is no specific registration designation for schools, some of the programs registered in the Yoga Alliance are specifically school based (e.g., see Kripalu Yoga at https:// kripalu.org/kyis-teacher-training or Little Flower's Yoga School Project at http://littlefloweryoga.com/programs/the-school-yoga-project). There are also programs such as Yoga Foster (www.yogafoster.org) that offer online training and support for school personnel. Currently, there is no research pointing to the best type of training for persons teaching yoga in schools, but in the field, there seems to be a preference for individuals with both education and yoga credentials. Those with only a yoga training background may need supervision and/or training to help them navigate school culture as well as the many nuances of working within the educational system and within the context of student diversity and student needs. Finally, although there is no specific research to date, many practitioners in the field argue that those who most effectively teach yoga skills to students should have an active personal yoga practice (Cook-Cottone 2017).

Core Yoga Interventions

Yoga in schools includes four core practices: postures, breath work, relaxation exercises, and mindful meditations (Cook-Cottone 2017). Programs offer these four core practices in varying sequences and intensities, often supplementing the core practices with psychoeducation and/or engagement in curricular content intended to increase well-being (Cook-Cottone 2017). Supplemental content is often aligned with social and emotional learning standards and goals (Childress and Harper 2015; Cook-Cottone 2017).

Physical Postures

Yoga postures (asanas) have many benefits, such as increased flexibility, strengthened muscles, enhanced balance, an improved immune system, better posture, enhanced lung function, slower and deeper breathing, enhanced oxygenation of tissues, and relaxation of the nervous system (for a review of benefits, see Cook-Cottone 2017). Yoga postures stretch and tone muscles and are typically done along with deep, diaphragmatic breath. Connection to the present moment is cultivated through alignment of breath, attention, and intention as students move through and stay in the yoga poses (Cook-Cottone 2017). For a detailed overview of poses that are a good fit for schools, see Cook-Cottone (2017).

Breath Work

According to Yogis in Service, a not-for-profit group that provides training in trauma-informed yoga for schools (see www.yogisinservice.org), your breath is your most powerful tool in stress management and self-regulation (Cook-Cottone et al. 2017a). In yoga, the breath is used to calm and strengthen the nervous system, engage in the present moment, negotiate distress, and enhance concentration (Cook-Cottone 2017; Cook-Cottone et al. 2017a). The rate of breath can vary throughout the day in service of your autonomic nervous system (ANS) as well as with intentional direction of the breath. The normal range is 12–20 breaths per minute for students 6 years and older; slow breathing averages about 16 breaths a minute. Critically, breath is considered the only function of the ANS that can be accessed in an intentional manner (Cook-Cottone 2017). Applying breath work to self-regulation, students can learn to notice and work with their breathing. Yoga breath work helps students understand that changes in breathing can indicate internal distress; relaxed, deep, diaphragmatic breathing can restore the nervous system to a coordinated, integrated functioning; and equalizing the length of inhalation and exhalation can help students bring their minds and bodies into balance (Cook-Cottone et al. 2017a).

In yoga, there are various types of breathing exercises to help students work with breath to create calm and active engagement. For example, diaphragmatic breathing involves breathing deep into the belly. It is believed that stress and the development of bad breathing habits can result in a shallow, restricted breathing. As another example, whole-body breathing uses your whole body in the inhalation and exhalation of breath. Students can scan their bodies and notice any tensions and see if they can begin to soften tension with their breath. Last, grounding and calming breath is a great breathing exercise for students and school personnel (Cook-Cottone 2017). The time to use this breath is when the student is presenting as overstimulated, anxious, wound up, or upset (see the practice script and homework in the following subsections).

PRACTICE SCRIPT: GROUNDING AND CALMING BREATHS

Today we are going to practice grounding and calming breaths. Grounding and calming breaths are a good way to cope when you feel overwhelmed or like you might react in a way that you won't be proud of later. Grounding and calming breaths help you to calm down, slow down your heartbeat and your breathing, soften your feelings, and make better choices. There are two steps to grounding and calming breaths: step one, ground. Step two, breathe.

Step one, ground: Check in with your body. Sometimes it helps to place one hand on your belly and one hand over your heart. This way you can feel your belly breath and your heartbeat. Notice any tension you might feel in your muscles or your face, maybe in your jaw. Now, press your feet into the ground. It might be helpful to imagine that your feet can root deeply into the earth like a tree. Keep your knees just a tiny bit bent, or softened. Notice your body from your feet, through your belly, all the way to the crown of your head. Your job right now is to work on feeling really grounded in your feet, like a tree that has deep roots.

Step two, breathe. Now, bring your awareness to your breath. At first simply notice your breath. You can feel your belly and your chest move as you breathe and maybe feel the air moving in or out of your nose or your mouth. If it feels OK, see if you can breathe through your nose. Bring the air in through your nose and let the air out through your nose. Now, slowly slow your breath, and on your next inhale, count to four as you breathe in air. Now, exhale and count to five as you let all of the air go. Do this three more times: in, 1, 2, 3, 4, and out, 1, 2, 3, 4, 5. Breathe in, 1, 2, 3, 4, and out, 1, 2, 3, 4, 5. And last one: breathe in, 1, 2, 3, 4, and out, 1, 2, 3, 4, 5.

Now just breathe, letting the air come in and go out as you'd like. Notice your breathing; notice your heart beat. Notice whatever you might be feeling. Notice any tensions. Now, notice your feelings and thoughts. Notice how grounding your feet and breathing deeply helps soften your feelings and thoughts, giving you room and space to make your best choices. Good work!

HOMEWORK: GROUNDING AND CALMING BREATH HOME PRACTICE

For homework, practice grounding and calming breaths once each day.

- You can try it when you are alone, maybe writing down in your journal what you notice in your body, feelings, and thoughts before and after you practice.
- You can try it during yoga if you are doing a really hard pose. See what you notice.
- You can try it when you feel stressed or upset. Notice if you think it might help you make better choices.
- Teach one of your parents or a caring grown-up how to do grounding and calming breaths and see what both of you notice.

Relaxation

Relaxation exercises create a bridge from the more active, external practices of yoga to the internal, meditative practices (Cook-Cottone 2017). There are many ways to engage students in relaxation. For example, in systematic relaxation, awareness is guided across the length of the body from the head to the toes and back to the crown of the head. Throughout the practice, students are guided to maintain deep, diaphragmatic breathing while bringing a release and relaxation to the muscle. To provide contrast, students can be guided to engage and then relax muscles in each area. Another type of relaxation is the body scan, in which awareness is brought to each area of the body.

Guided visualization is the use of imagery to create calm and relaxation. In this practice, students are guided through an imaginary journey. They may visualize rising in flight on a giant bird, floating down a river in a canoe, riding a whale in the ocean, or hiking up a mountain filled with flowers and trees. It is important to note that within the context of trauma-informed practice, guided visualization without a grounding physical practice can lead to dissociation for some students (Cook-Cottone 2004; Cook-Cottone et al. 2017a). Therefore, it is recommended that the yoga instructor keep bringing students' focus to the physical sensation of the body and the breath (Cook-Cottone 2004; Cook-Cottone et al. 2017a).

Meditation

Meditation is the practice of mindful awareness. This process involves three steps: 1) present-moment attention (i.e., mindful awareness of thoughts, emotions, physical sensations, and/or a focus on an object); 2) noticing, recognizing, and allowing wandering thoughts with compassion and without judgment; and 3) self-regulating (i.e., returning attention gently and effectively back to the first step (Cook-Cottone 2017). The student practices a mindful awareness of thoughts, emotions, and body sensations by going through the process of attention, noticing, and self-regulating.

In concentration meditation, students focus on an object (e.g., glitter in a meditation jar, an object on their desk, breath, the sensation of their feet on the floor in walking meditation, a scarf in mindful movement). In this form of meditation, they can also move through the three steps of attending, noticing, and self-regulating. It can be very helpful for students, especially young students and those new to meditation, to verbally guide them through this process. Often, new meditators need reminders that it is natural for them to think and for the mind to become distracted. Meditation is the practice of noticing this process and continuously bringing the mind back to mindfulness awareness with compassion and without judgment. It is believed that over time, students who practice meditation come to learn the habits of their own mind and can more easily self-regulate when needing to focus on school or work. For a variety of meditation scripts for students, see Cook-Cottone (2017).

Implementing Yoga in Schools

Yoga can be implemented in a variety of ways in schools, ranging from a more traditional yoga class to quick yoga breaks and games in the classroom. Some schools offer yoga after school for students, teachers, and parents. Many districts integrate yoga into their physical education, health and wellness, and/or social and emotional learning programs. Also, districts integrate yoga into their three-tier prevention and intervention programs for students in need of self-regulation skills (Cook-Cottone 2017).

Yoga Sessions and Breaks

Yoga sessions can be offered almost anywhere, including outside, in the gymnasium, or in a classroom. For guidance, ideally, about 12 square feet is needed for each 2×6 foot yoga mat. In terms of space needs, for 30 students, you will need 360 square feet (a 20×18 foot space in the middle of the room). The length of a yoga class can be anywhere from 30 minutes for younger children to an hour or more for adolescents (Cook-Cottone 2017).

A yoga session can be broken down into the following segments: setting up the room (5 minutes), quieting and calming exercises (e.g., seated breath work and guided meditation, 3–5 minutes), warm-up exercises (e.g., simple physical poses and movements, 8–10 minutes), challenging and vigorous poses (10–15 minutes), learning and trying time (e.g., introduction to new and challenging poses, 15–20 minutes), grounding and recentering time (e.g., practice of stable standing poses and gradual movement to floor-based stretches, 10–15 minutes), and relaxation and closing (e.g., meditation and relaxation, 5–10 minutes).

A yoga break is a 5- to 10-minute break to stretch or do a few poses or breathing exercises between academic tasks. A yoga break may allow students time to assimilate academic content delivered in class, build a positive mood state, and support physical health (Cook-Cottone 2017). Types of yoga breaks include 1) breathing breaks, 2) taking a few moments to coordinate breath with movement (e.g., raising and lowering arms, opening and closing arms, stretching side to side, or folding forward and standing up), and 3) active practice breaks that invigorate the students in order to increase active engagement (e.g., engaging in a short sequence of poses). There are also a variety of yoga games that can be delivered during yoga breaks. Many of these games integrate yoga poses and practices into traditional games (e.g., Red Light, Green Light is played with the traditional or familiar rules but adding a yoga pose when the students freeze).

Social and Emotional Learning and Trauma-Informed Yoga: Yogis in Service

Children who have experienced, or are currently experiencing, trauma (e.g., abuse, neglect, neighborhood violence, ongoing community stress) can manifest outcomes that substantially affect their learning, emotion regulation, attentional systems, and relationship behaviors. These include traumatic adaptations that may manifest as behavioral challenges within the school setting. With increasing awareness of the broad exposure to and impact of adverse childhood events (Felitti et al. 1998), school personnel often seek trauma-informed practices (Cook-Cottone 2017). School-based yoga can help students learn skills to self-regulate and bring themselves to calm (Butzer et al. 2016; Childress and Harper 2015; Cook-Cottone 2017; Cook-Cottone et al. 2017a).

The Yogis in Service trauma-informed yoga approach directly aligns the yoga interventions with the specific domain of trauma symptoms (Cook-Cottone et al. 2017a). First, it is critical for school personnel and yoga teachers to be trained on the symptoms and effects of trauma and how to refer students of concern for social and mental health support (Table 16–1) (Cook-Cottone 2017).

Specifically, the hyperarousal and reactivity and dissociation (i.e., disconnection from mental processes) symptoms are addressed through the physicality of the asana practice and cues for interoceptive awareness (i.e., awareness of internal body sensations). Avoidance of trauma-reminiscent stimuli and reexperiencing of trauma memories and feelings is addressed through yoga, relaxation, and meditation practices that promote engagement in the present moment. Posttrauma alterations in cognitions that leave individuals at risk for anxiety or depressive thinking patterns are addressed through the promotion of 12 empowering themes, or self-statements, that are aligned with yoga and trauma research (see Tables 16–1 and 16–2). Last, relational disconnection is addressed through the yoga teacher's presence and responsiveness to the physical and mental experiences of the students as they practice. The goal is two-pronged: First, yoga helps the students move from deregulation and reaction to self-regulation using the tools practiced in classes and sessions. Second, yoga helps teachers see student behaviors within the context of trauma exposure and a need to provide support and tools for self-regulation.

Developmental Adaptations

Yoga can be easily adapted for students of different ages and grade levels (Childress and Harper 2015; Cook-Cottone 2017). Overall, the length of the yoga session; use of props, concrete examples, and demonstrations; and need for routine vary by age. Younger children respond positively to using animal names for yoga poses; integrating story and literature; and using props, such as breathing buddies (e.g., bean bags with googly eyes) and scarves. Middle school students need structure, emotional support, and tools for emotion regulation. Middle and high school students are more sensitive to scheduling issues, such as yoga being offered at the same time as competitive sports. For this age group, scheduling is an important aspect of program implementing. Middle and high school students respond well to opportunities for leadership as they are asserting their autonomy and responding more to peer influence. Note that high school students

TABLE 16–1. Reactions to traumatic exposure and the Yogis in Service trauma-informed yoga approach

Symptoms related to trauma exposure	Elements
Hyperarousal and dissociation	Embodied practice (physicality and interceptive awareness)
Avoidance and reexperiencing	Engagement in the present moment (yoga and mindfulness practices)
Alterations in cognitions	Intentional, empowered thinking (12 cognitive intentions)
Relational disconnection	Yoga teacher presence and responsiveness (relational attunement)

Source. Adapted from Cook-Cottone et al. 2017a.

TABLE 16–2. Yogis in Service trauma-informed yoga 12 empowering themes

Theme	Self-statement
Part I: Inner resources	
Empowerment	I can.
Worth	I am worth the effort.
Part II: Physical basics	
Safety	I deserve to be safe.
Breath	My breath is my most powerful tool.
Presence	I work toward presence in my body.
Feeling	I feel so I can heal.
Part III: Self-regulation	
Grounding	My body is a source for connection, guidance, and coping.
Choice	I can find choice in the present moment.
Ownership	I can create the conditions for safety and growth.
Sustainability	I can create a balance between structure and change.

TABLE 16–2. Yogis in Service trauma-informed yoga 12 empowering themes *(continued)*

Theme	Self-statement
Part IV: Mindful grit	
Compassion	I honor the individual path of recovery and growth.
Self-determination	I work toward the possibility of effectiveness and growth in my own life.

Source.   Adapted from Cook-Cottone et al. 2017a.

can handle longer yoga sessions and generalize skills more easily into their lives, whereas younger children will need more in-the-moment guidance and reminders. See Table 16–3 and Cook-Cottone (2017) for more developmental guidance.

Secularity and Religion as They Relate to Yoga in Schools

Yoga instruction should follow several key grounding principles (Cook-Cottone 2017): 1) it should prioritize access and inclusion, 2) it should be aligned with legal imperatives and secular ethics and should not be religious, and 3) it should be research based. First, yoga instruction in school approaches should prioritize access and inclusion for all students (Cook-Cottone 2017; Cook-Cottone et al. 2017b). This is done by respecting diverse religious and nonreligious beliefs, maintaining separation of church and state in both principle and practice, and recognizing religious equality before the law (Cook-Cottone 2017; Cook-Cottone et al. 2017b). The yoga curriculum should be consistent with legal requirements of the First Amendment, which maintains religious neutrality in public schools and their associated activities (Cook-Cottone 2017; Cook-Cottone et al. 2017b). Second, yoga in school programs should take a secular approach. The approach in schools should not be religious or spiritual and should not comprise practices, symbols, or narratives from historically religious traditions (Cook-Cottone 2017; Cook-Cottone et al. 2017b). Integrating cultural artifacts that are often associated with traditional yoga (e.g., mandalas, chanting om, Sanskrit terms) can be risky because concerned parents may view these objects as reflecting religious values (Cook-Cottone 2017; Cook-Cottone et al. 2017b). See Cook-Cottone et al. (2017b) for a case study of a school district that was involved in a lawsuit positing that yoga is a religion and therefore should not be taught in schools. In 2013, the court system agreed

TABLE 16–3. Yoga practice by age group

Grade level	Yoga practice tips
Grades K–2	• Yoga sessions should be 15–45 minutes (the younger and less experienced the participants, the shorter the session). • Use clear and simple language. • Use guided relaxation and meditation more than silence. • Use props, such as breathing buddies or feathers (maximum of one prop per session). • Use themes and stories (link to language arts and literature). • Use animals, elements of nature, and shapes to describe poses. • Establish rituals and routines. • Be consistent and predictable. • Use repetition and predictability to establish a sense of safety. • Make it fun, safe, and warm. • Use play to support learning. • Engage all senses in fun activities, moving to stillness and inward focus. • Don't explain everything; let them experience it. • Take time to spell out rules and expectations for participation. • Remember that all behavior communicates a need; listen to how students behave and be responsive. • Help them see cause and effect. • Use music intentionally, allowing for quiet time for reflection. • Note that younger students can become overwhelmed or distracted by too much stimuli. • Offer options for students to close their eyes (e.g., choose a focus point).

TABLE 16–3. Yoga practice by age group (*continued*)

Grade level	Yoga practice tips
Grades 3–5	• Yoga sessions should be 20–40 minutes. • Integrate yoga games and songs. • Can spend more time in silent practices. • Can increase depth of breathing and relaxation exercises. • Use visualization techniques (e.g., images, stories) during relaxation exercises. • Use yoga journals. • Embodied games and practices are still important; engage through play. • Routine is still important. • Can begin to move toward a more typical, formal yoga class. • Increase focus on alignment in poses. • Consider introducing more challenging poses. • Introduce longer, flowing sequences. • Use partner work. • Allow students to learn through experience rather than telling them. • Give students opportunities to lead. • Give them the rational reason for learning a lesson. • Be mindful of placement of males behind females in class.

TABLE 16–3. Yoga practice by age group *(continued)*

Grade level	Yoga practice tips
Grades 6–8	• Yoga sessions should be 45–60 minutes.
	• Silent and reflective practice can extend to 20 minutes.
	• Encourage proper alignment in poses.
	• Model proper alignment and suggest adjustments.
	• Let students try poses together using photos and description of poses.
	• Integrate the Internet in the exploration of new poses and techniques.
	• Explain benefits of exercises and poses, bringing in science and health curriculum.
	• Teach lessons along with explanations of the benefits of the practice.
	• Connect yoga tools to developmental challenges (e.g., moodiness, achievement, social stress, emotional sensitivity).
	• Allow appropriate expression of emotions.
	• Keep a steady pace in sessions.
	• Use variety in poses, discussions, relaxation, and meditations.
	• Use sharing and partner work to allow time for peer support and bonding.
	• Teach how lessons can be integrated into lives outside school.
	• Emphasize emotional safety, creating a judgment-free space.
	• Do not allow negative body talk directed toward self or others.
	• Shift "I can't" statements to "I'll try" statements.
	• Use team work to deal with implementation challenges from rotating class schedules.
	• After-school yoga clubs, yoga-based interventions, and yoga should be integrated into wellness and physical education class to create accessibility.
	• Be mindful of placement of males behind females in class.
	• Offer time during and after class for clarifying questions and working through poses.

TABLE 16–3. Yoga practice by age group (*continued*)

Grade level	Yoga practice tips
Grades 9–12	• Yoga sessions should be 60–90 minutes.
	• Yoga sessions are more aligned with formal yoga class structure.
	• Model proper alignment and suggest adjustments.
	• Present new concepts and practice tools and allow for dialogue and reactions.
	• Use body-positive talk.
	• Emphasize emotional safety, creating a judgment-free space.
	• Foster a sense of belonging.
	• Be discerning when doing partner work.
	• Do not allow negative body talk directed toward self or others.
	• Shift "I can't" statements to "I'll try" statements.
	• Practices can be used before tests, athletic events, and other potential stressful experiences.
	• Encourage proper alignment in poses.
	• Consider integrating yoga teacher training programs into school curriculum.
	• Model proper alignment of yoga poses and suggest adjustments.
	• Use team work to deal with implementation challenges from rotating class schedules.
	• After-school mindfulness clubs, yoga-based interventions, and yoga integrated into wellness and physical education class create accessibility.
	• Journals can be useful tools of self-reflection and growth.
	• Integrate sharing and partner work.

TABLE 16–3. Yoga practice by age group (*continued*)

Grade level	Yoga practice tips
Grades 9–12 (*continued*)	• Support self-determination. • Be mindful of placement of males behind females in class. • Offer time during and after class for clarifying questions and working through poses. • Integrate the principles of embodied growth and learning. • Teach how lessons can be integrated into lives outside school. • Encourage a self-directed practice.

Source. Reprinted and adapted from Cook-Cottone 2017. Used with permission.

with the school district, ruling that the practice of yoga in schools neither endorses nor inhibits any religion (Cook-Cottone et al. 2017b). There was an appeal, and in 2015, the California Court of Appeals upheld the lower court's ruling that the school district's program was constitutional. Secular yoga for schools should be informed by research into the legality of such programs in the school district (Cook-Cottone et al. 2017b).

Safe, Inclusive, and Accessible Programs

In alignment with traditional school values, it is important for school-based yoga teachers to emphasize safety, inclusion, and accessibility (Childress and Harper 2015; Cook-Cottone 2017). In order to emphasize safety, select basic poses and focus on self-regulation above working toward advanced poses (Cook-Cottone 2017). Yoga teachers should be very attentive when students are attempting poses. Offering students choice when it comes to poses and variations is a trauma-informed best practice. Accordingly, teachers should remind students that if something does not feel right, they should not continue doing it. The teacher can offer students options for each pose that may feel safer or more grounded.

The pace of the class contributes to safety and quality. The pace should allow for time to carefully build and practice poses, practice breath work, and engage in meditations and activities. Teachers who focus on quantity over quality often lead a rushed class, missing the point of mind and body integration and connection with the present (Cook-Cottone 2017). For more on best practices for yoga in schools, see Childress and Harper (2015).

Inclusion and access are critical. Consultation with school physical therapists, occupational therapists, special education teachers, and school mental health professionals (i.e., school psychologist, school counselor, and school social workers) can help the individuals teaching yoga in schools create an inclusive yoga class through the development of lesson plans with appropriate accommodations and supports (Cook-Cottone 2017). Lois Goldberg (2013) wrote a wonderful book titled *Yoga for Children With Autism and Special Needs* that serves as a how-to manual for yoga for kids in classrooms and therapeutic settings. Culturally responsive practices are also a critical aspect of inclusion (see Grant and Ray 2018). Chapter 10, "Immigrant Youth," includes more information on cultural adaptation.

Research Support

Research on yoga in schools reveals an array of interventions using various forms, aspects, and dosages of yoga and a few manualized yoga interventions

(Cook-Cottone 2017; Serwacki and Cook-Cottone 2012). Until recently, there were too few studies to validly compare outcomes across studies or to meaningfully aggregate outcomes using systematic reviews or meta-analyses (Cook-Cottone 2017). To date, there have been three major reviews of the research on yoga in schools: Serwacki and Cook-Cottone (2012), Ferreira-Vorkapic et al. (2015), and Khalsa and Butzer (2016) (see Table 16–4).

In 2012, Serwacki and Cook-Cottone identified 12 published studies of yoga in schools (see Table 16–4). Samples for which yoga was implemented as an intervention included youth with autism, intellectual disability, learning disability, and emotional disturbance, as well as typically developing youth (Serwacki and Cook-Cottone 2012). For children with special needs, effects of participating in school-based yoga programs appeared to be beneficial in reducing stress, improving cognitive functioning, increasing self-confidence and social confidence, improving communication and contribution to the classroom, and improving attention and concentration (Serwacki and Cook-Cottone 2012). For typically developing students, participation was associated with decreased body dissatisfaction, anxiety, negative behaviors, cognitive disturbances, impulsivity, and emotional and physical arousal, as well as increased perceived self-concept and emotional balance (Serwacki and Cook-Cottone 2012). The methodological limitations included lack of randomization, small samples, limited detail regarding the intervention, and statistical ambiguities, which curtailed the ability to provide definitive conclusions or recommendations. These findings speak to the need for greater methodological rigor and an increased understanding of the mechanisms of success for school-based yoga interventions (Cook-Cottone 2017; Serwacki and Cook-Cottone 2012).

In 2015, using strict selection criteria emphasizing controlled trials and not including research on students with special needs, Ferreira-Vorkapic and colleagues conducted a meta-analysis based on 9 studies, with 7 studies depicted in a plot of general effect size (Ferreira-Vorkapic et al. 2015). The types of yoga used included Vinayasa, Ashtanga, Yoga Ed, Kripalu yoga, Niroga, Mindful Girls Yoga, and Hatha yoga. The dosages of yoga ranged from 15 to 90 minutes one to five times a week for 10–18 weeks. Five of the studies used an active control group (physical education or physical activity), and the other studies used a waitlist or no intervention (Ferreira-Vorkapic et al. 2015). The general plot of the outcomes indicated divided results, with half of the studies favoring yoga and the other half favoring controls. In aggregate, the overall effect for yoga was not found to be significant because of the heterogeneity of the variables (see Table 16–4).

In 2016, Butzer and Khalsa published their review of 47 studies, with a total sample size of 4,522 participants. Their review included research in 19 elementary and preschools, 6 middle schools, 7 middle and high schools, and 13 high

TABLE 16–4. Comprehensive research reviews of yoga in schools

Study	Scope and method	Outcomes
Serwacki and Cook-Cottone 2013	The authors reviewed and evaluated 12 published studies using Sackett's level-of-evidence strategy.	There were generally positive outcomes for typical youth and youth with special needs. Low scientific quality was found across studies. Increased methodological rigor is needed.
Ferreira-Vorkapic et al. 2015	The authors identified 48 published studies that included a yoga-based intervention and reviewed 9 studies with control groups restricted to school settings. Studies of yoga-based programs for children with learning disabilities or any diagnosed mental disorder were excluded. The authors reviewed literature, conducted a meta-analysis, and depicted 7 of the 9 studies in an effect size plot.	There were mixed results, with some studies favoring yoga and others favoring controls. Effects calculated for each outcome suggested that results favored yoga for mood indicators, tension and anxiety, self-esteem, and memory. The overall effect for yoga was found not to be significant, likely because of the heterogeneity of the variables and the low number of studies used in the analysis. More high-quality studies are needed.
Khalsa and Butzer 2016	The authors performed a systematic review of 47 studies that explicitly incorporated yoga-based postures and/or breathing exercises. They excluded studies of students with special educational needs or disabilities or emotional, behavioral, or learning difficulties.	There has been a rapid increase in the amount of research on yoga in schools. Studies have numerous design limitations. There is a high degree of variability in yoga intervention characteristics. Overall, yoga in the school setting is a viable and potentially effective strategy for increasing student health and well-being.

schools. The sample sizes ranged from 20 to 660 participants. The review included 25 randomized controlled trials, 7 nonrandomized controlled trials, 9 uncontrolled trials, and 4 qualitative studies (Khalsa and Butzer 2016). The studies were conducted primarily in the United States ($n=30$) and India ($n=15$). Most of the studies (85%) were conducted within the school curriculum. Further, most (62%) were implemented as formal school-based yoga programs (Khalsa and Butzer 2016).

Specific positive student self-report outcomes noted by Khalsa and Butzer (2016) included improved mood state, self-esteem, self-control, self-regulation, and emotion regulation; increased feelings of happiness, relaxation, and social and physical well-being; and decreased aggression, social problems, rumination, emotional arousal, intrusive thoughts, and alcohol use. Teacher-rated outcomes included improved classroom behaviors, emotion regulation skills, independence, attention skills, transition skills, self-regulation, concentration, mood, ability to function under pressure, attention, adaptive skills, and social skills. Teacher ratings also indicated reductions in performance impairments, hyperactivity, behavioral symptoms, internalizing symptoms, and maladaptive behaviors (Khalsa and Butzer 2016). Objective data collected from school records and academic tests showed positive intervention improvements in student grades and academic performance (Khalsa and Butzer 2016). Finally, physiological and cognitive outcome measures showed decreased cortisol concentrations as well as improved breathing patterns, micronutrient absorption, strength, flexibility, heart rate variability, and stress reactivity as indicated by skin conductance response (Khalsa and Butzer 2016). Khalsa and Butzer (2016) observed that many positive outcomes were trends ($P<0.1$) rather than statistically significant ($P<0.05$). Ultimately, the authors concluded that yoga in the school setting is a viable and potentially efficacious strategy for improving child and adolescent health and therefore is worthy of continued research. They also emphasized the importance of and need for more high-quality research (Khalsa and Butzer 2016)

There are many research questions yet to be answered (Cook-Cottone 2017). For example, researchers have yet to explore the effects of various types of yoga; the ideal dosage; and the effects of engagement in other mind and body practices such as tae kwon do, previous yoga practice, or home practice. Further, the field has yet to identify a best practices active control group methodology; physical education class and waitlist control have been found to be problematic (Cook-Cottone 2017). To date, no study has explored the ideal qualification of a yoga teacher for schools (e.g., school personnel trained as yoga teachers vs. yoga teachers trained to teach in schools). Many studies do not use a manual, do not detail the yoga program used in the study, and do not report treatment fidelity or assess the effects of attendance and student engagement (Cook-Cottone 2017).

Many of the researched programs do not describe inclusion of at-risk youth, diverse populations, or adaptations for students with special needs.

Conclusion and Future Directions

Overall, yoga is an easy-to-implement, affordable, and likely effective tool for helping students connect to and engage in the present moment. Yoga in schools is a secular practice that includes yoga postures, breathing exercises, relaxation techniques, and meditation. Its key mechanisms are believed to be increased mind and body awareness, self-regulation, and physical fitness. Yoga, vis-à-vis these mechanisms, appears to help students with mood and well-being and leads to decreased risk for psychological disorders, improved behavior, enhanced academic performance, better management of stress and trauma, improved relationships, and increased quality of life. Yoga is suitable for trauma-informed schools and can be easily adapted for students with special needs and for children across developmental levels. Yoga research has been rapidly increasing, with promising results across age levels. There are now ample resources and training to help you learn effective ways to bring yoga to your school. There is a need for continued increase in the quality of research conducted in schools and for schools to enthusiastically and effectively engage with researchers.

KEY POINTS

- School-based yoga teachers should receive highly skilled training and ongoing continuing education and should pursue a regular personal practice.

- In the delivery of yoga in schools, schools should adopt or create a secular and inclusive style of yoga that is easily adapted for students with special needs and across all developmental levels.

- Yoga promotes self-regulation of physiological, emotional, and cognitive systems and therefore is an ideal fit for a trauma-informed school approach.

- High-quality studies can be conducted only if researchers and school personnel forge a positive, collaborative approach in designing and implementing research, such as randomized controlled trials.

Discussion Questions

1. What do you think is meant by the statement "Teachers cannot give what they do not embody, and embodiment requires practice"? How might a teacher's personal practice, or lack of practice, affect how he or she delivers a yoga program in school?

2. What differences do you notice in how yoga is taught across age groups? How is this similar to developmental considerations in the delivery of academic content? How is it different? What additional considerations are there when delivering yoga?

3. What is the importance of a secular approach to yoga in the schools? What is the relationship between inclusion and keeping yoga secular? Who might feel excluded if the yoga is not delivered in a secular manner? Describe why.

4. How can yoga help meet the demand for trauma-informed practices? What aspects of yoga are a good fit? What aspects of yoga might be problematic and require a nuanced approach?

Suggested Readings

Butzer B, Flynn L: Research Repository: Yoga and Meditation for Children and Adolescents. Dover, NH, Yoga 7 Classrooms, 2018. Available at: www.yoga4classrooms.com/supporting-research. Accessed August 22, 2018. Keep up on the research with this free organized reference list of peer-reviewed published studies and research review articles. This resource provides links to abstracts and full-text publications when available and is updated quarterly.

Cook-Cottone CP: Mindfulness and Yoga in Schools: A Guide for Teachers and Practitioners. New York, Springer, 2017. This text is a comprehensive guide to implementing a yoga program in schools.

Childress T, Harper JC: Best Practices for Yoga in the Schools. Best Practices Guide, Vol 1. Atlanta, GA, YEC-Omega Publications, 2015. This is an easy-to-read guide to the best practices in implementing yoga in schools.

Kripalu Center for Yoga & Health, www.kriplau.org. Attend the Yoga in the Schools Symposium offered at Kripalu.

References

Bryant EF: The Yoga Sutras of Patanjali: New Edition, Translation, and Commentary. New York, North Point Press, 2015

Butzer B, Ebert M, Telles S, et al: School-based yoga programs in the United States: a survey. Adv Mind Body Med 29(4):18–26, 2015 26535474

Butzer B, Bury D, Telles S, et al: Implementing yoga within the school curriculum: a scientific rationale for improving social-emotional learning and positive student outcomes. J Child Serv 11(1):3–24, 2016

Childress T, Harper JC: Best Practices for Yoga in the Schools. Best Practices Guide, Vol 1. Atlanta, GA, YEC-Omega Publications, 2015

Cook-Cottone C: Childhood posttraumatic stress disorder: diagnosis, treatment, and school reintegration. School Psych Rev 33(1):127, 2004

Cook-Cottone C: Dosage as a critical variable in yoga therapy research. Int J Yoga Therap 23(23):11–12, 2013 24165519

Cook-Cottone CP: Mindfulness and Yoga in Schools: A Guide for Teachers and Practitioners. New York, Springer, 2017

Cook-Cottone CP, LaVigne M, Travers L, et al: Trauma-informed yoga: an embodied, cognitive-relational framework. Int J Complement Altern Med 9(1):00284, 2017a

Cook-Cottone CP, Lemish E, Guyker W: Interpretative phenomenological analysis of a lawsuit contending that school-based yoga is religion: a student of school personnel. Int J Yoga Therap 27(1):25–35, 2017b

Cook-Cottone CP, Talebkhah K, Guyker W, et al: A controlled trial of a yoga-based prevention program targeting eating disorder risk factors among middle school females. Eating Disorders 25(5):392–405, 2017c

Felitti VJ, Anda RF, Nordenberg D, et al: Relationship of childhood abuse and household dysfunction to many of the leading causes of death in adults: the Adverse Childhood Experiences (ACE) Study. Am J Prev Med 14(4):245–258, 1998 9635069

Ferreira-Vorkapic C, Feitoza JM, Marchioro M, et al: Are there benefits from teaching yoga at schools? A systematic review of randomized control trials of yoga-based interventions. Evid Based Complement Alternat Med 2015:345845, 2015 26491461

Frank JL, Kohler K, Peal A, et al: Effectiveness of a school-based yoga program on adolescent mental health and school performance: findings from a randomized controlled trial. Mindfulness 8:544–553, 2017

Goldberg L: Yoga Therapy for Children With Autism and Special Needs. New York, WW Norton, 2013

Grant KB, Ray JA (eds): Home, School, and Community Collaboration: Culturally Responsive Family Engagement. Thousand Oaks, CA, SAGE, 2018

Khalsa SBS, Butzer B: Yoga in school settings: a research review. Ann N Y Acad Sci 1373(1):45–55, 2016 26919395

Serwacki ML, Cook-Cottone C: Yoga in the schools: a systematic review of the literature. Int J Yoga Therap 22(22):101–109, 2012 23070680

Chapter 17

Mindfulness and Technology

Tara Cousineau, Ph.D.
Bridget Kiley, M.Sc.
Zev Schuman-Olivier, M.D.

The App Generation

Digital Natives and Digital Immigrants

Today's modern youth are raised squarely in digital playgrounds. One might say that youth born in twenty-first-century industrial countries are figuratively tethered to technology. From ages 0 to 20, young people are exposed to, and engaged with, a variety of digital technologies. They have not known life without them. Popularly referred to as *digital natives* (Prensky 2012), this savvy population born into an unprecedented era of tech gadgetry can be captured by a panoply of descriptive terms: App Generation, Google Generation, iGen, Net Gen, and Y Gen, among others. Social media scholar danah boyd [sic] describes contemporary youth as living *networked lives* in which the physical and digital spaces are entangled. On the basis of her field research with youth across the United States, boyd frames the digital behavior of young people from their perspective: as mundane daily practices that repurpose technology to fulfill their desires, goals, and emerging identities (boyd 2014). If there is any word to describe the engagement of youth with digital technology it would be *variety*. Teens especially are adept at consuming a diverse menu of digital media simultaneously and often passively, such as listening to music, playing games, surfing social media, or texting, while also doing homework or chores or socializing. Increasingly, digital gadgets serve as a young person's preferred medium with which to "chill" and relax in an overscheduled and demanding daily routine. Smartphones serve much like contemporary transitional objects of desire and safety, and many young people claim they could not live without them.

In contrast, the adults raising these youth have been referred to as *digital immigrants*, reflecting their later arrival to technology and more functional needs (e.g., managing work, staying in touch with family, GPS navigation). However, the gap is rapidly narrowing as families, educators, and health providers become more deeply engaged with digital tools, mobile devices, and social media. Educator Marc Prensky, who originally coined the terms digital natives and digital immigrants, notes that such a generational distinction is increasingly irrelevant. He posits that we imagine instead a concept of *digital wisdom* that refers "both to wisdom arising from the use of digital technology to access cognitive power beyond our usual capacity and the wisdom in the use of technology to enhance our innate capabilities" (Prensky 2012, p. 202). We find a conceptual framework of digital wisdom apt for a discussion about how the interaction of technology and mindfulness might inform youth's daily practices in contemporary ways.

With more than 18 million practitioners of meditation in the United States, it is no surprise that a multitude of digital mindfulness applications have sprung up for consumption, ranging from tools intended to augment attention and focusing skills, provide biofeedback, offer guided audio recordings for relaxation, and build virtual communities and meditation centers. There is growing evidence that mindfulness-based interventions (MBIs) for youth are beneficial in clinical and nonclinical samples (see Chapter 3, "State of the Research on Youth Mindfulness"), and it is natural to infer that other modes of delivery for MBIs would also be promising. Digitally supported mindfulness programs are increasingly the subject of health promotion interventions among adults (Fish et al. 2016; Plaza et al. 2013), although the potential benefits for youth are yet to be determined. We approach this nascent field of mindfulness applications for youth, primarily adolescents and emerging adults, with excitement and caution because our digital wisdom is just emerging.

Downsides of Technology and Opportunities for Mindfulness

Youth and their families are more "connected" than ever. On average, 90% of U.S. households have three or more Internet-connected devices such as smartphone, desktop or laptop computer, and tablet or streaming media device, with the median American household containing five of them (Pew Research Center 2017). Further, mobile phone use has neared saturation levels; more than 95% of Americans own a cell phone, and smartphone owners have increased from 35% of Americans in 2011 to 77% in 2017. Even though disparity gaps remain, the use of mobile devices for communicating and to access the Internet is ubiquitous.

It is now almost cliché to see images of families eating out for dinner or vacationing on a beach, each member glued to his or her technology gadget of choice. The educational nonprofit group Common Sense Media regularly surveys the media habits of children and families across age groups (e.g., ages 0–8, tweens, teens, and parents). Even 5 years ago, 72% of children ages 8 and younger accessed some kind of mobile device daily, and almost 40% of children younger than age 2 years used a mobile device for media (Common Sense Media 2018). These rates are likely increasing. Unsurprisingly, teenagers drive mobile media usage. A high-school senior spends an average of 6 hours daily with new media during leisure time, excluding time spent at school or for homework (Common Sense Media 2015; Twenge 2017a). Their younger cohort of tweens is close behind: the average eighth grader spends about 5 hours daily on a mobile device. Although this may seem physically impossible given time spent in school, doing sports, and sleeping, today's youth are fervently multitasking with media, listening to music, playing video games, texting, or group chatting. Additionally, virtually all public spaces in which youth interact are now networked because teachers and educational settings, just like health providers and medical practices, have adopted digitally enhanced learning tools, and most public institutions have adopted technology as essential for work flow and communication.

The immersion in information technology and new media also has downsides, potentially contributing to a more distracted, less connected, less empathic, and even potentially harmful social milieu. Social scientists are noting trends worthy of caution: parallel increases in consumption of multimedia and mobile ownership and increasing rates of unhappiness for teens who spend more time than average on screen activities. For instance, psychologist Jean Twenge, who studies cultural trends, cautions that the presence of technology in teens' lives has caused some dramatic shifts, including that "12th-graders in 2015 are going out less often than *eighth-graders* did as recently as 2009" (Twenge 2017a, p. 19) and that "the number of teens who get together with their friends nearly every day has been cut in half in just fifteen years" (Twenge 2017a, p. 71). Twenge has asserted in a controversial *Atlantic* article (Twenge 2017b) that today's youth are more vulnerable than their millennial predecessors: "Rates of teen depression and suicide have skyrocketed since 2011. It's not an exaggeration to describe iGen as being on the brink of the worst mental-health crisis in decades. Much of this deterioration can be traced to their phones." Although this statement is potentially alarmist, the trends highlight a need for mindful consumption and restraint. On the other hand, there are many positive associations with innovative technologies, such as augmenting human cognitive capabilities, igniting movements for social change, and deepening social ties (boyd 2014; Thompson 2014). Thus, there is a sensible call for finding a middle way or maintaining a balanced media diet.

Naturally, youth are shaped by their environments, as are their brains, which poses the serious question of just how are youth navigating their identity and well-being amid rapid digital innovations? At the same time, the potential for technology-enhanced approaches to mindfulness and mind-body skills also poses the potential for creative and scalable means for positive skill building, including biofeedback, calming and emotion regulation skills, and practices in mindfulness and self-compassion. Digital mindfulness tools may be an acceptable approach for youth in educating, or punctuating, their daily lives with health-promoting opportunities. Moreover, these tools may offer health providers a nonpharmacological option for stress management. It may seem ironic that apps may be an ideal mode for young people to build mastery for practice, not to mention potentially offsetting a typical complaint among youth that mindfulness is boring. At the least, a mindfulness app may insert a "sacred pause" in the course of a busy and networked life.

Mindful Technology for Youth: Baby Steps

Increasingly, the therapeutic frameworks for empirically derived Web or mobile interventions are inspired by the very off-line MBIs shown to improve well-being, such as mindfulness-based stress reduction and mindfulness-based cognitive therapy. These emergent digital MBI approaches focus largely on the delivery, via audio, video, or animation, of the essential components of mindfulness, such as awareness of bodily sensations, breath focus, observance and acceptance of thoughts and feelings, and lovingkindness meditation. Technology adaptations also offer a variety of features, such as daily tips or reminders via text messages or push notifications and self-report tracking of progress or mood states.

A literature review of self-directed technology-based mindfulness interventions identified 10 studies for analysis, primarily targeting university students and adult populations experiencing a variety of conditions, including anxiety, depression, cancer, or chronic pain, from which we can extrapolate the potential of mindfulness interventions for youth (Fish et al. 2016). Overall, the digital interventions ranged from 2 to 12 weeks and showed some benefits, including reports from participants of an overall benefit; symptom reduction for stress, anxiety, and depressive symptoms; and reduced rumination. As well, it was demonstrated that the technology helped support sustained practice after the intervention through reminder e-mails and digital tracking of practice. This is encouraging because sustaining practice and mental training fosters the development of new habits and builds confidence.

Evidence-based interventions are in the early stages, but the marketplace for technology-based mindfulness is outpacing scientific evaluation. Consumer apps are largely geared toward adults, and mindfulness digital platforms are increasingly offered as an employee benefit in workplaces, although a number of children's games and tools are available for pediatric audiences (Culbert 2017). As of this writing, there are more than 1,300 mindfulness-based mobile applications (MB-MAs). It is likely that self-selected youth who are interested in mindfulness will download apps intended for adults or use their parents' devices to access them. As such, it helps to understand the quality of MBMAs as they become mainstream and may increasingly be incorporated into school programs or medical settings.

Two published reviews not only indicated the growing popularity of MBMAs but evaluated their features and usability (Mani et al. 2015; Plaza et al. 2013). In general, these reviews found that the available functionalities were limited and there was no clear, cohesive meaning or description of mindfulness. One analysis found that about half (56%–61%) of the apps were devoted to meditation, which is a core practice for engaging in mindfulness. Some offered reminders or tracking (e.g., 37% offered daily, weekly, or monthly personal statistics), and 28% provided access to social networks. Relatively few apps offered basic psychoeducation: 13% included mindfulness training, 11% offered assessments, and 9% demonstrated attention focus skills (Plaza et al. 2013). Further, only 13.9% of the MBMAs included audio tracks, a primary mode of sharing guided meditations. Roughly 20% of the apps were found to be difficult to use because of background color or lack of exit buttons. None of the apps was specifically geared to health professionals as a potential resource, and the product descriptions did not indicate or report on evaluations of biological or psychological health outcomes.

In another review, Mani et al. (2015) used the Mobile Application Rating Scale (MARS) and found that only 23 apps (roughly 4% of 606 identified apps) met their criteria for inclusion as mindfulness training, that is, the mobile application included *both* educational instruction in the practice of mindfulness (the what, why, and how-to) and guided meditations, music, and audio relaxations. Of these apps, virtually all offered mindful breathing and body scan exercises, and many offered such features as timers or reminders. Included in the overall review were app titles that typically can be found in online recommendation lists for teenagers, such as Headspace, Smiling Mind, Buddhify, Stop Breathe and Think, and Take a Chill. Although many apps scored in the acceptable range for engagement, functionality, aesthetics, information quality, and user satisfaction, few apps scored high. Only one product, Headspace, was subject to a preliminary test of efficacy, and it showed improvement in positive affect and reduced depressive symptoms in a relatively small sample over 10 days.

In other words, there is a paucity of evidence regarding the benefits of commercially available mindfulness apps for well-being. In the literature, cohesive descriptions of mindfulness training and content related to mindfulness, indications of proof-of-concept evaluations, rigorous assessments, and randomized clinical reviews were lacking. On the whole, there is limited to little research evaluating the efficacy of MBMAs, suggesting a buyer-beware approach even if the apps appear to "do no harm."

It may be wise for professionals trained in mindfulness to evaluate and curate the available options. In other words, it's best for educators, clinicians, and parents to be familiar with mindfulness apps and evaluate any potential negative effects before suggesting their use for youth in their charge. Digital wisdom would also suggest that we adopt an adventurous attitude in meeting youth where they are currently engaged and be open to learning from their expertise, creativity, and experiences in how MBMAs could support their preferences and needs.

Bridging Mindfulness Training in the Real World With Digital Means

Over the past two millennia, mindfulness practices have been adapted to be integrated into the cultural context of each time period and culture. The concept of *skillful means* has developed to describe nontraditional, counterintuitive, or unexpected ways in which people can act that turn out to be the most appropriate and wise action for a given situation. As such, seemingly unconventional methods (such as technology-based tools) may be the most sensible way to teach mindfulness. These methods may offer a way to skillfully help meet people where they are. Consider a person who may be reluctant to engage in a traditional, time-intensive mindfulness learning process. When technology is used as a digital form of skillful means, it may offer novel approaches (e.g., apps, games) or engage familiar modes of communication (e.g., text reminders, push notifications) that provide a nontraditional, but very wise, way to raise awareness and enhance engagement in new and unfamiliar skills.

For tweens and teens in particular, MBMAs may serve as a form of skillful means for introducing and practicing mindfulness and compassion. Given that mobile devices are teens' primary communication tool, smartphones (and other Internet-enabled mobile devices) have the potential to serve as an ideal portal for health communication with the least resistance. Further, according to Twenge (2017a), the introduction of smartphones has virtually closed the Internet access gap by social class, which potentiates the reach and impact of digital health promotion initiatives and interventions. In the spirit of digital wisdom, we believe mindfulness-based technology tools have the potential to be digital means for engaging today's youth.

Although research on the efficacy of technology-based mindfulness engagement is limited, the encouraging results from MBIs (see Chapter 3) in traditional youth settings may inform developmentally appropriate digital MBI programs. A recent meta-analysis (Parsons et al. 2017) demonstrated that the frequency of home practice of mindfulness is associated with the beneficial effects of MBIs, yet most studies do not adequately assess the length of time participants spend practicing mindfulness skills over the course of an intervention or follow-up period. This is due in part to a wide variation in quality of MBI research designs, which frequently lack control groups with adequate dose-matched training requirements (e.g., 45 minutes of daily physical exercise or reading). These studies also are limited by self-report and recall bias, as well as the very practical challenge of tracking duration of mindfulness practice (formal and informal) to arrive at a measure of intervention dosage (i.e., total minutes of mindfulness practice).

Nevertheless, the data supporting the importance of practice suggest the possibility that mobile devices, with their capability for repeated engagement, gamification, tracking, and reminders, could have an impact on supporting sustained practice of mindfulness taught in face-to-face to encounters, groups, and digital tutorials. Although this is highly speculative, it is generally understood that the more time people spend practicing mindfulness skills, the better the positive outcomes, and digital heath apps may serve as a potentiator. Further research is needed to know if mobile device–assisted practice and remotely generated reminders have a beneficial impact by enhancing practice dose or, paradoxically, whether they actually hinder the development of the full complement of self-regulative functions (e.g., internalized motivation, mindfulness self-efficacy, remembering to attend to the moment) because of an overreliance on technology for practice and reminders.

Potential Benefits of Emerging Applied Technologies for Youth

In spite of the current paucity of evidence-based mindfulness apps, lessons learned from other areas of digital health prevention or intervention programs for youth with a larger evidence base may be a helpful corollary.

Mobile Technology in Adolescent Health Promotion and Prevention

Young people find health apps useful, at least when they are asked to try them. Systematic and meta-analytic reviews of text messaging interventions for the promotion of healthy lifestyle and behavior change among adolescents and young adults show that interventions using mobile phones are effective, in cost and usability, and should be further developed to support positive health outcomes and prevention of risky behavior (Badawy and Kuhns 2017; Mason et al. 2015; Militello et al. 2012). Areas studied in these reviews cover a vast array of important adolescent health issues, including oral contraceptive use, human papillomavirus vaccinations, tobacco and alcohol prevention and cessation, sun protection, and sexual health. In general, text messaging was used as a tool for education, positive reinforcement or personalized feedback, and goal setting, and some mobile programs offered incentives or gamified reward systems.

Apps for Youth With Chronic Physical Conditions

A systematic review of literature published on mobile- and tablet-based apps for teens with chronic illnesses or long-term conditions found 4 eligible studies (pretest and posttest evaluation and one randomized controlled trial) out of 19 that evaluated apps supporting young people (10–24 years) with asthma, cancer, and type 1 diabetes (Majeed-Ariss et al. 2015). The review looked at apps that could be considered as a self-management intervention for five core skills for physical health conditions: problem solving, decision making, resource utilization, forming patient–health professional relationships, and taking action. These technologies were aimed at helping adolescents with self-management of the conditions, such as blood glucose monitoring, improved asthma management and self-efficacy, and improving the chemotherapy and recovery experience. As proof-of-concept studies, the samples were small, ranging from 4 to 18 participants, with a combined sample of 46 teenage participants, and therefore were not generalizable. Even so, these feasibility studies highlighted important findings, such as the need for participatory design (i.e., gathering expertise from health professionals and enlisting adolescents as co-creators in designing or adapting apps in developmentally meaningful ways), especially if the shared goal is to promote adherence and engagement, knowledge and skills, and support as teens transition to adult-centered care.

Evidence for Mobile-Based Mindfulness Technologies for Youth

Overall, among the emergent field of mobile apps in mindfulness, the few studies with adolescents do suggest feasibility and potential benefits for well-being, and adverse effects have not been reported. For instance, Turner and Hingle (2017) recently evaluated an MBMA developed for helping adolescents ages 14–18 become more aware of weight-related behaviors by focusing attention on breath, using guided practice for mindful eating and physical movement, and watching videos that encourage self-observation skill-building and increasing awareness of hunger and satiety cues. The pilot study found that the app, called b@Ease Mindfulness, was highly acceptable and useful, with participants reporting increased time spent in mindfulness states, such as mindful eating, as well as high adherence to physical activity from the first week to the third week. Overall, the app was found to support weight-related behaviors as a health-based performance program supporting improved eating behaviors and physical activity practices and aided in sleep for overall improved well-being. The research team concluded that future enhancements might include increased practice for sustained mindfulness states, enhanced video streaming and tracking of video use, and bigger sample sizes to improve development of the app and reporting of outcomes.

A larger, randomized controlled study with college students and young adults used an Internet-based mindfulness and cognitive-behavioral therapy (CBT) training program that incorporated telephone support (Mak et al. 2017). This study compared an 8-week Web-based mindfulness training program called iMIND ($N=604$) with a cognitive-behavioral training program called iCBT ($N=651$). The results were promising and showed positive results for both programs in improving mental and physical health measures, including psychological distress, life satisfaction, sleep disturbance, and pain and energy levels, which were sustained at the 3-month follow-up. However, the attrition or dropout rates were high, suggesting room for improvement in sustaining interest and engagement.

Even less is known about the potential for MBMAs to support self-compassion training. One randomized controlled study of a mobile app called BodiMojo with 273 adolescents (age range 14–19 years) compared the app group with a waitlist control (Rodgers et al. 2017). The 6-week program included guided relaxation and mindfulness audios, mood tracking and supportive feedback messages, self-assessments, a daily behavioral tip, and push notification reminders. In addition, the teens were asked to record their mood in the app once a day and to keep a daily gratitude journal. At baseline and posttest, participants completed measures of body esteem, social comparison, and self-compassion. Compared with the control group, the teens in the app group showed increases in body esteem and self-compassion. Therefore, MBMAs grounded in self-compassion theory may have the potential to promote positive body image and overall well-being by targeting the negative self-evaluations that are common in this age group.

This fledgling research suggests that positive behavior change among adolescents through mobile-based interventions is feasible and must continue to be developed using high-quality study designs with larger samples sizes, as well as input from adolescents, parents, and health professionals.

Mindful Education and Parenting

There are an emerging evidence base for and interest in fostering prosocial behaviors and skills among youth. As mindfulness becomes more widespread among adults with children and trickles down to early education, one wonders if apps might be useful for addressing the growing demand. Educators, media outlets, and software designers are incorporating new digital methods that support social and emotional learning (SEL), character building, and mindfulness.

Young Children

With teenagers and emerging adults driving mobile usage, the majority of MBMAs target this age group for obvious reasons. As families and schools become more immersed in technology and multimedia, however, younger children are being increasing exposed to technology tools. As Common Sense Media reported, children as young as age 2 are using media devices for interactive storytelling, games, and video (Common Sense Media 2018). The World Economic Forum (2016) released a report that highlights *noncognitive competencies* as key areas for growth. In a similar vein, the nonprofit Collaborative for Academic, Social, and Emotional Learning (htpps://CASEL.org), includes five core competencies for effective SEL models, in two of which mindfulness practices squarely align: self-management and self-awareness (the other core areas are responsible decision making, relationship skills, and social awareness). In the context of early childhood, it makes sense to consider MBIs as a subtype of socioemotional learning interventions.

Younger children from prekindergarten to grade 8 can benefit from technology tools used in intentional ways under the guidance of caregivers or educators (Culbert 2017). Given that digital health tools for youth are just emerging, empirical studies with younger children tend to include not mobile devices per se but rather classroom use of audio recordings or social and emotional learning games and cartoons viewed on computers or tablets. Animations and digital games that teach emotional regulation, breathing, and kindness are increasingly available. Most are inspired by the emerging social and neuroscience evidence regarding the benefits of mindfulness and SEL and draw on expert advice, but very few are rigorously evaluated for efficacy.

For example, *Sesame Street* considers social and emotional learning core to its programming and offers an app called Breathe, Think, Do with Sesame that engages children ages 4 and older to help the characters breathe and to select coping strategies in various stressful situations. The educational nonprofit Committee for Children and the creator of the Second Step social and emotional learning series offer a tablet game for 7- to 9-year-olds called ParkPals: Kindness Rules, which engages children in a virtual playground and gives them the responsibility to make the right choices while teaching four qualities of kindness: fair play, responsibility, safety, and respect. The organization also released an app for children ages 5–12, parents, and teachers called Mind Yeti. This app encourages mindfulness skills and supports guided audio practices in calming down, falling asleep, focusing, and various prosocial behaviors, including gratitude and kindness. Such technology-based programs offered in safe spaces can augment SEL curricula and introduce essential elements of mindfulness, such as breathing awareness, naming of emotions, perspective taking, and kind behavior.

Evidence for multimedia components in early school learning environments is emerging. For instance, one controlled study assessed the effects of a daily audio-guided mindfulness intervention for elementary school students and teachers and found a significant positive effect on grade point average (Bakosh 2013). In a randomized controlled study, Lisa Flook (coauthor of Chapter 14, "Mindfulness in Schools") and colleagues at the University of Wisconsin–Madison evaluated the Kindness Curriculum, a 12-week prekindergarten classroom program taught by mindfulness instructors (Flook et al. 2015). The curriculum (which can be downloaded for free from the Center for Healthy Minds, https://centerhealthyminds.org) included two 20-minute sessions per week, with various activities in mindfulness-based prosocial skills, including mindful movement, breathing exercises, and kindness practices (sharing, empathy, and gratitude). One activity used a CD audio in an exercise called Belly Buddy Breathing. Children were asked to notice the sensations of a Beanie Baby toy placed on their bellies as they lay on the floor and to observe the rise and fall as they breathed. The results of this study showed higher grades for the children exposed to the Kindness Curriculum compared with the control group in the areas of approaches to learning, health and physical development, and social and emotional development (there were no differences in cognition, general knowledge, or language and communication).

Parents and Caregivers

It may come as some surprise that parents of tweens and teens spend significant time on their devices, *on par* with that of their children. This fact in itself is worthy of discussion in understanding the modern family milieu and the potential for mindfulness interventions for caregivers. According to a recent national survey of more than 1,700 parents conducted by Common Sense Media and the Center on Media and Human Development at Northwestern University, moms and dads of tweens and teens spend an average of 9 hours daily on screens (including time watching TV or DVDs, browsing websites, using e-readers, and social networking, not accounting for simultaneous use) (Common Sense Media 2016). Moreover, 82% (7 hours, 43 minutes) of parents' use is devoted to personal screen time, in contrast to work-related media screen time (1 hour, 39 minutes). Like their children, parents multitask with media, with more than half (58%) reporting that they use media while working, including engaging in such activities as listening to music, watching TV, using social media, and texting.

Today's parents are positive and confident about technology, according to the Common Sense Media (2016) survey: Nearly 80% of parents surveyed believe they are good media and technology role models for their children. Most parents (94%) believe technology has a positive influence in education and that it helps develop a variety of positive skills, creativity, personal expression, and preparation for twenty-first-century jobs. A majority of parents (77%) have rules about the content that their tweens and teens can view, as well as rules about not using technology during family meals (78%) or at bedtime (63%). Of course, it's not easy being a parent in the digital age, and it may be no surprise that 37% reported that negotiating media use causes parent-child conflicts. An adolescent's age likely influences these kinds of negotiations, with more parents of tweens (34%) reporting enforcing house rules for technology use compared with parents of teens (21%).

This also suggests a potential rhetoric gap between what parents say about technology use and what they allow. It may also reflect a lack of public awareness regarding emerging cultural trends on poorer emotional well-being factors among American youth (e.g., less sleep, more stress) and what to do about it (Twenge 2017a). As the divide between digital natives and digital immigrants is narrowing and confidence levels among parents are increasing, a question arises: As parents' comfort levels with their own technology consumption grow, are they inadvertently communicating an acceptance of or overreliance on technology-enabled activities and deprioritizing essential social and emotional skills; basic needs for play, quiet time, and rest; or time spent in prosocial activities and volunteering?

No doubt, parents would benefit from mindfulness and mindful parenting skills. As mindfulness programs increase in school settings, mindfulness education and books for parents are on the rise in parallel. Guiding parents to use MBMAs might be an ideal pathway for the introduction of mindfulness to youth. Anecdotally, our (T.C. and Z.S.-O.) clinical experience with parents reveals that parents are seeking alternative ways to reduce their children's anxiety and insomnia (e.g., showing the child an animated tutorial on breathing techniques). Parents are increasingly downloading apps with audio relaxations and mindfulness tracks to help their children calm down before doing homework or taking a test, learn problem solving in tricky social situations, or go to sleep.

In this emerging area of digital mindfulness tools, parents seeking relief for their children are likely ahead of mental health practitioners in experimentation and adoption of MBMAs (although we could not find confirmation of this assertion other than our clinical experience). Practical consumer guidance and reviews from health experts are needed to support a digital wisdom approach so that vulnerable parents and children are not swayed by quick fixes and false hopes that a mindfulness app can solve various afflictions. Further research is needed to examine the possibility that overreliance on technology instead of more traditional time-tested parental modes of providing a soothing presence that can enhance secure attachment could instill in children a dependency on their parents' smartphone as the source of warmth, comfort, and guidance.

In general, we find that there is currently a paradox when it comes to mindfulness-based mobile apps and other digital health tools. Many consumer apps that claim to be "scientifically inspired" or "research based" provide little evidence. On the other hand, the relatively few evidence-based tools with scientific validation are not sold commercially. Even though the literature on technology-based MBMAs for youth is relatively scarce, a picture is emerging on which technology resources may be beneficial to youth in general (Table 17–1).

TABLE 17–1. Mindfulness-based mobile technologies: strengths and opportunities

Current strengths	Areas of opportunity
• Offer a means to introduce mindfulness in daily life • May serve to augment practice in daily life • Convenience • Affordability • May enhance adolescents' interest and lower barriers to mindfulness practice • May engage youth with gamification and mindfulness buddies via social interaction and group engagement • May also increase wise use of technology	• Increase scientific evidence for effectiveness and efficacy • Evaluate safety and developmentally tailored skills education • Assess the risks for attrition and competition for attention (e.g., boredom with mindfulness, limited diversity of learning tools) by using mobile technology • Attend to cultural differences and accessibility (e.g., socioeconomic status, language) • Understand the barriers to technology access and resources (e.g., broadband)

Digital Wisdom in Practice

We offer two hypothetical scenarios that would allow clinicians, educators, or parents to integrate a mindfulness-based mobile application in a simple and practical way. *The example apps are not endorsements of particular commercial products*, and the provider or caregiver may swap in any quality mindfulness app. Ideally, providers should be familiar with the mindfulness application they recommend, preferably using it on a regular basis personally or professionally, and should feel confident that the skills in the app support the therapeutic goals and the basic teachings of mindfulness practice. These cases assume that each child has a basic set of technology skills and familiarity with mobile devices appropriate for his or her age.

Case Example 1

Danny is an 8-year-old boy who has trouble focusing in class and tends to get anxious with math homework. His parents, who are divorcing, get frustrated with each other. They have different opinions about how Danny can structure his time after school and on weekends, including playtime, sports, video games, and extra practice math activities his teacher sends home. The third-grade teacher, Ms. Rondo, tries to support Danny with clear instructions. She posts tutorial links on the online parent-teacher portal but notices that neither parent has engaged with the portal. The guidance counselor, Mr. Gilbert, has been brought in to help Danny's family get on the same page, and one of his recommendations is to use Mind Yeti, a mindfulness app geared for both children and parents. In a family meeting, he suggests that Danny and his parents use the free version of the app together for 10 minutes at the end of the day for the next 2 weeks before the next parent meeting. First, Mr. Gilbert explains what mindfulness is, and then he shows the app to Danny and his parents. He invites them to try a 3-minute slow breathing exercise together, which is one of the "Yeti Powers" that can help with the "hubbub." Mr. Gilbert asks if they are game to try this at home. They agree. Mr. Gilbert explains that Danny can pick which Yeti Power he'd like to try first but says that he would like Danny to try all of them over the next 2 weeks. These powers include breath, thoughts, feelings, body, senses, gratitude, and kindness. Mr. Gilbert also asks the parents to participate as much as possible and to engage with Danny in a reflection conversation after listening to an audio: *What do you like about this Yeti power? How do you think it can help you at school? At home? When playing baseball? I wonder how it could help me, too?* Mr. Gilbert or Danny's parents may even suggest that Danny eventually show his little sister how to use the app as well, as a way to empower Danny with his newfound skills. Mr. Gilbert also lets Ms. Rondo know that Danny can come down to his office and use the app.

Case Example 2

Carolina is a 15-year-old girl with low self-esteem and anxiety. She was a chubby and carefree girl in elementary school, but she experienced an early growth spurt and shot up taller than all of her friends. Her self-esteem suffered. An avid athlete skilled in a number of sports, Carolina also experienced two concussions in the prior year. These events temporarily took her out of sports, the one arena where she felt confident. When her mood plummeted and social anxiety set in, leading to isolation and suicidal ideation, she was placed in a therapeutic day program. It was here that Carolina learned mindfulness skills as a way to sit with her unpleasant thoughts and feelings, learning to expand her "window of tolerance" and calm her nervous system. The mindfulness group leader in the program, Margey, suggested that Carolina use the Stop, Breathe, and Think app on her smartphone on a daily basis and whenever she felt triggered or in a low mood. She advised Carolina to track her *weekly settledness* on the basis of the minutes she spent practicing the meditations. Carolina could also use the app's check-in feature to name the top emotions before and after the meditation, as a simple way to reflect on her moods. In addition, Margey suggested that Carolina could use her own journal to write out her experiences. In this way, she could also remember and share her observations with the group and her therapist. Over time, Carolina found that she likes using the app feature that allows her to create her own custom meditation times with her preferred soundscapes. She now uses it regularly as a means for informal mindfulness practice whenever she needs it.

Not all children or teens have access to smartphones or tablets, and there is no one-size-fits-all approach in using technology to encourage a positive wellness habit. Technology can support and be used in conjunction with mindfulness skills that are ideally reinforced and modeled by counselors, teachers, and parents. For those wary or resistant to using technology, it can be helpful to frame the use of digital mindfulness apps as simply another item in the toolkit. It can be helpful to reduce commonplace barriers for a less technology-fluent adult by showing him or her how to access an app store, set up a username and password, and download an app and then practicing a mindfulness skill together. The initial time spent up front can alleviate anxiety and encourage practice at home. Of course, the likelihood is that children will pick up the app instructions fairly quickly. Using a curious and playful approach in experimenting with which digital mindfulness tools work best can augment the likelihood of adoption.

Conclusion and Future Directions

Overall, youth instructed in traditional mindfulness and social and emotional learning skills show better self-regulation, prosocial behavior, school success, and well-being. It remains to be seen whether technology-based mindfulness tools will evince similar results. Because of the ubiquity of digital technology in the lives of youth, mobile apps are ideally positioned as a form of skillful means to engage youth in mindfulness practices and may serve as a useful adjunct to mindfulness interventions. An intriguing question for future study is whether the use of mindfulness-based mobile apps may lead youth and their caregivers to mindfully engage not only in their digital playgrounds but in real-world interactions. Could there be spillover effects from the use of mindfulness apps? We can imagine, or perhaps hope, that young people might regularly practice mindful moments—whether triggered by a push notification or because they simply remembered to notice their thoughts and feelings through a new habit of mindfulness. A pocketful of mindfulness just might be the trick that nudges a young person to refrain from sending an impulsive text or from taking a social media post too personally; to appreciate the beauty in the natural world; or to recognize the common humanity among family, friends, and strangers. Indeed, mindfulness technologies may play a role in helping youth and their caretakers cultivate digital wisdom one ping at a time.

KEY POINTS

- Technology tools can serve as an adjunct to real-world practices.
- With efficacy of mindfulness-based interventions currently unproven, it is wise to take a buyer-beware approach, seeking recommendations from mindfulness experts and health consumer reviews.
- Enlist youth as experts and consumers in the development of mindfulness-based technologies.
- Parents, educators, and clinicians should be familiar with the programs they recommend.
- Seek apps that offer mindfulness psychoeducation as well as practices and skills.

Discussion Questions

1. What does digital wisdom mean to you? And how can you support children to identify what digital wisdom means to them?
2. How might technology-based mindfulness tools be integrated into your program or practice?
3. In what ways can you support patients and/or students so they can use technology as a skillful means for mindfulness in their daily life?

Suggested Readings

Books

boyd d: It's Complicated: The Social Lives of Networked Teens. New Haven, CT, Yale University Press, 2014

Steiner-Adair C: The Big Disconnect: Protecting Childhood and Family Relationships in the Digital Age, New York, Harper, 2013

Thompson T: Smarter Than You Think: How Technology is Changing Our Minds for the Better. New York, Penguin, 2013

Website

Common Sense Media (www.commonsensemedia.org) provides education and advocacy to families to promote safe technology and media for children.

References

Badawy SM, Kuhns LM: Texting and mobile phone app interventions for improving adherence to preventive behavior in adolescents: a systematic review. JMIR Mhealth Uhealth 5(4):e50, 2017 28428157

Bakosh LS: Investigating the effects of a daily audio-guided mindfulness intervention for elementary school students and teachers. Doctoral dissertation, Sofia University, Sofia University, Palo Alto, CA, 2013

boyd d: It's Complicated: The Social Lives of Networked Teens, New Haven, CT, Yale University Press, 2014, pp 211–212

Common Sense Media: The Common Sense Census: Media Use by Teens. San Francisco, Common Sense Media, November 3, 2015. Available at: www.commonsensemedia.org/research/the-common-sense-census-media-use-by-tweens-and-teens. Accessed May 17, 2018.

Common Sense Media: The Common Sense Census: Plugged-in Parents of Tweens and Teens. San Francisco, Common Sense Media, December 6, 2016. Available at: www.commonsensemedia.org/research/the-common-sense-census-plugged-in-parents-of-tweens-and-teens-2016. Accessed May 17, 2018.

Common Sense Media: Zero to Eight: Children's Media Use in America 2013. San Francisco, Common Sense Media, October 28, 2018. Available at: www.commonsensemedia.org/research/zero-to-eight-childrens-media-use-in-america-2013. Accessed May 17, 2018.

Culbert T: Perspectives on technology-assisted relaxation approaches to support mind-body skills practice in children and teens: clinical experiences and commentary. Children (Basel) 4(4):E20, 2017 28355179

Fish J, Brimson J, Lynch S: Mindfulness interventions delivered by technology without facilitator involvement: what research exists and what are the clinical outcomes? Mindfulness 7(5):1011–1023, 2016 27642370

Flook L, Goldberg SB, Pinger L, et al: Promoting prosocial behavior and self-regulatory skills in preschool children through a mindfulness-based kindness curriculum. Dev Psychol 51(1):44–51, 2015 25383689

Majeed-Ariss R, Baildam E, Campbell M, et al: Apps and adolescents: a systematic review of adolescents' use of mobile phone and tablet apps that support personal management of their chronic or long-term physical conditions. J Med Internet Res 17(12):e287, 2015 26701961

Mak WW, Chio FH, Chan AT, et al: The efficacy of Internet-based mindfulness training and cognitive-behavioral training with telephone support in the enhancement of mental health among college students and young working adults: randomized controlled trial. J Med Internet Res 19(3):e84, 2017 28330831

Mani M, Kavanagh DJ, Hides L, et al: Review and evaluation of mindfulness-based iPhone apps. JMIR Mhealth Uhealth 3(3):e82, 2015 26290327

Mason M, Ola B, Zaharakis N, et al: Text messaging interventions for adolescent and young adult substance use: a meta-analysis. Prev Sci 16(2):181–188, 2015 24930386

Militello LK, Kelly SA, Melnyk BM: Systematic review of text-messaging interventions to promote healthy behaviors in pediatric and adolescent populations: implications for clinical practice and research. Worldviews Evid Based Nurs 9(2):66–77, 2012 22268959

Parsons CE, Crane C, Parsons LJ, et al: Home practice in mindfulness-based cognitive therapy and mindfulness-based stress reduction: a systematic review and meta-analysis of participants' mindfulness practice and its association with outcomes. Behav Res Ther 95:29–41, 2017 28527330

Pew Research Center: Internet and technology mobile fact sheet. Washington, DC, Pew Research Center, January 12, 2017. Available at: www.pewinternet.org/factsheet/mobile. Accessed May 17, 2018.

Plaza I, Demarzo MM, Herrera-Mercadal P, et al: Mindfulness-based mobile applications: literature review and analysis of current features. JMIR Mhealth Uhealth 1(2):e24, 2013 25099314

Prensky M: From Digital Natives to Digital Wisdom: Hopeful Essays for 21st Century Learning. Thousand Oaks, CA, Corwin, 2012

Rodgers RF, Donovan E, Cousineau TM, et al: Preliminary findings from a randomized-controlled trial of BodiMojo: a mobile app for positive body image. Paper presented at the International Conference on Eating Disorders, Prague, Czech Republic, June 2017

Thompson C: Smarter Than You Think: How Technology is Changing Our Minds for the Better. New York, Penguin,

Turner T, Hingle M: Evaluation of a mindfulness-based mobile app aimed at promoting awareness of weight-related behaviors in adolescents: a pilot study. JMIR Res Protoc 6(4):e67, 2017 28446423

Twenge JM: iGen: Why Today's Super-Connected Kids Are Growing Up Less Rebellious, More Tolerant, Less Happy—And Completely Unprepared for Adulthood. New York, Atria, 2017a

Twenge JM: Have smartphones destroyed a generation? The Atlantic, September 2017b. Available at: www.theatlantic.com/magazine/archive/2017/09/has-the-smartphone-destroyed-a-generation/534198. Accessed May 16, 2018.

World Economic Forum: New Vision for Education: Fostering Social and Emotional Learning Through Technology. Geneva, Switzerland, World Economic Forum, March 10, 2016. Available at: www.weforum.org/reports/new-vision-for-education-fostering-social-and-emotional-learning-through-technology. Accessed May 16, 2018.

Chapter 18

Mindfulness and Creativity

Sayyed Mohsen Fatemi, Ph.D.
Ellen J. Langer, Ph.D.

IN this chapter we explain the important role of mindfulness that, when integrated with creativity, can promote critical thinking in youth. Additionally, we provide the reader an introduction to the work E.J.L. and colleagues have done over the past decades on mindfulness—or, more specifically, what is now called *Langerian mindfulness*—including ways to develop creativity and potential applications of mindfulness with youth.

Langerian mindfulness was the first author's (S.M.F.) introduction to *critical mindfulness* as a new paradigm in psychology (for more specifics, see Fatemi 2016). Critical mindfulness introduced a focus on intrapersonal, interpersonal, educational, social, and health implications of mindfulness (Langer 1993, 2000, 2009; Langer and Abelson 1972; Langer and Piper 1987; Langer et al. 1978; Rodin and Langer 1977). We propose that a perspective shift in the state of a youth's mind would potentially lead him or her to explore novelty, creativity, and innovation.

There have certainly been numerous studies on creativity in a wide variety of contexts, including everyday creativity, creativity and society, creativity and spirituality, creativity and art, and creativity and relationships (see Richards 2007). Our focus here is not to summarize the literature but to provide the reader with examples as to why creativity is vital to the developing mindfulness of youth. It also seems that modern education is highly concentrated on the science, technology, engineering, and mathematics (STEM) curriculum. Although these subjects are very important and are crucial to the intellectual development of youth, at the same time, we are witnessing decreasing support for the arts. We tend to wonder, as Gardner (2006) did,

> What sense would we make of the greatest work of art or literature, or the most important religious or political ideas, or the most enduring puzzles about the meaning of life and death, if we only thought of them in the manner of a scientific study or proof? If all we did was quantify? What political or business leader would be credible, at the time of crisis, if all he could do was offer scientific explanations or mathematical proofs, if he could not address the hearts of his audience? (p. 15)

We do not intend to lessen the focus on or argue against the emphasis on STEM or scientific knowledge in general, However, we do wish to remind the reader that the "complete" human being (i.e., a mental, emotional, physical, and, where applicable, spiritual being) at times, especially when suffering, needs a sense of hope that extends beyond what the scientific view may call empirical or rational knowledge. As human beings, we seek inspiration, and when we enter the role of therapist or healer, we enter a complex and creative therapeutic space that exists beyond mathematical proofs. Yet we must still strive to discover, to investigate and research with all our available tools and methods. The great physicist Niels Bohr once mused on this irony: "there are two kinds of truth, deep truth and shallow truth, and the function of Science is to eliminate the deep truth" (Gardner 2006, p. 15). In this chapter, we strive to restore this deeper truth of the human experience and call the reader's attention to what is creative and spontaneous in therapeutic work with youth.

Langerian mindfulness begins with an analysis of different modes of being in the world. Specifically, the automatic and passive state in which youth may become caught in their previously established perceptual, emotional, cognitive, and behavioral patterns is brought into awareness. This mode of being can give rise to feeling disconnected from the present moment and could result in the youth missing out on the many opportunities the moment could offer. When youth are operating on automatic pilot, their experience of the moment is subjected to distortion, circumscription, limitation, and constriction. In addition, the tyranny of the past overdetermines the present moment, and, accordingly, youth find themselves determined by history instead of by the here-and-now opportunities. This kind of automaticity can phenomenologically nurture a predisposition toward not paying attention to alternatives. Youth would therefore be cut off from their creativity because creativity relies on an ability to see novelty and have the courage to seek and express it.

A remedy to functioning on automatic pilot comes through an existential mode of mind that is characterized by an open, flexible, and proactive way of being in the world. This mode of being is transformational: youth engage in a search for possibilities, which provides the opportunity for a radical transformational process whereby youth can develop new ways of interacting with their learning, their peers, and the environment. We propose that "mindfulness is a flexible state of mind in which we are actively engaged in the present, noticing new things and sensitive to the context. When we are in a state of mindlessness, we act like automatons who have been programmed to act according to the sense our behavior made in the past, rather than the present" (Langer 2000, p. 220).

Mindful Creativity

Mindful creativity lies in a comfortable dissociation from the rigid mental structures that prescribe an obedience to what is known. The essence of creativity and critical mindfulness begins with questioning and challenging the frameworks of perception that were inherited from the past. Creativity moves beyond the ordinary and everyday routines, past conditioning, and away from the interference of what can be an unhelpful ruminative mind.

Creativity challenges the way things are and explores other ways things can be. Creativity inspires youth to transform the world for the better. Creativity is a path of discovery, much like the act of mindful meditation, and it can make the unknown known and move one closer to the unfamiliar and the unexplored parts of the self and the world.

Applications of Mindful Creativity

Educational systems that tend to underlie and promote preestablished mental frameworks may encourage learners to merely abide by expected outcomes. When youth are exposed to recursive modes of thinking and emotions through education and social interactions, they are likely to follow the priming of the suggested frameworks. As a result, they unquestionably accept these assumptions as being solid and reliable. Teachers operating in these systems may also pay less attention to the process. Therefore, when learners are exposed to cognitive, perceptual, and emotional mechanisms from the past, they may not be able to move beyond the familiar. The emphasis on preplanned learning agendas may also limit learners' access to the plethora of possibilities. The epistemological exploration of the content of learning induces mindlessness, with a focus on relationships that are fixed and accepted mindlessly.

In questioning the educational system and mainstream pedagogical policies, we argue that most of the existing teaching and learning approaches harbor mindlessness. As mindlessness increases, creativity and the act of drawing novel distinctions decrease. It is only in mindfulness that we can investigate alternative modes and notice novel things. When we are in a state of mindfulness, we can actively live in the present, situate ourselves in the moment, and think creatively about perspectives and possibilities. In contrast, when we are in a state of mindlessness, we unquestionably rely on our mindsets and ignore alternative approaches.

Langer (1993) challenges many of our beliefs about learning and argues that they have been learned mindlessly and work to our detriment. She recommends mindful learning and propounds its consequences, which can produce a great array of opportunities. When it comes to the art of self-expressiveness or general expressiveness, mindfulness can help learners seek avenues of possibilities beyond the learned modes of sensibility. Students who learn the art of looking for novelty amid the familiar can also learn to use creative modes of expressiveness.

Challenging Cognitive and Emotional Commitments

Mindfulness questions the unquestionability of cognitive and emotional frameworks from the past. When youth focus on constructs inherited from the past, they are not fully receptive to the present. The influence of learned reference points in both cognitive and emotional domains may limit youths' ability to view the immediate moment, and it restricts and limits their examination of alternative modes of possibilities. For instance, if you have used a label (such as calling someone "lazy") in the past, you are likely to apply the same label when encountering the person again. In school, if a youth has gotten the message that no one believes he or she will be successful, the youth may simply surrender to that label and stop trying. Essentially, the youth may become so entrenched in negative beliefs about himself or herself that he or she may not be able to detach from the label. Instead, the youth identifies with it.

Challenging Mindless Modes of Expressiveness

Modes of expressiveness fall into two categories: 1) mindless modes of expressiveness, which are connected to the schematic structures of preestablished belief systems, emotions, and behaviors and 2) mindful modes of expressiveness. The leading factor of mindlessness-based phenomenology is the notion of certainty. Within the stability of a mindlessly repeated schematic analysis, youth expressions resonate with the preexisting patterns. There is no space for development of a contextual and sensual cognitive and emotional phenomenology.

When youth acquire their beliefs mindlessly and without mindfully questioning them, their belief system is recursively controlling their mode of expressiveness, and the chance of mindless expressiveness increases. Mindlessness-based cognitive and emotional registration suggests a monolithic perspective that defines reliability and viability in the context of schematic structures of the past. When youth are encouraged to rely on single perspectives, their language is limited to the suggested reference points of those prescribed perspectives, and they are not able to express themselves in other ways. Although the schematic structures associated with scientific rigor have fruitful applications for wellness, these schemas can hinder youths' search for novelty because they impose a single mode of sensibility on both experiences and expression of those experiences.

One of the many helpful ways to break the tyranny of the schematic past is to use poetry. Poetry gives rise to both engagement and disengagement: engagement through involvement in multiple modes of expressiveness (e.g., language, emotions, interpretation, history) and disengagement through acting from a single perspective (i.e., the specific poem itself). Poetry espouses a shift from reductionism to richness: it brings about a flight from univocity to polysemy.

To understand the creation of possibilities through the act of poetry, one needs to disengage oneself from what Langer (1993) calls *premature cognitive commitment*. A poetics-based phenomenology opens the possibilities for new modes of expressiveness because one's sensibility is no longer limited to previous schematic analysis. This requires that one be mindful. This mindfulness, in Langerian terms (Langer 2009), requires noticing new things, paying attention to a flux distinct from the past, and exploring the layers of the unexpressed. The essence of Langerian mindfulness is engagement.

Engagement constitutes one of the main components of mindfulness. In mindless phenomenology, a youth's working memory keeps his or her thinking within established categories. Once the youth is locked into a particular category, he or she is not looking for alternative ways of understanding the experience. Propositions are considered absolute. However, in a mindfulness-based living experience, statements and propositions are presented in a conditional format, which allows youth to understand the tentativeness of the proposition. They are therefore open to investigating other possibilities. As youth become mindfully engaged in an experience, they are not only there, they also are *being there*. This engagement gives rise to living in the moment in a mindful manner.

In a revolutionary perspective on modes of thinking and expressiveness, Langer (2009) argued that operating from a position of *not* knowing provides us with more possibilities for expressing the unexpressed: it allows us to go beyond the preestablished discourses of thinking and promotes paying attention to novel things. Explaining this mindful phenomenology of creativity, Langer (2009) noted that

> [w]hen we learn mindlessly, we look at experience and impose a contingent relationship between two things—what we or someone else did and what we think happened as a result. We interpret that experience from a single perspective, oblivious to the other ways it can be seen. Mindful learning looks at experience and understands that it can be seen in countless ways, that new information is always available, and that more than one perspective is both possible and extremely valuable. It's an approach that leads us to be careful about what we "know" to be true and how we learn it. At the level of the experience, each event is unique. (pp. 29–30)

Challenging Certainty

Challenging the position of certitude and calling for the fluidity of living in the moment through observing new things, Langer (2009) suggested that

> [c]ertainty is a cruel mindset. It hardens our minds against possibility and closes them to the world we live in. When all is certain, there are no choices for us. If there is no doubt, there is no choice. When we are certain, we are blind to the uncertainties of the world whether we recognize it or not. It is uncertainty that we need to embrace. (pp. 24–25)

Mindful creativity openly creates possibilities and avidly looks for newness within the modes of expressiveness and the things that are being expressed. Art-based phenomenology can be one form of mindful expressiveness for youth, departing from mindlessness and proactively and mindfully creating possibilities, or it can be plagued with the tyranny of the prescriptive modes of schematic analysis, thus proceeding within the realm of mindlessness. Enhancing the possibilities in the heart of mindfulness would help youth explore the realm of sensibility beyond the predetermined scripts of certainty because when youth are mindful, they are able to think of several perspectives. This can facilitate the process of transcending the commonly accepted forms of sensation and perception.

The fluidity of creative mindfulness enriches the indeterminacy of creative expressiveness and promises the possibility of self-creation through the expansion of choices. When people embrace mindfulness, the certainty of an X being an X can be changed into a belief that an X can be an X while also being a Y. Political, personal, and cultural positions of youth can be enlivened through a discovery of the relationship between the modes of expressiveness and the search for new possibilities of exploration. When acting from a mindful perspective, people can think of perspectives other than own, with empathy, understanding, flexibility, and openness. This will help people bridge gaps and create values.

Therapeutic Applications

How can therapists and clinicians employ Langerian mindfulness in practice? The following techniques can be used in therapeutic contexts to encourage youth to work creatively with challenges and problems.

1. **Understand the difference between absolute propositions and conditional propositions.** Invite youth to explore the differences between certitude and contingency and their psychological implications. For example, looking at an object and then asserting that it is a bottle of water has quite different implications from articulating that it *can be* a bottle of water. The former freezes reality of the object, whereas the latter opens it up to numerous possibilities— the object can be many things, including a bottle of water, a pencil holder, or a vase. As another example, youth can be given words that are not conventionally related to one another and then are asked to connected the words in creative sentences. Alternatively, they can be given the same sentence in two modes, absolute mode and conditional mode, and then are asked to examine the differences between them. In the absolute mode, an X is identified as stable, unchanged, and definitive. In the conditional mode, an X can be a Y or many other things. Understanding the difference helps youth learn to examine the realm of possibilities beyond the given set of their assumptions and enables them to see how their choices can go beyond the established set of contexts in which the choices are embedded. This perceptiveness helps youth see how social construction of realities can be revisited and deconstructed. On a personal level, it allows them to see how they can revamp their narratives and discover their own voice by distancing themselves from absolutes and looking for alternative modes of composing new narratives.

2. **Pay attention to variability.** Youth are encouraged to learn about attention and its variability to help them see the power of managing their attention. When our attention is mindlessly fixed on one thing and is not flexibly moving toward other possibilities, we become locked into unquestioned positions. Questioning this unquestionability is at the heart of Langerian mindfulness. Encourage youth to see how paying attention to the temporary dimension of their experiences allows them to deal with stressful situations in a more effective manner. Langerian mindfulness argues that *no one is always anything*. For instance, no one is always depressed. Even if you have been labeled as depressed, there are times when you may be depressed or

semidepressed, but there are also times when you are not depressed. Ask the youth, "What are the circumstances that make you depressed, and what are the situations or factors that can be elicited to make you not depressed?" Of course, this type of therapeutic approach must be applied skillfully with respect to timing and in consideration of the strength of the therapeutic alliance. The therapist must take care to not invalidate the youth's experience.

3. **Exercise the power of choice.** From a Langerian mindfulness perspective, the experience of anxiety can be viewed to some extent as a choice. An increase in mindfulness and the resulting creativity help youth see how they can shift from an automatic mode or behavior, that is, anxiety in response to some stimulus, to a healthier behavioral response to the anxiety-provoking stimulus. This shift illustrates how choices can be sensibly celebrated through an act of mindfulness and its call for exploring novel perspectives. Clinicians using the Langerian model can help youth examine moment by moment the possibility of making choices instead of abiding by an automatically learned behavior (in this example, the anxious response). Therapists can teach youth to exercise the power of choice in how they interpret and respond to stimuli, which helps them see that choices are usually plentiful.

4. **Act with authenticity.** At times, youth can end up lost in the meanders of pretentiousness. Langerian studies have demonstrated that even animals, such as dolphins, can tell the difference between an ostentatious mode of being and an authentic presentation (Langer 1993, 2009). Teaching creative mindfulness helps youth to be in touch with themselves without being afraid or anxious. This helps youth discover the importance of their own agency rather than depending too much on the good opinion of others. Mindfulness increases a genuine sense of individuation to the effect that youth do not need to rely on the good opinion of others to feel good about themselves.

5. **Practice detachment from subjectivity.** If you take off your watch and place it in front of your eyes, this act of separation suggests that you are not equated with your watch. Langerian therapists using creative mindfulness teach youth to practice detaching their thoughts and sensations from themselves. This detachment helps youth see how indulging in their own recursive thoughts generates a subjective image where mindlessness resides. By increasing their creative mindfulness, youth learn how to mindfully experience detachment from their own subjectivity, including their thoughts, assumptions, and mindsets.

6. **Celebrate multiple perspectives.** A perspective defines and determines what one is looking at, and if a youth is exclusively embedded within a single perspective, he or she may not be able to see beyond that perspective. We may be so immersed in our own world that we may not be aware of the existence of many other worlds that lie beside our own. Youth are encouraged

to examine the possibilities of many other perspectives that are potentially available but may be unbeknownst to them. This can have numerous therapeutic benefits, including empathy and affect attunement for interpersonal relationships. A therapist practicing Langerian mindfulness might use different prompts, such as feature films, to promote multiple perspectives. For instance, the film *Beauty and the Beast* delineates how a shift in one's experience can bring about an orientation toward someone else's experience.

7. **Welcoming new information.** Mindlessness is characterized by a recalcitrant, dogmatic stance in which one is cognitively or emotionally stuck in a single position without displaying any sign of intentionality to reconsider the given position. In contrast, mindfulness fosters flexibility and openness. It helps youth open their minds in a curious and receptive state, allowing exploration of what may unfold in the immediate now. Receptiveness, openness, and flexibility facilitate the process of welcoming new information and knowledge. This will be of great benefit for youth, especially in encouraging them to look beyond the mindsets they take for granted.

8. **Learning sensitivity to context.** From a Langerian perspective, nothing is context free. By learning the importance and significance of context, youth will be able to mindfully address and manage any given context. When people act in a mindless manner, they merely recall laws and regulations in a universal sense, without any sensitivity to the situations in which those laws are applied. We are told not to raise our voices in the library, but what if no one is in the library except you and your friend and his car is going to be towed unless you shout at him to move it? Would you consider shouting to be appropriate or not? Learning the importance of sensitivity to context helps youth enhance their perceptiveness of contextual features in cultural, social, and psychological realms.

Conclusion and Future Directions

Langerian mindfulness as a distinct doctrine on mindfulness has significant implications for cultivating youth mindfulness. The 40-year-long research legacies of Langerian mindfulness and its empirical and experimental substantiation indicate that there is much to gain from applying a Langerian perspective for youth mindfulness and creativity (e.g., Langer 1993).

In closing, we remind the reader that mindfulness, just like any technology, must be used appropriately and precisely. We reiterate the words of Spariosu (2004):

We might posse the "best" scientific theory, such as deep ecology, the "best" information and communication technology, such as digital and quantum computers, or the "best" political system, such as democracy. And yet, we may end up putting them all to inappropriate and counterproductive uses, as we have seen happen repeatedly throughout the history of scientific and technological development, as well as the history of world politics. (p. 21)

Mindfulness is not only about a change of cognition and emotion; it entails a shift in one's being. It is a radical transformation of consciousness. When we are in a mindful state, we choose to increase our competencies in how we direct and manage our attention. This art of perspective management intrinsically gives rise to the art of shifting our attention as well. In every single moment of our encounter with the immediate now, we are able to consciously and deliberately choose to move our attention from one subject to another subject. Mindfulness, thus, has a lot to do with the quality of attention and awareness. It is an elevated sense of awareness that can be learned and practiced. The elevation presupposes a focus on the moment of now, which is also associated with a liberation from the past. The past does not cease to operate. It operates in its own domain, but it does not own the mind.

KEY POINTS

- Langerian mindfulness suggests that to be mindful, one needs to seek novelty.

- Seeking novelty helps one live in the moment and experience the present more effectively and proactively.

- We can teach youth to reflect on the implications of mindfulness and understand how a mindful way of living can help them become aware of different choices in life.

- Youth can learn how creativity can encompass daily activities, including their interactions with others.

Discussion Questions

1. Think of a situation that has recently brought you anxiety and stress. What shift in perspective might help you manage the situation in a healthier way?
2. Think of an unavoidable stressful situation that gave you difficulty. How might your understanding of a creative and a mindful choice help you cope with the situation in a more effective manner?

3. You invite your friends to a party. It is getting late but they have not arrived yet, and your anxiety starts to increase. How can mindful creativity help you manage your anxiety?

Suggested Readings

Langer EJ: Mindfulness. Reading, MA, Addison-Wesley, 1989

Langer EJ: On Becoming an Artist: Reinventing Yourself Through Mindful Creativity. New York, Ballantine, 2005

Langer EJ: Counterclockwise: Mindful Health and the Power of Possibility. New York, Ballantine, 2009

References

Fatemi SM: Critical Mindfulness: Exploring Langerian Models. New York, Springer, 2016

Gardner H: Five Minds for the Future. Boston, Harvard Business School Press, 2006

Langer EJ: A mindful education. Educ Psychol 28(1):43–50, 1993

Langer EJ: Mindful learning. Curr Dir Psychol Sci 9(6):220–223, 2000

Langer E: Counterclockwise: Mindful Health and the Power of Possibility. New York, Ballantine, 2009

Langer EJ, Abelson RP: The semantics of asking for a favor: how to succeed in getting help without really dying. J Pers Soc Psychol 24(1):26–32, 1972

Langer EJ, Piper AI: The prevention of mindlessness. J Pers Soc Psychol 53(2):280–287, 1987

Langer EJ, Blank A, Chanowitz B: The mindlessness of ostensibly thoughtful action: the role of "placebic" information in interpersonal interaction. J Pers Soc Psychol 36(6):635–642, 1978

Richards R (ed): Everyday Creativity and New Views of Human Nature: Psychological, Social, and Spiritual Perspectives. Washington, DC, American Psychological Association, 2007

Rodin J, Langer EJ: Long-term effects of a control-relevant intervention with the institutionalized aged. J Pers Soc Psychol 35(12):897–902, 1977 592095

Spariosu MI: Global Intelligence and Human Development: Toward an Ecology of Global Learning. Cambridge, MA, MIT Press, 2004

Index